Blood, Blood Products and AIDS

Blood, Blood Products
— and AIDS —

Edited by

R. Madhok, MD, C. D. Forbes, MD
University Department of Medicine, Royal Infirmary, Glasgow, UK

and

B. L. Evatt, MD
Centers for Disease Control, Atlanta, USA

Springer-Science+Business Media, B.V.

Originally published by Chapman and Hall in 1987.
MyCopy version of the original edition 1987

DOI 10.1007/978-1-4899-3394-2

British Library Cataloguing in Publication Data

Blood, blood products and AIDS.
1. AIDS (Disease) 2. Epidemiology
I. Madhok, R. II. Forbes, Charles D.
III. Evatt, B.
614.5′993 RC607.A26

www.springer.com/mycopy

Contents

Contributors

Louis M. Aledort, MD
The Mount Sinai Medical Center, New York, USA

Graeme R. D. Catto, MD
University of Aberdeen, Aberdeen, UK

Terence L. Chorba, MD
Centers for Disease Control, Atlanta, USA

James W. Curran, MD, MPH
Centers for Disease Control, Atlanta, USA

Roger Detels, MD
University of California, Los Angeles, USA

Ulrich Desselberger, MD, MRCPath, MRCP
University of Glasgow, Glasgow, UK

Roger Y. Dodd, PhD
Transmissible Diseases Laboratory, American Red Cross, Rockville, Maryland, USA

Bruce L. Evatt, MD
Centers for Disease Control, Atlanta, USA

John L. Fahey, MD
University of California, Los Angeles, USA

Charles D. Forbes, DSc, FRCP
University of Glasgow, Glasgow, UK

Michael S. Gottlieb, MD
University of California, Los Angeles, USA

Andrew Innes, MB, MRCP
University of Aberdeen, Aberdeen, UK

Janine M. Jason, MD
Centers for Disease Control, Atlanta, USA

Gordon D. O. Lowe, MD, FRCP
University of Glasgow, Glasgow, UK

Alison M. MacLeod, MD, MRCP
University of Aberdeen, UK

Rajan Madhok, MD, MRCP
University of Glasgow, Glasgow, UK

Alison Mawle, MD
Centers for Disease Control, Atlanta, USA

D. B. L. McClelland, FRCPath
Edinburgh and South-East Scotland Regional Blood Transfusion Service, Edinburgh, UK

J. Steven McDougal, MD
Centers for Disease Control, Atlanta, USA

Philip P. Mortimer, FRCPath
Public Health Laboratory Service, London, UK

Janet K. A. Nicholson, MD
Centers for Disease Control, Atlanta, USA

Patricia Wilkie, PhD
University of Stirling and Glasgow, Glasgow, UK

Acknowledgements

Chapter 3 The author is grateful to Dr Richard M. Elliot for critical reading of this chapter.

Chapter 4 The authors thank Drs B. Evatt and J. Curran for reviewing their chapter.

Chapter 5 This chapter is supported by grants AI20672 and AI32511 from the National Institutes of Allergy and Infectious Disease and a grant from the AIDS Clinical Research Center from the University of California Task Force on AIDS.

Chapter 8 This chapter is contribution number 721 from the American Red Cross Biomedical Research and Development Laboratories.

Chapter 12 This chapter is supported in part by a contract from the National Heart, Lung and Blood Institute; by Health Services Administration grant number MCB–360001–04–01; by Health and Human Services grant number HL–30567–02; by the Regional Comprehensive Hemophilia Diagnostic and Treatment Center; the Margie Boas Fund; the International Hemophilia Training Center of the World Federation of Hemophilia, Polly Annenberg Levee Hematology Center, Department of Medicine, Mount Sinai School of Medicine of the City University of New York, NY 10029.

Foreword

When the history of AIDS comes to be written, the chapters devoted to the spread of the disease among haemophiliacs and the recipients of blood transfusions may be relatively brief in comparison with those describing the disastrous epidemic in Africa and the effect that the threat of infection had on the sexual mores of the developed world. I doubt, however, whether any chapters will be more poignant than those describing the tragedy of the thousands who lived in anticipation of developing a lethal disease as a consequence of the treatment that they had previously regarded as a key to health.

If scientists are unable to develop an effective antidote in time to help those who have become infected they must, at least, try to make the maximum use of the tragic experience of the victims to learn the most effective means of preventing the spread of the disease to others. Much has already been learnt, as is described here by 23 of the leading experts in Great Britain and the United States, and many advances have already been made that will improve medical care in the future; but there remains an urgent need for more research and more collaboration between clinicians and scientists in a wide variety of disciplines if further unnecessary misery is to be avoided. If this book helps to bring that about it will have repaid the efforts of the contributors many times over.

Richard Doll

1

The epidemiology of AIDS

—— *Janine M. Jason and James W. Curran* ——

1.1 INTRODUCTION

Cases of the acquired immune deficiency syndrome (AIDS) were first reported in June and July of 1981, as clusters of Kaposi's sarcoma and *Pneumocystis carinii* pneumonia among homosexual men (CDC, 1981, a, b). Since then, epidemiologic surveillance has been used by investigators and public health professionals to identify that an outbreak existed, to characterize the outbreak, and to determine and predict its extent and course. Surveillance and epidemiologic studies will be used increasingly to ascertain the effects of interventions. In addition to surveillance, epidemiologic methods are used to provide essential data about the pathogenesis of AIDS, and about the transmission, disease spectrum, and cofactors involved in human immunodeficiency virus (HIV) infection.

In this chapter we will review the current characteristics of the AIDS epidemic, with emphasis on the United States (US) cases associated with blood product usage. We will then discuss how modelling techniques have been applied to surveillance data to estimate disease incubation period and incidence trends. Epidemiologic data linking AIDS and immune defects to the infection will be reviewed. Evidence suggesting that virus is transmitted through sexual, blood, and maternal-fetus/infant routes, and not through casual contact, will be presented. Finally a variety of prevention strategies and their early outcomes will be described.

1.2 CHARACTERISTICS OF THE EPIDEMIC

As of May 12, 1986, 20 531 cases of AIDS were reported to the Centers for Disease Control (CDC). This figure includes 20 240 adults and 291 children, the latter being defined as persons under 13 years of age at the time of their AIDS diagnosis. Of all reported patients 93% were male, 7% were female.

Males predominate in all risk group categories except 'heterosexual contacts', including the categories 'intravenous drug user' and transfusion-associated AIDS; this gender difference is not present in paediatric cases. Of all cases, 89% are between the ages of 20 and 49 years, an age group at low risk for most other causes of morbidity and mortality. The distribution of risk groups has not changed markedly since 1982–83 (Tables 1.1 and 1.2). There were 58% cases diagnosed on the basis of *Pneumocystis carinii* pneumonia, 17%, Kaposi's sarcoma, and 5% both. The overall case-fatality rate is 54%; 86% of patients diagnosed prior to January 1982 have died.

Table 1.1 US adult AIDS cases, by risk group* and sex (Centers for Disease Control, May 12, 1986)

	Males (%)	*Females (%)*	*Total (%)*
Homosexual or bisexual men†	14 842 (79)	— (—)	14 842 (73)
Intravenous (IV) drug user	2 776 (15)	704 (52)	3 480 (17)
Haemophilia/coagulation disorder	153 (1)	4 (0)	157 (1)
Heterosexual contact‡	57 (0)	244 (18)	301 (1)
Transfusions with blood/blood products	205 (1)	121 (9)	326 (2)
None of the above/other§	866 (5)	268 (20)	1 134 (6)
Total	18 899 (100)	1 341 (100)	20 240 (100)

*Groups listed are ordered hierarchically; cases with multiple characteristics are tabulated only in the group listed first.

†1616 (11%) of homosexual men also reported having used IV drugs.

‡With a person with AIDS or at risk for AIDS.

§Includes 459 persons born in countries in which most AIDS cases have not been associated with known risk factors.

Table 1.2 US paediatric* AIDS cases, by risk group† and sex (Centers for Disease Control, May 12, 1986)

	Males (%)	*Females (%)*	*Total (%)*
Haemophilia/coagulation disorder	12 (8)	0 (0)	12 (4)
Parent with AIDS or at increased risk for AIDS‡	108 (68)	111 (85)	219 (75)
Transfusion with blood/blood products	29 (18)	15 (11)	44 (15)
None of the above/other	11 (7)	5 (4)	16 (5)
Total	160 (100)	131 (100)	291 (100)

*Includes patients under 13 years of age at the time of diagnosis.

†Groups listed are ordered hierarchically; cases with multiple characteristics are tabulated only in the group listed first.

‡Epidemiologic data suggest transmission from infected mother to child before, at, or shortly after the time of birth.

Two circumstances may have affected national AIDS surveillance other than the epidemic itself. First, reports of AIDS go to state public health agencies, which in turn provide information to CDC. This leads to reporting lags between AIDS diagnosis and Federal inclusion of a given patient's data in surveillance information (Curran *et al.*, 1985). Second, in June 1985 the case definition of AIDS used for national reporting was changed to include a small number of additional diagnoses and to take into consideration the results of serologic testing for antibody to HIV (CDC, 1982, 1986a). It was estimated that this change would result in reclassification of less than 1% of cases previously reported to CDC and the number of additional new cases reportable as a result of the revision would be small (CDC, 1982). In the case of haemophilia-AIDS, this change has thus far resulted in the addition of 10 cases (6% of all cases) that would have previously not been classified as AIDS.

1.3 HAEMOPHILIA AND TRANSFUSION-ASSOCIATED AIDS

1.3.1 Haemophilia-AIDS

Haemophilia-AIDS surveillance is done through haemophilia treatment centres (HTC), in cooperation with the National Hemophilia Foundation, as well as through state health departments. Because the vast majority of haemophiliacs requiring factor therapy have some contact with HTC, this system provides more complete surveillance than is possible for other risk groups (Johnson *et al.*, 1985). This situation, in combination with the manner in which this community was exposed to the AIDS virus, make the haemophiliac population an ideal one for evaluating disease pathogenesis and transmission.

The number of persons with haemophilia-associated AIDS reported to CDC was 175 as of May 18, 1986. Of these persons 170 were male, 5 were female. The median age was 33.5 years (range 2–81 years). There were 71% of cases with *Pneumocystis carinii* pneumonia and 33% well-documented oesophageal candidiasis. Only 4 persons had Kaposi's sarcoma. The case-fatality ratio was 57%, with only one person surviving 2 years following his AIDS diagnosis. This case-fatality ratio is identical to that for all cases of AIDS associated with opportunistic infections, and higher than that for all cases of AIDS in which Kaposi's sarcoma was the sole AIDS-related diagnosis (43%). Of the haemophilia-AIDS patients 160 (92%) had haemophilia A, 8 (5%) had haemophilia B, 5 (3%) had von Willebrand's disease, and 1 had factor V deficiency.* Factor VIII concentrate was used by 72 as their only blood product and 6 used factor IX. Using denominators extrapolated from a national survey (DHEW, 1977), the incidence of AIDS for the year 1985 was

*This information was unavailable for one case still under investigation.

6.4 per 1000 (80 cases) for persons with haemophilia A and 1.6 per 1000 (5 cases) for persons with haemophilia B.

1.3.2 Transfusion-associated AIDS

HIV serologic screening of blood donors was instituted in spring of 1985 (CDC, 1985a). The latest summary of transfusion-associated AIDS cases was published in November, 1985 and included cases reported up to 15 August, 1985 (Peterman *et al.*, 1985a). At that time 194 cases had been reported to CDC; 60% were male. Ages ranged from 0 (newborn) to 82 years. Infants appeared to be disproportionately represented (10% of cases), given the number of units of blood they received; however, the analysis could not take into consideration the volume of transfusion received in relation to the individual's body size or blood volume. Out of 21 children 14 received transfusions for problems associated with prematurity. The reasons for transfusion in 173 adult cases were unknown in 46% of them; known causes included cardiac surgery (27%), other surgery or trauma (22%), and other medical reasons (6%). As with haemophilia-AIDS, the vast majority of patients were diagnosed as having AIDS on the basis of opportunistic infections; only 4 adults had Kaposi's sarcoma.

1.3.3 Incidence rates and incubation period

While the number of haemophiliacs in the US can be reliably estimated (DHEW, 1977), this is not the case for other groups at risk for AIDS. One study used estimated denominators to calculate AIDS incidence figures for various risk groups within geographic areas known to have a large number of AIDS cases, as well as for the entire US, for the year June 1983–May 1984 (Hardy *et al.*, 1985). These calculations suggest that rates for single men and intravenous drug abusers in San Francisco and New York City may be in the range of 175–269 per 100 000. These rates were therefore similar to that calculated for all US haemophilia A patients (estimated at 199 per 100 000 in this report).

Investigators at CDC recently completed a statistical evaluation of the incubation period for transfusion-associated AIDS, i.e. the time between transfusion and AIDS diagnosis, based on the 100 adult cases that had been reported to CDC as of April 1, 1985 (Lui *et al.*, 1986). The distribution of these data was found to most closely fit the Weibull family of curves. Based on this distribution it was estimated that the predicted mean incubation period for transfusion-associated AIDS would be 4.5 years (90% confidence interval: 2.6–14.2 years), although the observed mean incubation period was only approximately 2.5 years. This prediction is consistent with the observation from cohort studies that the risk of AIDS persists for many years and that HIV is likely to persist for the life of the human host. This has important implications in regard to the projected extent and duration of the AIDS epidemic (Marx, 1986). For example, current prevention measures may not have a visible impact upon the AIDS epidemic curve until years after they are instituted. For that reason, special studies to determine the incidence of HIV infection *per se* are needed.

1.4 INTERNATIONAL SURVEILLANCE

Surveillance techniques and the intensity of surveillance for AIDS vary greatly from one country to another, just as they do for other causes of morbidity and mortality. This makes it difficult to compare incidence figures on an international level. The case numbers for each country individually are of interest, but it must be realized that they may reflect an awareness or non-awareness of the disease, as well as the actual disease occurrence. As of September 30, 1985, 1573 cases of AIDS were reported to the World Health Organization European Collaborating Centre on AIDS, by the 21 countries corresponding with that Centre (CDC, 1986b). Males represented 92% of cases; 42% of all cases reported were 30–39 years of age. Homosexual men accounted for 60–100% of cases in 12 of 16 countries providing this information. The largest numbers of reported cases have been Belgium (118), the United Kingdom (225), the Federal Republic of Germany (295), and France (466).

In the Americas, 778 cases have been reported from 14 countries other than the US, including Brazil (182), Canada (190), and Haiti (340) (Curran *et al.*, 1985). Cases have been reported among residents of 25 African countries. Studies in Zaire suggest that the male-to-female ratio, at 1.1 to 1, differs greatly from that found in the US or Europe (Curran *et al.*, 1985), due in part to an increased risk for both men and women from heterosexual transmission and a relative lack of cases in the male-predominant risk groups of the US and Europe (i.e. homosexual men, intravenous drug abusers, and haemophiliacs).

1.5 PATHOGENESIS AND COURSE OF DISEASE

HIV has been isolated from lymphocytes and tissues of persons with AIDS or at risk for AIDS (Ho *et al.*, 1985a; Barré-Sinoussi *et al.*, 1983; Gallo *et al.*, 1984; Levy *et al.*, 1984). This virus is tropic and cytopathic for T helper cells *in vitro* (Klatzmann *et al.*, 1984; McDougal *et al.*, 1985a). Epidemiologic studies have provided strong evidence of an association between AIDS and HIV infection and also the best means of evaluating the spectrum and course of disease. Epidemiologic work includes seroprevalence surveys (Levy *et al.*, 1984; Brun-Vezinet *et al.*, 1984; Safai *et al.*, 1984; Des Jarlis *et al.*, 1984) and several studies have in addition shown an association between HIV seropositivity and (a) decreased numbers of T helper cells and (b) degree of exposure to certain blood products, number of sexual partners, or certain sexual activities (Jason *et al.*, 1985; Groopman *et al.*, 1985).

A large number of epidemiologic studies are currently underway to investigate the spectrum, course, and cofactors involved in HIV infection. These projects are preliminary, given the long incubation period for this disease (Lui *et al.*, 1986) and the recency of seroconversion for most at-risk populations. For example, two independent studies suggest that over half of the factor concentrate recipients in the US acquired antibody to HIV between 1981 and the end of 1983 (Evatt *et al.*, 1985; Eyster *et al.*, 1985). Given these limitations, based on 6875 members of a hepatitis B study cohort in San Francisco, it has been estimated that by 1985 serologic evidence of HIV exposure was 28 times more common than AIDS itself and that 500 000–1 000 000 Americans had been infected as of September 1985 (Curran *et al.*, 1985).

Infection with HIV appears to be prolonged, if not permanent, in most instances. The virus has been isolated as much as 69 months after an individual was known to be antibody-positive; this is true of asymptomatic, as well as symptomatic, individuals (Barré-Sinoussi *et al.*, 1983; Gallo *et al.*, 1984; Jaffe *et al.*, 1985). Virus isolation may be more frequently possible from symptomatic individuals. In one study, 5 of 6 seropositive haemophilic children with lymphadenopathy had virus isolated from their peripheral blood lymphocytes, compared with 1 of 13 asymptomatic, seropositive children ($p=0.003$, two-tailed Fisher's Exact Test) (Gomperts *et al.*, 1985). However, this finding may not be universally true, since in another study virus was isolated from 8 of 12 (67%) of asymptomatic homosexual males who had been seropositive for HIV 4–69 months (Jaffe *et al.*, 1985).

Longitudinal studies are extremely difficult to compare to one another because of differing, or unstated: (1) seroprevalence rates in the populations studied, (2) seroconversion patterns, (3) time periods since seroconversion and time intervals examined, and (4) the presence or absence of, and duration of, symptomatic illness at the time of enrolment. One cohort of 42 homosexual males with lymphadenopathy was enrolled in New York City in February 1981. Ten (24%) had developed AIDS at 42 months after enrolment (Mathur-Wagh *et al.*, 1985). In the San Francisco cohort discussed above, 2 of 31 (7%) individuals who were seropositive in 1978–80 had developed AIDS within 6 years of their entry into the study (Jaffe *et al.*, 1985). Over the 6-year period, two-thirds of the cohort had antibody to HIV and nearly a third had some clinical abnormality thought to be related to the virus. In a third study, 5 independent cohorts were evaluated for approximately 3 years, including 3 groups of homosexual men, 1 group of haemophiliacs, and 1 group of intravenous drug abusers. No individual had

AIDS at enrolment, but the location and date of enrolment differed for each group, as did HIV seroprevalence rates at the time of each cohort's enrolment (Goedert *et al.*, 1986). The 3-year incidences of AIDS ranged from 34% for the New York City homosexual cohort to 8% for the Danish homosexual cohort who were enrolled. In another paper concerning one of the above five cohorts, consisting of a group of Philadelphia haemophiliacs, researchers found that 70% of individuals who were seropositive more than 3 years had lymphadenopathy, compared to 10% of those seropositive 3 years or less (Eyster *et al.*, 1985).

1.6 TRANSMISSIBILITY OF THE VIRUS

As discussed above, many antibody-positive individuals appear to be actively infected for prolonged periods (Barré-Sinoussi *et al.*, 1983; Gallo *et al.*, 1984; Jaffe *et al.*, 1985; Gomperts *et al.*, 1985). HIV has been isolated from semen, cervical secretions, saliva, tears, and blood; virus particles have been found in fetal organs of an abortus of an infected mother (Groopman *et al.*, 1984; Ho *et al.*, 1984; Zagury *et al.*, 1984, 1985; Fujikawa *et al.*, 1985; Vogt *et al.*, 1986; Wofsy *et al.*, 1986; Jovaisas *et al.*, 1985). Concerns have therefore been expressed about the risks associated with interactions with infected individuals. These concerns have been addressed by a number of epidemiologists using both surveillance and research techniques.

Blood transmission of HIV is strongly supported by the presence of intravenous drug use, haemophilia, and the receipt of transfusion as risk factors for AIDS (Tables 1.1 and 1.2). Epidemiologic studies have shown an association between AIDS or HIV and: (1) sharing of needles among IV drug users (Curran *et al.*, 1985), (2) factor concentrate dosage of haemophilia A patients (Jason *et al.*, 1985), and (3) the receipt of various blood components, including cells, platelets, plasma, and whole blood (Peterman *et al.*, 1985; Curran *et al.*, 1984).

The current data also support that HIV is transmitted sexually, but fail to support interpersonal transmission through non-sexual contacts. To date, 6 of 46 (13%) of sex partners participating in CDC haemophilia household studies have antibodies to HIV. These participants all had a haemophilic sex partner with AIDS, AIDS-related complex (ARC), or clinically asymptomatic HIV infection documented by the presence of antibody. The seroprevalence rate was highest for partners of haemophiliacs with ARC (2 out of 9 or 22%), but this rate was not significantly different from that for partners of other infected haemophiliacs (4 out of 37 or 11%). Two seropositive sex partners have developed AIDS, as did their spouses; 2 developed ARC; and 2 are clinically well. Researchers at Walter Reed Army Medical Center included 7 female spouses in an evaluation of 27 index patients with ARC and 14 index patients with AIDS (Redfield *et al.*, 1985a). Two of the 4 spouses of

AIDS patients themselves had HIV antibodies and ARC symptoms. Three of 3 spouses of ARC patients had antibody or virus isolated from their blood; one of these herself had ARC. Risk, therefore, exists for sex partners of both homosexual men and heterosexual men and women; further studies will help quantify this risk (Redfield *et al.*, 1985a; Jason *et al.*, 1986). Risk is not limited to those having rectal intercourse (Jason *et al.*, 1986; Redfield *et al.*, 1985b); it is unclear whether risk varies with the clinical status of the antibody-positive individual.

Transplacental transmission of HIV has been documented (Jovaisas *et al.*, 1985; Vilmer *et al.*, 1984; Lapointe *et al.*, 1985; Stewart *et al.*, 1985). Although HIV has been isolated from breast milk (Thiry *et al.*, 1985), it is not known if it is transmissible through this route (Stewart *et al.*, 1985; Thiry *et al.*, 1985). Early postnatal transmission from a mother to her infant appears to have occurred in at least one instance. The mother had been delivered by caesarean section and had received a blood transfusion post-delivery from a donor who later developed AIDS. The mother and infant both subsequently developed HIV antibodies and symptoms of AIDS. The types of contact leading to maternal-child transmission could not be determined; however, the mother was breast feeding (Ziegler *et al.*, 1985). For that reason, at the present time breast feeding by an antibody-positive mother should be strongly discouraged. The incidence of AIDS in infants of infected mothers is reportedly high (personal communication, M. Rogers, CDC, 1986). From one study, it would appear that asymptomatic, infected mothers of infants with AIDS may themselves frequently develop symptoms following pregnancy. Twelve of 16 mothers evaluated over an average of 30 months went on to have symptoms: 5 developed AIDS and 7, AIDS-related complex. This study suggests that the risk of subsequently born infants developing AIDS is also high: 4 infants developed AIDS in 12 subsequent pregnancies of 11 mothers (Scott *et al.*, 1985). Interpretation of these data are limited by the selection procedure, i.e. to instances in which a mother has already delivered a child diagnosed as having AIDS.

The risk associated with other forms of household and casual contacts appear to be minimal. Although the virus has been isolated from saliva, the isolation rate is low (Ho *et al.*, 1985b) and saliva does not appear to be an effective route of transmission (Saviteer *et al.*, 1985; Schechter *et al.*, 1986). In 2 studies of haemophiliac patients' households, no one who was not a sex partner was found to have HIV antibodies (Jason *et al.*, 1986; Lawrence *et al.*, 1985). In one of these studies it was possible to determine that household members had experienced 44 person-years of assisting in factor concentrate administration without developing antibodies (Lawrence *et al.*, 1985). To date, none of 128 non-sex partner household members participating in CDC haemophilia household studies have antibody to HIV; 37 of these participants were 5–17 years of age. Results of other studies also support that non-

sex contact transmission is rare, if it exists at all (Friedland *et al.*, 1986). In all but one instance (Ziegler *et al.*, 1985), infection has occurred in children of an infected parent only when a transplacental route was possible (Redfield *et al.*, 1985b; Friedland *et al.*, 1986; Ragni *et al.*, 1985). Child-to-child transmission has not been documented.

1.7 POLICY IMPLICATIONS

It is extremely difficult to quantify the economic impact of AIDS upon the US medical system, government, and society. One estimate, based upon a number of extrapolations, suggests that the first 10 000 patients with AIDS will require 1.6 million days in the hospital and incur over $1.4 billion in in-patient expenditures. Losses incurred from disability and premature death are estimated at over $4.8 billion (Hardy *et al.*, 1986). Cost of care may vary widely from one location to another; however, this estimate provides a reminder of the potentially overwhelming impact of the AIDS epidemic (CDC, 1985b).

The most obvious strides in preventing HIV transmission have been made in the area of blood product safety. Enzyme immunoassay (EIA) serologic test kits for antibody to HIV were licensed in March 1985 and are being used throughout the US and in an increasing number of other countries. One US-based survey showed that 0.9% of blood units tested were initially reactive and 0.08–0.32% were repeatedly reactive; reactivity rates varied by region of the country (CDC, 1985a). Overall, approximately 0.25% of blood units have been found to be repeatedly reactive (CDC, 1985b). In two series, samples that were strongly reactive in EIA tests had a 94% and 97% rate of positivity in Western blot testing (CDC, 1985b). The sensitivity and specificity of various test kits, indirect immunofluorescence, Western-blot, and radio immunoprecipitation techniques, in relation to one another, have been evaluated (Weiss *et al.*, 1985a; NBTS, 1985; Courouce, 1986; Mortimer, Parry and Mortimer, 1985; Sandstrom *et al.*, 1985). All kits appear to be adequate screening tools, although improved versions will likely be developed. The low HIV seroprevalence rates of US blood donors indicate that the risk associated with blood products will be minimized without affecting the US blood supply adversely.

Heat-treated clotting factor concentrates were developed several years ago with the unfulfilled goal of decreasing hepatitis infectivity of factor concentrates. These products have been commercially available, but were not widely used until two studies showed that HIV is heat-sensitive (McDougal *et al.*, 1985b; Spire *et al.*, 1985). The virus was non-detectable when treated according to commercial manufacturers' various specifications (McDougal *et al.*, 1985b). The National Hemophilia Foundation currently recommends that all haemophiliac patients requiring factor therapy be treated with heat-treated products only (NHF, 1985). Preliminary studies have indicated no seroconversion in persons receiving only heat-treated products (Felding *et al.*, 1985; Mosseler *et al.*, 1985; Rouzioux *et al.*, 1985). Two cases of seroconversion possibly associated with heat-treated factor have been reported (White *et al.*, 1986; van den Berg *et al.*, 1986). Both were associated with products produced prior to the initiation of donor screening. One reported individual had a past history of intravenous drug abuse; this patient was lost to follow-up (White *et al.*, 1986). The second patient seroconverted 4 months following his last usage of the implicated concentrate (personal communication, W. van den Berg, 1986). Virus was not isolated from either patient; it is therefore unknown if these seroconversions represent infection or exposure to inactive viral components. However, donor screening, in addition to heat treatment, should virtually ensure the safety of currently produced concentrates.

While heat treatment and donor screening appear to be highly effective means of minimizing HIV transmission through blood products, because of the long incubation period of AIDS, cases in blood product recipients will continue to occur. Furthermore, more than 74% of US factor VIII concentrate recipients have been infected with the virus and may have sex partners at risk for HIV virus transmission (Jason *et al.*, 1985, 1986). Studies of household members are underway to determine the extent of this risk. The CDC and the National Hemophilia Foundation have recommended that factor recipients refrain from genital intercourse and oral sex, or at least use condoms during intercourse, and that they and their spouses defer pregnancy until these studies are completed. Similar recommendations had been made by the Public Health Service (PHS) for all infected persons and for members of all risk groups (CDC, 1983, 1985c).

Antedating recommendations and policies involving blood product recipients, in March 1983, the PHS recommended that members of high-risk groups reduce the number of their sexual partners (CDC, 1983). Condoms theoretically would provide some protection against HIV and transmission (Conant *et al.*, 1986); components of some spermicides have been effective *in vitro* in inactivating HIV (Hicks *et al.*, 1985; Voeller, 1986). The safest means of protection, however, remains abstinence from sexual activities involving the exchange of body fluids. In December 1985, PHS recommended that pregnant women or women who may become pregnant, who may be at risk for HIV infection, be offered counselling and antibody testing (CDC, 1985d). Infected women should be advised to consider delaying pregnancy.

Risk of transmission in work, school, and hospital settings appears minimal (Jason *et al.*, 1986; Ho *et al.*, 1985b; Saviteer *et al.*, 1985; Friedland *et al.*, 1986; Weiss *et al.*, 1985b; Hirsch *et al.*, 1985). The PHS has published guidelines emphasizing that antibody-positive individuals should not be excluded from ordinary school and workplace activities (CDC, 1985e, f). Hospital precautions do not require the routine use of isolation, gown, or mask but do include the use of non-sterile gloves if contact with blood, body fluids, secretions, or excretions is anticipated (AHA, 1986).

Until a vaccine becomes available, prevention of transmission through sexual contact and intravenous drug abuse depends upon effective education. Education will require the cooperation of federal and local agencies, local community groups, health professionals, and both structured and unstructured social networks, with a unified goal of diffusing unreasonable fears; providing counsel and support concerning difficult, reasonable fears; and fostering avoidance of behaviours associated with virus transmission and acquisition. Evaluation of the effectiveness of educational programmes will be essential. For example, in one study assessing what haemophilic patients understood about the meaning of their own HIV antibody status, 18 of 18 providers indicated that they gave explanations consistent with CDC recommendations. However, one-third of the patients thought having HIV antibody protected them from AIDS and 31% did not know that antibody meant they had contact with the AIDS virus (Hargraves *et al.*, in press). An example of evaluation on a broader scale, is the determination that following the 1983 recommendations by the PHS and others to reduce the number of sexual partners (CDC, 1983), the number of reported sexually transmitted infections in homosexual men in New York City greatly declined (CDC, 1984). While the relation between the information/education and this finding could not be directly evaluated, the finding is compatible with a positive effect.

In conclusion, our understanding of AIDS has increased exponentially in the past five years. The ultimate resolution to the AIDS epidemic will come with the development of a vaccine and specific antiviral therapies. Epidemiology will have an important role in the evaluation of vaccine and therapeutic efficacy, just as it continues to serve a vital role determining the nature, characteristics, and extent of the AIDS epidemic and in educating the public to minimize disease transmission.

REFERENCES

AHA (1986) Management of HTLV-III/LAV infection in the hospital. The recommendation of the advisory committee on infections within hospitals. American Hospital Association, January, 1986.

Barré-Sinoussi, F., Chermann, J. C., Rey, F. *et al.* (1983) Isolation of T-lymphotropic retrovirus from a patient at risk for acquired immune deficiency syndrome (AIDS). *Science*, 220, 868–71.

Brun-Vezinet, F., Rouzioux, C., Barre-Sinoussi, F. *et al.* (1984) Detection of IgG antibodies to lymphadenopathy-associated virus in patients with AIDS or lymphadenopathy syndrome. *Lancet*, i, 1253–6.

CDC (1981a) *Pneumocystis* pneumonia – Los Angeles. *MMWR*, 30, 250–2.

CDC (1981b) Kaposi's sarcoma and *Pneumocystis* pneumonia among homosexual men – New York City and California. *MMWR*, 30, 305–8.

CDC (1982) Update on acquired immune deficiency syndrome (AIDS) – United States. *MMWR*, **31**, 507–14.

CDC (1983) Prevention of acquired immune deficiency syndrome (AIDS): Report of inter-agency recommendations. *MMWR*, **32**, 101–4.

CDC (1984) Declining rates of rectal and pharyngeal gonorrhea among males – New York City. *MMWR*, **33**, 295–7.

CDC (1985a) Results of human T-lymphotropic virus type III test kits reported from blood collection centers – United States, April 22 – May 19, 1985. *MMWR*, **34**, 375–6.

CDC (1985b) Update: Public Health Service workshop on human T-lymphotropic virus type III antibody testing – United States. *MMWR*, **34**, 477–8.

CDC (1985c) Provisional Public Health Service Inter-Agency recommendations for screening donated blood and plasma for antibody to the virus causing acquired immunodeficiency syndrome. *MMWR*, **34**, 1–5.

CDC (1985d) Recommendations for assisting in the prevention of perinatal transmission of human T-lymphotropic virus type III/lymphadenopathy-associated virus and acquired immunodeficiency syndrome. *MMWR*, **34**, 721–6, 731–2.

CDC (1985e) Education and foster care of children infected with human T-lymphotropic virus type III/lymphadenopathy-associated virus. *MMWR*, **34**, 517–21.

CDC (1985f) Recommendations for preventing transmission of infection with human T-lymphotropic virus type III/lymphadenopathy-associated virus in the work place. *MMWR*, **34**, 681–86, 691–5.

CDC (1986a) Revision of the case definition of acquired immunodeficiency syndrome for national reporting – United States. *MMWR*, **34**, 373–5.

CDC (1986b) Update: acquired immunodeficiency syndrome – Europe. *MMWR*, **35**, 35–8, 43–6.

Conant, M., Hardy, D., Sernatinger, J. *et al.* (1986) Condoms prevent transmission of AIDS-associated retrovirus (letter). *JAMA.*, **255**, 1306.

Courouce, A.-M. (1986) Evaluation of eight ELISA kits for the detection of anti-LAV/HTLV-III antibodies (letter). *Lancet*, **i**, 1152–3.

Curran, J. W., Lawrence, D. N., Jaffe, H. *et al.* (1984) Acquired immunodeficiency syndrome (AIDS) associated with transfusions. *N. Engl. J. Med.*, **310**, 69–75.

Curran, J. W., Morgan, W. M., Hardy, A. M. *et al.* (1985) The epidemiology of AIDS: current status and future prospects. *Science*, **229**, 1352–7

Des Jarlis, D. C., Marmor, M., Cohen, H. *et al.* (1984) Antibodies to a retrovirus etiologically associated with acquired immunodeficiency syndrome (AIDS) in populations with increased incidences of the syndrome. *MMWR*, **33**, 377–9.

DHEW (1977) Study to evaluate supply–demand relationships for AHF and PTC through 1980. NIH publication 77–1274, US Department of Health, Education, and Welfare.

Evatt, B. L., Gomperts, E. D., McDougal, J. S. and Ramsey, R. B. (1985) Coincidental appearance of LAV/HTLV-III antibodies in hemophiliacs and the onset of the AIDS epidemic. *N. Engl. J. Med.*, **312**, 483–6.

Eyster, M. E., Goedert, J. J., Sarngadharan, M. G. *et al.* (1985) Development and early natural history of HTLV-III antibodies in persons with hemophilia. *JAMA* **253**, 2219–23.

Felding, P., Nilsson, I. M., Hansson, B. G. and Biberfeld, G. (1985) Absence of antibodies to LAV/HTLV-III in haemophiliacs treated with heat-treated factor VIII concentrate of American origin (letter). Lancet, **ii**, 832–3.

Friedland, G. H., Saltzman, B. R., Rogers, M. F. *et al.* (1986) Lack of transmission of

HTLV-III/LAV infection to household contacts of patients with AIDS or AIDS-related complex with oral candidiasis. *N. Engl. J. Med.*, **314**, 344–9.

Fujikawa, L. S., Salahuddin, S. Z., Palestine, A. G. *et al.* (1985) Isolation of human T-lymphotropic virus type III from the tears of a patient with the acquired immunodeficiency syndrome. *Lancet*, **ii**, 529–30.

Gallo, R. C., Salahuddin, S. Z.Popovic, M. *et al.* (1984) Frequent detection and isolation of cytopathic retroviruses (HTLV-III) from patients with AIDS and at risk from AIDS. *Science*, **224**, 500–3.

Goedert, J. J., Biggar, R. J., Weiss, S. H. *et al.* (1986) Three-year incidence of AIDS in five cohorts of HTLV-III-infected risk group members. *Science*, **231**, 992–5.

Gomperts, E. D., Feorino, P., Evatt, B. L. *et al.* (1985) LAV/HTLV-III presence in peripheral blood lymphocytes of seropositive young hemophiliacs. *Blood*, **65**, 1549–52.

Groopman, J. E., Salahuddin, S. Z., Sarngadharan, M. G. *et al.* (1984) HTLV-III in saliva of people with AIDS-related complex and healthy homosexual men at risk for AIDS. *Science*, **226**, 447–9.

Groopman, J. E., Mayer, K. H., Sarngadharan, M. G. *et al.* (1985) Seroepidemiology of human T-lymphotropic virus type III among homosexual men with the acquired immunodeficiency syndrome or generalized lymphadenopathy and among asymptomatic controls in Boston. *Ann. Intern. Med.*, **102**, 334–7.

Hardy, A. M., Allen, J. R., Morgan, W. M. and Curran, J. W. (1985) The incidence rate of acquired immunodeficiency syndrome in selected populations. *JAMA*, **253**, 215–20.

Hardy, A. M., Rauch, K., Echenberg, D. *et al.* (1986) The economic impact of the first 10,000 cases of acquired immunodeficiency syndrome in the United States. *JAMA*, **255**, 209–11.

Hargraves, M. A., Jason, J. M., Chorba, T. L. *et al.* (In press) Hemophiliac patients' knowledge and educational needs concerning AIDS. *Amer. J. Hematol.*

Hicks, D. R., Martin, L. S., Getchell, J. P. *et al.* (1985) Inactivation of HTLV-III/LAV-infected cultures of normal human lymphocytes by nonoxynol-9 in vitro (letter). *Lancet*, **ii**, 1422–3.

Hirsch, M. S., Wormser, G. P., Schooley, R. T. *et al.* (1985) Risk of nosocomial infection with human T-cell lymphotropic virus III (HTLV-III). *N. Engl. J. Med.*, **312**, 1–4.

Ho, D. D., Schooley, R. T., Rota, T. R. *et al.* (1984) HTLV-III in the semen and blood of a homosexual man. *Science*, **226**, 451–3.

Ho, D. D., Rota, T. R., Schooley, R. T. *et al.* (1985a) Isolation of HTLV-III from cerebrospinal fluid and neural tissues of patients with neurologic syndromes related to the acquired immunodeficiency syndrome. *N. Engl. J. Med.*, **313**, 1493–7.

Ho, D. D., Byington, R. E., Schooley, R. T. *et al.* (1985b) Infrequency of isolation of HTLV-III virus from saliva in AIDS (letter). *N. Engl. J. Med.*, **313**, 1606.

Jaffe, H. W., Darrow, W. W., Echenberg, D. F. *et al.* (1985) The acquired immunodeficiency syndrome in a cohort of homosexual men. A six year follow-up study. *Ann. Intern. Med.*, **103**, 210–14.

Jason, J., McDougal, J. S., Holman, R. C. *et al.* (1985) Human T-lymphotropic retrovirus type III/lymphadenopathy-associated virus antibody. Association with hemophiliacs' immune status and blood component usage. *JAMA*, **253**, 3409–15.

Jason, J. M., McDougal, J. S., Dixon, G. *et al.* (1986) HTLV-III/LAV antibody and immune status of household contacts and sexual partners of persons with hemophilia. *JAMA*, **255**, 212–5.

Johnson, R. E., Lawrence, D. N., Evatt, B. L. *et al.* (1985) Acquired immunodeficiency syndrome among patients attending hemophilia treatment centers and mortality experience of hemophiliacs in the United States. *Am. J. Epidemiol.*, **121**, 797–810.

Jovaisas, E., Koch, M. A., Schafer, A. *et al.* (1985) LAV/HTLV-III in a 20-week fetus (letter). *Lancet*, **ii**, 1129.

Klatzmann, D., Barre-Sinoussi, F., Nugeyre, M. T. *et al.* (1984) Selective tropism of lymphadenopathy associated virus (LAV) for helper-inducer T-lymphocytes. *Science*, **225**, 59–63.

Lapointe, N., Michaud, J., Pekodic, D. *et al.* (1985) Transplacental transmission of HTLV-III virus. *N. Engl. J. Med.*, **312**, 1325–6.

Lawrence, D. N., Jason, J. M., Bouhasin, J. D. *et al.* (1985) HTLV-III/LAV antibody status of spouses and household contacts assisting in home infusion of hemophilia patients. *Blood*, **66**, 703–5.

Levy, J. A., Hoffman, A. D., Kramer, S. M. *et al.* (1984) Isolation of lymphocytopathic retroviruses from San Francisco patients with AIDS. *Science*, **225**, 840–2.

Lui, K.-J., Lawrence, D. N., Morgan, W. M. *et al.* (1986) A model-based approach for estimating the mean incubation period of transfusion-associated acquired immunodeficiency syndrome. *Proc. Natl Acad. Sci, USA*, **83**, 3051–5.

Marx, J. L. (1986) The slow, insidious natures of the human T lymphotropic retroviruses. *Science*, **231**, 450–1.

Mathur-Wagh, U., Mildvan, D., Spigland, I. *et al.* (1985) Longitudinal assessment of persistent generalized lymphadenopathy (PGL) in homosexual men. *Adv. Exp. Med. Biol.*, **187**, 93–6.

McDougal, J. S., Mawle, A., Cort, S. P. *et al.* (1985a) Cellular tropism of the human retrovirus HTLV-III/LAV. I. Role of T cell activation and expression of the T4 antigen. *J. Immunol.*, **135**, 3151–62.

McDougal, J. S., Martin, L. S., Cort, S. P. *et al.* (1985b) Thermal inactivation of the acquired immunodeficiency syndrome virus, human T-lymphotropic virus-III/ lymphadenopathy-associated virus, with special reference to antihemophilic factor. *J. Clin. Invest.*, **76**, 875–7.

Mortimer, P. P., Parry, J. V. and Mortimer, J. Y. (1985) Which anti-HTLV-III/LAV assays for screening and confirmatory testing? *Lancet*, **ii**, 873–7.

Mosseler, J., Schimpf, K., Auerswald, G. *et al.* (1985) Inability of pasteurised factor VIII preparations to induce antibodies to HTLV-III after long-term treatment (letter). *Lancet*, **i**, 1111.

NBTS (1985) Study Subgroup of the National Blood Transfusion Society. Evaluation of 3 immuno-enzyme kits for the detection of anti-LAV antibodies. Comparison with confirmation tests (French). *Rev. Fr. Transfus. Immunohematol*, **28**, 325–44.

NHF (1985) The National Hemophilia Foundation Medical and Scientific Advisory Council. Recommendations concerning AIDS and the treatment of hemophilia. Hemophilia Information Exchange, AIDS Update, Feb. 14, 1985, New York, NY.

Peterman, T. A., Jaffe, H. W., Feorino, P. M. *et al.* (1985) Transfusion-associated acquired immunodeficiency syndrome in the United States. *JAMA*, **254**, 2913–7.

Ragni, M. V., Urbach, A. H., Kiernan, S. *et al.* (1985) Acquired immunodeficiency syndrome in the child of a haemophiliac. *Lancet*, **i**, 133–5.

Redfield, R. R., Markham, P. D., Salahuddin, S. Z. *et al.* (1985a) Frequent transmission of HTLV-III among spouses of patients with AIDS-related complex and AIDS. *JAMA*, **253**, 1571–3.

Redfield, R. R., Markham, P. D., Salahuddin, S. Z. *et al.* (1985b) Heterosexually acquired HTLV-III/LAV disease (AIDS-related complex and AIDS). Epidemiologic evidence for female-to-male transmission. *JAMA*, **254**, 2094–6.

Rouzioux, C., Chamaret, S., Montagnier, L. *et al.* (1985) Absence of antibodies to AIDS virus in haemophiliacs treated with heat-treated factor VIII concentrates (letter). *Lancet*, **i**, 271–2.

Safai, B., Sarngadharan, M. G., Groopman, J. E. *et al.* (1984) Seroepidemiological studies of human T-lymphotropic retrovirus type III and acquired immunodeficiency syndrome. *Lancet*, **i**, 1438–40.

Sandstrom, E. G., Schooley, R. T., Hodd, T. *et al.* (1985) Detection of human anti-HTLV-III antibodies by indirect immunofluorescence using fixed cells. *Transfusion*, **25**, 308–12.

Saviteer, S. M., White, G. C., Cohen, M. S. and Jason, J. (1985) HTLV-III exposure during cardiopulmonary resuscitation (letter). *N. Engl. J. Med.*, **313**, 1606–7.

Schechter, M. T., Boyko, W. J., Douglas, B. *et al.* (1986) Can HTLV-III be transmitted orally? (letter). *Lancet*, **i**, 379.

Scott, G. B., Fischl, M. A., Klimas, N. *et al.* (1985) Mothers of infants with the acquired immunodeficiency syndrome. Evidence for both symptomatic and asymptomatic carriers. *JAMA*, **253**, 363–6.

Spire, B., Dormont, D., Barre-Sinoussi, F. *et al.* (1985) Inactivation of lymphadenopathy-associated virus by heat, gamma rays, and ultraviolet light. *Lancet*, **i**, 188–9.

Stewart, G. J., Tyler, J. P., Cunningham, A. L. *et al.* (1985) Transmission of human T-cell lymphotropic virus type III (HTLV-III) by artificial insemination by donor. *Lancet*, **ii**, 581–5.

Thiry, L., Sprecher-Goldberger, S., Jonckheer, T. *et al.* (1985) Isolation of AIDS virus from cell-free breast milk of three healthy virus carriers (letter). *Lancet*, **ii**, 891–2.

van den Berg, W., ten Cate, J. W., Breederveld, C. and Goudsmit, J. (1986) Seroconversion to HTLV-III in haemophiliac given heat-treated factor VIII concentrate (letter). *Lancet*, **i**, 803–4.

Vilmer, E., Fischer, A., Griscelli, C. *et al.* (1984) Possible transmission of a human lymphotropic retrovirus (LAV) from mother to infant with AIDS (letter). *Lancet*, **ii**, 229–30.

Voeller, B. (1986) Nonoxynol-9 and HTLV-III (letter). *Lancet*, **i**, 1153.

Vogt, M. W., Witt, D. J., Craven, D. E. *et al.* (1986) Isolation of HTLV-III/LAV from cervical secretions of women at risk for AIDS. *Lancet*, **i**, 525–7.

Weiss, S. H., Goedert, J. J., Sarngadharan, M. G. *et al.* (1985a) Screening test for HTLV-III (AIDS agent) antibodies. Specificity, sensitivity, and applications. *JAMA*, **253**, 221–5.

Weiss, S. H., Saxinger, W. C., Rechtman, D. *et al.* (1985b) HTLV-III infection among health care workers. Association with needle-stick injuries. *JAMA*, **254**, 2089–93.

White, G. C. II, Matthews, T. J., Weinhold, K. J. *et al.* (1986) HTLV-III seroconversion associated with heat-treated factor VIII concentrate (letter). *Lancet*, **i**, 611–12.

Wofsy, C. B., Cohen, J. B., Hauer, L. B. *et al.* (1986) Isolation of AIDS-associated retrovirus from genital secretions of women with antibodies to the virus. *Lancet*, **i**, 527–9.

Zagury, D., Bernard, J., Leibowitch, J. *et al.* (1984) HTLV-III in cells cultured from semen of two patients with AIDS. *Science*, **226**, 449–51.

Zagury, D., Fouchard, M., Cheynier, R. *et al.* (1985) Evidence of HTLV-III in T-cells from semen of AIDS patients: expression in primary cell cultures, long-term mitogen-stimulated cell cultures, and cocultures with a permissive T-cell line. *Cancer Res.*, **45**(9 Suppl), 4595s–7s.

Ziegler, J. B., Cooper, D. A., Johnson, R. O. *et al.* (1985) Postnatal transmission of AIDS-associated retrovirus from mother to infant. *Lancet*, **i**, 896–8.

2

Transfusion-associated AIDS

—— *Terence L. Chorba and Bruce L. Evatt* ——

2.1 INTRODUCTION

Soon after the epidemic of acquired immune deficiency syndrome (AIDS) began in the United States the preponderance of cases was found to be in two groups of individuals, homosexual men (CDC, 1981) and intravenous drug abusers (Wormser *et al.*, 1983). This unusual distribution suggested hepatitis B as a possible model of transmission for proposed infectious agents. The occurrence of this syndrome in patients who had received blood products soon added additional support to that model. The Centers for Disease Control (CDC) received the first report of a haemophilia patient with *Pneumocystis carinii* pneumonia in January of 1982 and the second and third patients were found by the CDC through routine surveillance of requests in June and July of 1982 for drugs available only from CDC to treat *P. carinii* pneumonia (CDC, 1982a). Inquiries concerning these initial patients' sexual activities, drug usage, ethnicity and travel or residence provided little evidence that the disease could have been acquired by contact with homosexuals, illicit drug abusers or Haitian immigrants. The hypothesis that AIDS developed in these patients as a result of an infectious agent transmitted by the blood products' administration seemed logical and research for the occurrence of disease in transfusion recipients intensified. Soon it became clear that AIDS was a major problem for blood banks and the plasma industry.

By mid-June 1987 over 37 000 US patients with AIDS have been reported to the CDC (1987). Of these patients, the principal risk factors for developing AIDS have included transfusion with blood or blood products for 1166 (364 with haemophilia and 802 who were transfused with blood or blood products for other reasons). In this chapter we will review the topic of transfusion-associated AIDS and its implications for transfusion practices.

2.2 INFECTIOUS CONSIDERATIONS IN BLOOD-PRODUCT TRANSFUSIONS

After the initiation of the widespread use of blood transfusion in the 20th century, data soon accumulated that implicated blood as a vehicle for transmission of infectious organisms. In 1943, Beeson first reported jaundice occurring in patients 1–4 months after transfusion with blood or plasma, and suggested an infectious aetiology (Beeson, 1943). The list of infectious agents transmitted by blood has gradually expanded (Table 2.1) and now many post-transfusion viral, bacterial and parasitic diseases are well-described entities (Soulier, 1984). The appearance of the retroviruses have added new problems and concerns on the safety of the various blood products. The approaches investigators took to reduce the risk of transmitting infectious agents have all but eliminated most as transfusion problems in countries where good medical care and screening procedures have been available. For instance, until the retroviruses appeared, only hepatitis and cytomegalovirus (CMV) created much concern for transfusionists in the United States.

In most instances the approach to reduction of risk for infection related to transfusions has been successful when the physician has considered both the nature of the organism and the type of transfusion component in question. Some components may be safe, others not, depending upon the biology of the organism, the ability of laboratories to screen easily for infected elements, the methods of component storage, and the application of inactivating procedures for infective agents. Both cellular and non-cellular preparations such as cryoprecipitate, fresh frozen plasma, and non-heat-treated plasma factor preparations have been associated with the transmission of several known viral agents, including CMV, human parvovirus B19, hepatitis B virus, and the virus(es) of non-A, non-B hepatitis (Soulier, 1984; Enck *et al.*, 1979). Another cell-associated virus, Epstein–Barr virus (EBV) has been transmitted by fresh blood, platelets, and leukocyte transfusions but not by fresh-frozen plasma or factor VIII or factor IX concentrates. Because of their biology the

Table 2.1 Infectious agents transmitted by transfusion

Viral	Parasitic
Hepatitis A	Malaria
Hepatitis B	Filariasis
Hepatitis non-A, non-B	Trypanosomiasis
Cytomegalovirus	Toxoplasmosis
Epstein–Barr virus	Babesiosis
Serum parvoviruses	Bacterial
HTLV-I/HIV	Multiple organisms
Treponemal	
Syphilis	

newly discovered retroviruses, human T-lymphotropic virus type I (HTLV-I) and human immunodeficiency virus (HIV), also carry a wider and divergent risk for cellular and non-cellular products. HIV has been transmitted by transfusion of blood and components, non-heat-treated factor concentrates and the exclusive use of cryoprecipitate (Koeper, Kammsley and Levy, 1985; CDC, 1985a). On the other hand, HTLV-I transmitted by blood transfusion with whole blood or cellular blood components has been reported, but this retroviral agent may be much more difficult to transmit with cell-free blood products (Okochi, Sato and Hinuma, 1984; Chorba *et al.*, 1985) and transmission by factor concentrate does not seem to be a problem (Chorba *et al.*, 1985). This may be explained to some extent because HTLV-I is not shed in large numbers into the plasma surrounding the infected lymphocytes (Gallo *et al.*, 1982) as is HIV (Palmer *et al.*, 1985).

2.3 HIV INFECTION AND CELLULAR BLOOD PRODUCTS

2.3.1 Epidemiological data

The first case of AIDS reported in association with cellular blood product transfusion (Ammann *et al.*, 1983; Curran *et al.*, 1984) was a 20-month-old infant who, in 1982, developed severe cellular immune deficiency and multiple opportunistic infections after receiving several blood component transfusions for erythroblastosis fetalis. Subsequently, the investigation of 3 adults who had the onset of *P. carinii* pneumonia between June and July 1982 strengthened the hypothesis that a potentially transmissible agent was producing AIDS in transfusion recipients (Curran *et al.*, 1984). Investigations of other transfusion-related AIDS cases demonstrated a consistent pattern. The ratio of male to female was 10:8 and the age range of the patients was from 19 to 67 years (median 54 years). The geographic distribution of cases was similar to those seen with other risk groups and was consistent with the source of the blood donations. Of the first 18 cases, 83% had received transfusions in association with surgery and 50% had been cardiac surgeries. Initially, the median time between transfusion and onset of illness was 24.5 months (range 10–43 months) and between transfusion and diagnosis of *P. carinii* pneumonia 27.5 months (range 15–57 months). (More recent data have shown an increase in incubation time to a mean of 54 months (Lui *et al.*, 1986).) All recipients had received more than one type of blood product ranging from packed cells, fresh frozen plasma, whole blood and platelet concentrates. When the donors of the first 7 cases were tracked down and investigated with extensive interviews and immunologic investigations, none of the donors had AIDS at that time (an observation that subsequently changed). However, 8 high risk donors to the 7 cases were identified by history or abnormal immunologic evaluations. Six of the 7 patients who had developed AIDS were exposed to at least one donor from a group at increased risk for AIDS and all 7 were exposed to a donor with decreased T helper/T suppressor ratio, a common finding in patients suffering with AIDS or related disorders. As an outcome of these studies, the US Public Health Service in March 1983 recommended that persons with symptoms suggestive of AIDS or members of groups at increased risk for AIDS refrain from donating blood or plasma.

2.3.2 Laboratory data

Epidemiologic work by Jaffe *et al.* (1984) demonstrated a higher prevalence of antibodies to the membrane antigens (MA) of cells infected with HTLV-I (which has limited antigenic cross-reactivity and genetic homology with HIV) in serum of donors of blood to transfusion-associated AIDS patients than among a control group of blood donors. These antibodies appear to have been directed against HIV-encoded glycoproteins that cross-react with HTLV-I antigens (Groopman *et al.*, 1984). Isolation of a retrovirus (the lymphadenopathy virus (LAV)) in a haemophiliac patient and subsequently similar virus to LAV from AIDS patients identified the possible aetiological agents for AIDS. This group of viruses, LAV and HTLV-III, later became known collectively as human immunodeficiency virus (HIV). When an assay for antibodies to HIV became available, similar work was important in supporting the hypothesis that HIV causes AIDS and is potentially transmissible from an infective blood donor to a susceptible recipient (Feorino *et al.*, 1984; Jaffe *et al.*, 1985a). Isolation of the virus from blood donor–recipient pairs convinced physicians and investigators that the aetiological agent for transfusion AIDS had been found.

2.4 APPROACH TO SAFETY OF CELLULAR PRODUCTS

2.4.1 Screening for HIV

HIV has been isolated from at least a single peripheral blood specimen in 67–95% of persons with specific antibody to HIV (Feorino *et al.*, 1985; Jaffe *et al.*, 1985b). Because HIV infection has been demonstrated in asymptomatic persons, the presence of antibody should be considered presumptive evidence of current infection and thus a potential carrier state. A number of 'surrogate' laboratory assays have been evaluated to distinguish potentially infectious blood donors from non-infected blood donors, including determination of T helper/T suppressor cell ratio, antibody to hepatitis B core antigen, and immune complexes, but none has proven as sensitive and as specific as the available assays for antibody to HIV (McDougal *et al.*, 1985a) (Table 2.2). With the development of inexpensive, commercially available enzyme-linked

Table 2.2 Screening tests for donors of blood products to transfusion-associated AIDS

Test	*Suspected donors* (n=*18*) *No. positive/no. tested*	*(%)*
Low T_4/T_8 Ratio	15/18	83.3
α-HBc	10/16	62.5
SBA	15/18	83.3
α-LAV p25 RIP	14/18	77.8
α-HTLV-III ELISA	15/16	93.8
α-HTLV-III blot	18/18	100.0
α-LAV blot	18/18	100.0

immunosorbent assay (ELISA) kits for detection of antibodies to HIV, identification of potentially infectious donors has helped to limit the risk of AIDS transmission by blood donors attending blood banks. Another laboratory method, the Western blot assay for HIV, has also proven effective in detecting antibodies to HIV but has not been easily adaptable for mass screening (Carlson *et al.*, 1985). Currently available commercial assays for antibody to HIV are reasonably accurate with high positive and negative predictive values (functions of prevalence or pretest probability of disease) in populations at increased risk for HIV infection. The performance characteristics of available ELISA and other HIV serologic tests are reviewed elsewhere (Carlson *et al.*, 1985; Schorr *et al.*, 1985; CDC, 1985b) and in Chapter 7.

2.4.2 Donor screening

On January 11, 1985, the CDC recommended that all blood used for transfusion or the manufacture of blood products be screened for HIV. On March 2, 1985, the Secretary of the Department of Health and Human Services (DHHS) Margaret Heckler, announced the licensure by the Food and Drug Administration (FDA) of the ELISA test as a screening test to be used in blood and plasma centres. By July 1985, FDA reported data from a survey of more than 1.1 million units of blood collected and tested for HIV antibody by 155 centres up to mid-June using the licensed ELISA tests (Kuritsky, 1985). Of this total, 2831 units (0.25%) were reactive for HIV antibody. CDC and the Atlanta region of the American Red Cross also reported data from the survey of 51 000 blood donors of whom 0.23% were repeatedly reactive for HIV antibody by ELISA (Allen *et al.*, 1985). Of 106 repeatedly reactive units, 34 (32%) demonstrated strong reactivity by ELISA; 94% of these 34 were also positive by Western blot tests, and 56% had positive cultures for HIV. None of 220 donors whose tests were initially reactive but subsequently negative had a positive Western blot assay for HIV and none had a positive HIV culture. Of repeatedly reactive donors with strong reactive tests, 89% were found on interview to have identifiable risk factors for HIV infection. None of those with weakly reactive tests had risk factors, and it is thought that this may reflect the non-specificity of the ELISA test.

Since March 1985, a two-phase screening procedure has been used by blood and plasma collection centres in the United States to decrease the transmission of HIV through transfusion of blood or blood products. First, potential donors are informed that if they have a risk factor for AIDS they should not donate; second, the blood or plasma accepted from donors is screened for an antibody to HIV. In September 1985, these criteria were broadened so that donor deferral recommendations included any men who had had sex with another man since 1977, including those who may have only had a single contact and who do not consider themselves homosexual or bisexual. This addition was the result of the observation that many individuals with confirmed positive HIV antibody test results were homosexual or bisexual males who did not perceive themselves as being in a risk group (CDC, 1985c; Schorr *et al.*, 1985).

Measures of sensitivity of the ELISA test have been very encouraging. Of all high risk persons attending a sexually transmitted diseases clinic in San Francisco, none of 70 men with negative HIV antibody tests had a positive virus culture, whereas 43 (60%) of 72 with repeatedly reactive tests were culture positive. Of these 72 antibody positive individuals, 70 (97%) were highly reactive for HIV by ELISA and 97% of those tested had a positive Western blot test as well (FDA, 1985).

The risk of contracting AIDS by blood transfusion has now been all but eliminated with the application of the ELISA test together with the use of self-exclusion criteria for high-risk donors by blood banks. In general, blood banks try to obtain confirmation of ELISA reactive tests by Western blot prior to notifying donors, and plasmapheresis facilities usually notify donors when a repeatedly reactive ELISA test result is obtained.

New cases of transfusion-associated AIDS will nonetheless probably continue to appear for two reasons: (1) since the incubation period for AIDS can exceed 5 years, some persons infected with HIV prior to the availability of the ELISA test may be expected to develop clinical manifestations including AIDS; (2) HIV transmission has now been reported from a person whose blood tested negative for HIV antibody at the time of blood donation. This donor appears to have had a recent infection through a single homosexual contact three months prior to blood donation, underscoring the importance of donor-deferral programmes in excluding blood from donors with very recent infections who do not have detectable antibody (CDC, 1986a).

2.5 HIV INFECTION AND CELL-FREE PRODUCTS

2.5.1 Factor concentrates – epidemiological data

The first haemophilia patient with AIDS was reported to CDC in January 1982. By the end of 1982, investigators suspected that non-heat-treated factor VIII preparations were the potential vehicle of HIV transmission. Evidence continued to accumulate that implicated the factor VIII preparations. (1) Cases had occurred who had no known risk factor and who had received only non-heat-treated factor VIII preparation. (2) AIDS cases initially had occurred among haemophilia patients who were heavy users of factor VIII concentrate. (3) Immune abnormalities and symptoms of the AIDS Related Complex were found to be associated with high factor concentrate use. (4) Finally, the distribution of cases were not related to the distribution of cases in other risk groups as had been the transfusion cases, but were similar to the distribution of the factor concentrates.

2.5.2 Laboratory data

As with AIDS patients whose risk factor was cellular blood product transfusion, a high prevalence of antibodies to HTLV-MA was found in the serum of haemophiliacs treated with non-heat-treated factor concentrates (Evatt *et al.*, 1983). Isolates of HIV were soon made from haemophiliacs with AIDS. When an assay for antibodies to HIV became available, HIV seropositivity was demonstrated in the majority of asymptomatic haemophilia patients (Ramsey *et al.*, 1984) and a temporal relationship between seroconversion and the epidemic of AIDS among haemophilia patients was demonstrated (Evatt *et al.*, 1985). Although HIV has not been isolated from factor concentrate preparations, most investigators are now convinced that the factor concentrate is the vehicle responsible for the transmission of HIV in most patients with haemophilia.

2.5.3 Viral inactivation studies

As noted above, the occurrence of AIDS cases with no known risk factor or exposure other than the use of non-heat-treated factor VIII preparations implicated non-heat-treated factor concentrates as potential vehicles of HIV transmission. Depending on the manufacturer, any given lot of commercially prepared factor VIII concentrate may contain plasma from between 2500 and 25 000 blood or plasma donors (Levine, 1985), and if not heat-treated, could present the patient with a greater chance of exposure to an infectious agent than would cryoprecipitate. However, HIV was found to be very heat labile; when HIV is added to lyophilized antihaemophilic factor and the mixture is heated to 60°C, 90% of virus is inactivated in about 30 min (McDougal *et al.*, 1985b). Heat treatment of factor concentrates in lyophilized form for 30h at 60°C effectively inactivates HIV without significantly altering the plasma recovery or plasma half-life (Heldebrant *et al.*, 1985). Several studies have documented a lack of HIV seroconversion state in haemophilia patients treated with American heat-treated factor VIII concentrates, indicating that proper heat-treatment reduces the potential risk of HIV transmission (Rouzioux *et al.*, 1985; Mosseler *et al.*, 1985; Felding *et al.*, 1985). However, the transmission of non-A, non-B hepatitis may still occur with heat-treated factor concentrates (Colombo *et al.*, 1985), and there have been reports of prolonged HIV seroconversion in at least three persons treated strictly with heat-treated intermediate- and/or high-purity factor VIII concentrate from a single manufacturer (van den Berg *et al.*, 1986; White *et al.*, 1986; HIE, 1986), which has resulted in concern that in some circumstances heat treatment may fail to inactivate the virus. No viral isolates were obtained from these patients; one individual had a drug abuse history and two others had received previously recalled lots of concentrates known to have contained plasma from a donor with AIDS. Several possible explanations have been offered to account for these observed seroconversions (HIE, 1986) including: (1) the particular heat-treatment process used by the manufacturer may not be completely effective in eliminating all infectious HIV particles; (2) seroconversions may reflect immunization by killed virus; (3) seroconversion may reflect passive receipt of immune globulin in factor concentrate; (4) seroconversions may have occurred years after viral infection from a non-heat-treated product; and (5) the patient(s) may have had another risk factor for developing AIDS. Because of frequent use of factor concentrates by many persons with coagulation disorders, additional efforts to guarantee viral inactivation without disrupting proteins in plasma-derived products are warranted. Accordingly, the manufacturer involved in this instance has voluntarily recommended the return of their lots of heat-treated factor VIII concentrate manufactured from plasma collected prior to donor screening for HIV antibody (HIE, 1986).

2.5.4 Other methods of viral inactivation

Other methods of viral inactivation in blood products are receiving intensive investigation. Present methods of heat treatment vary significantly (temperatures from 60 to 78°C on preparations varying from liquid to freeze-dried forms). These methods have been effective against HIV virus but the inactivation of non-A, non-B hepatitis (NANB) viruses in preparations has only been partially successful at best. NANB hepatitis remains a serious threat to patients; serial liver biopsies on patients who have been treated with factor VIII and factor IX concentrates have shown a considerable risk of chronic liver disease (Aledort *et al.*, 1985; Hay *et al.*, 1985; Colombo *et al.*, 1985). Thus many investigators are exploring alternative ways of viral inactivation aimed specifically at NANB hepatitis.

Ultraviolet light and beta-propiolactone will inactivate virus but the carcinogenic potential of beta-propiolactone and reduced yields of clotting factor has somewhat discouraged this methodology (Prince, Horowitz and Brotman, 1986). Other investigators have also shown the ability of tri-N-butyl phosphate (TNBP)/sodium cholate to inactivate viruses having lipid containing envelopes. This method appears to be useful on HIV, one strain of NANB hepatitis virus and hepatitis B virus (Colombo *et al.*, 1985).

Other researchers using novel ways of affinity chromatography purification to achieve highly purified products are also exploring these methods as ways to eliminate virus contaminants. For example, variations and combinations of inactivation procedures are being explored. Some companies are evaluating the use of increased temperature with increased purity of product. All of these methods still need field trials before final assessment can be made.

Presently, the safest commercially available product is heat-treated material that has been obtained from HIV-screened donors. For AIDS infection and the risk of NANB hepatitis will continue to remain a problem until future methods of inactivation are developed or fully assessed.

2.6 FUTURE OF BIO-FREE RECOMBINANT FACTOR CONCENTRATES

Investigators working independently at two separate companies, Genentech and Genetics Institute, have succeeded in isolating and cloning the gene for factor VIII (Wood *et al.*, 1984; Vehar *et al.*, 1984; Toole *et al.*, 1984). The gene has been found to be 186 000 kilobases long and the coding information for circulating factor VIII is spread among 26 exons. The extreme length of the gene and the necessity for extensive post translational modification discouraged the use of recombinant bacteria, such as *E. coli*, for the manufacture of this protein and thus initial attempts to produce the protein in culture systems have been with using mammalian cells. Recombinant factor VIII was successfully produced in cell lines and has been shown to be fully functional in that it corrects the defect caused by the missing protein in haemophiliac plasma and, when injected into haemophiliac dogs, has been found to correct the clotting and to circulate with a half-life similar to that of native factor VIII. Thus, the evidence accumulating suggests that bio-engineered factor VIII is equivalent to the blood derived protein. Progress is also being made on bioengineered factor IX. The gene for factor IX has been cloned and several biotechnology companies are trying to develop the bioengineered factor IX product (Kurachi and Davie, 1982; Jaye *et al.*, 1983). Bioengineered factor IX has an additional complication in that it requires gamma carboxylation of a glutamyl side chain. Because factor VIII deficiency is nine times as prevalent in the population as factor IX deficiency, bioengineering factor VIII is more viable commercially and is thus predicted to be available at an earlier date. There are no definite predictions as to when such products will be widely available; most investigators indicate that a several years' delay is probable.

2.6.1 Immunoglobulin preparations

When produced by plasma fractionation methods approved for use in the United States, immunoglobulin preparations, e.g. immunoglobulin (IG), hepatitis B immunoglobulin (HBIG), and intravenous immunoglobulin (IVIG), have not been implicated in transmission of HIV or other infectious agents (CDC, 1986b). Several studies have evaluated recipients of HBIG and IG, including recipients of lots subsequently found to be positive for HIV antibody (CDC, 1986b; Tedder, Uttley and Cheingsong-Popov, 1985). Although transient low levels of passively acquired HIV antibody have been detected after receiving HBIG that was strongly positive for HIV antibody, long-term seroconversion to HIV antibody-positivity or development of signs or symptoms suggestive of HIV infection in persons receiving IG, HBIG, and IVIG has not be observed (CDC, 1986b). HIV seropositivity has been observed in one HBIG recipient of 183 IG and/or HBIG recipients enrolled in CDC long-term follow-up studies of persons having needlestick exposures since August 1983, but no pre-exposure serum was available from this individual, and seropositivity may have predated the needlestick exposure and prophylaxis (CDC, 1986b).

The basic Cohn–Oncley fractionation processes (Cohen *et al.*, 1946; Oncley *et al.*, 1949) used in the production of immune globulins result in partitioning or inactivation at individual steps of from 10^{-1} to more than 10^{-4} of *in vitro* infectious units (IVIU)/ml (CDC, 1986b). It is estimated that the partitioning and inactivation processes result in HIV removal of in excess of 1×10^{15} IVIU/ml, whereas concentrations of infectious HIV in plasma of infected persons have been estimated to be less than 100 IVIU/ml (CDC, 1986b). In one study, the geometric mean titre of plasma from 43 HIV infected persons was 0.02 IVIU/ml (Wells *et al.*, 1986), demonstrating that the fractionation processes result in a considerable margin of safety with respect to removal of infectious HIV virus. In addition, since April 1985, all donor units used in making immune globulin products have been screened for antibodies to HIV, and all repeatedly reactive units have been discarded.

2.7 RECOMMENDATIONS TO PREVENT TRANSFUSION-ASSOCIATED DISEASE TRANSMISSION

The US Public Health Service has established recommendations for reducing potential risk of transmitting AIDS to recipients of blood, blood products, organs, and other tissues (CDC, 1982b, 1983, 1984, 1985c and d). Summarized, these include:

1. All donated blood and plasma, and blood or serum from donors of organs, tissues, or semen intended for human use, should be screened for HIV antibodies.
2. All individuals in high-risk groups for AIDS, including sexual partners of persons at high risk, and persons with positive tests, should refrain from donating plasma and/or blood. Persons in high-risk groups should not donate organs, tissues, or semen, regardless of the result of antibody testing.
3. Blood or plasma that is reactive for HIV should not be transfused or used for manufacture into injectable products capable of transmitting infectious agents.
4. An individual likely to have an HIV infection should be advised to refrain from donating blood, plasma, body organs, other tissue, or sperm. Devices that have punctured the skin, such as hypodermic and acupuncture needles, should be safely discarded or steam sterilized by autoclave before re-use, and whenever possible, disposable needles and equipment should be used.

2.8 THE FUTURE

Much additional information will be gathered with the widespread application of the ELISA test, and adjustments will undoubtedly be made in interpretations of the test in various laboratories as with any assay. The development of recombinant factor VIII from supernatants of cells transfected with the factor VIII gene (reconstructed using oligonucleotide probes based on partial amino acid sequence analysis) (Wood, *et al.*, 1984; Vehar *et al.*, 1984; Gitschier *et al.*, 1984) holds promise of another factor product that will provide an infection-free therapy for individuals with haemophilia A.

Until such time as a cure and/or a vaccine become available, attention to proper medical procedure and to behavioural restraint will remain the principal modalities for preventing further spread of the HIV agent.

REFERENCES

Aledort, L. M., Levine, P. H., Hilgartner, M. *et al.* (1985) A study of liver biopsies and liver disease among haemophiliacs. *Blood*, **66**, 367–72.

Allen, J. R. *et al.* (1985) HTLV-III antibody screening in a blood bank: Laboratory and clinical correlations. *Proceedings of Workshop on Experience with HTLV-III Antibody Testing*, sponsored by FDA, NIH and CDC, July 31.
Ammann, A. J., Cowan, M. J., Wara, D. W. *et al.* (1983) Acquired immunodeficiency in an infant: possible transmission by means of blood products. *Lancet*, **i**, 956–8.
Beeson, P. B. (1943) Jaundice occurring one to four months after transfusion of blood or plasma: report of seven cases. *JAMA*, **121**, 1332–4.
Carlson, J. R., Bryant, M. L., Hinrichs, S. H. *et al.* (1985) AIDS serology testing in low- and high-risk groups. *JAMA*, **253**, 3405.
CDC (1981) Kaposi's sarcoma and pneumocystis pneumonia among homosexual men – New York City and California. *MMWR*, **30**, 305.
CDC (1982a) *Pneumocystis carinii* pneumonia among persons with hemophilia A. *MMWR*, **31**, 365–7.
CDC (1982b) Acquired immune deficiency syndrome (AIDS): Precautions for clinical and laboratory staffs. *MMWR*, **31**, 577.
CDC (1983) Acquired immunodeficiency syndrome (AIDS): Precautions for health-care workers and allied professionals. *MMWR*, **32**, 450.
CDC (1984) Update: Acquired immunodeficiency syndrome (AIDS) in persons with hemophilia. *MMWR*, **33**, 589.
CDC (1985a) Changing patterns of acquired immunodeficiency syndrome in hemophilia patients – United States. *MMWR*, **34**, 241.
CDC (1985b) Update: Public Health Service workshop on human T-lymphotrophic virus type III antibody testing – United States. *MMWR*, **34**, 477.
CDC (1985c) Testing donors of organs, tissues, and semen for antibody to human T-lymphotropic virus type III/lymphadenopathy-associated virus. *MMWR*, **34**, 294.
CDC (1985d) Education and foster care of children infected with HTLV-III/LAV. *MMWR*, **34**, 517.
CDC (1986a) Transfusion-associated human T-lymphotropic virus type III/lymphadenopathy-associated virus infection from a seronegative donor – Colorado. *MMWR*, **35**, 389–91.
CDC (1986b) Safety of therapeutic immune globulin preparations with respect to transmission of human T-lymphotropic virus type III/lymphadenopathy-associated virus infection. *MMWR*, **35**, 231–3.
CDC (1987) Acquired immunodeficiency syndrome (AIDS) weekly surveillance report – United States, June 15.
Chorba, T. L., Jason, J. M., Ramsey, R. B. *et al.* (1985) HTLV-I antibody status in hemophilia patients treated with factor concentrates prepared from U.S. plasma sources and in hemophilia patients with AIDS. *Thromb. Haemostas.*, 180–2.
Cohen, E. J., Strong, L. E., Hughes, W. I. Jr *et al.* (1946) Preparation and properties of serum and plasma proteins. IV: A system for the separation into fractions of protein and lipoprotein components of biological tissues and fluids. *J. Am. Chem. Soc.*, **68**, 459–75.
Colombo, M., Mannucci, P. M., Carnelli, V. *et al.* (1985) Transmission of non-A, non-B hepatitis by heat-treated factor VIII concentrate. *Lancet*, **ii**, 1–4.
Curran, J. W., Lawrence, D. N., Jaffe, H. W. *et al.* (1984) Acquired immunodeficiency syndrome (AIDS) associated with transfusions. *N. Engl. J. Med.*, **310**, 69–75.
Enck, R. E., Betts, R. F., Brown, M. R. *et al.* (1979) Viral serology (hepatitis B virus, cytomegalovirus, Epstein–Barr virus) and abnormal liver function tests in transfused patients with hereditary hemorrhagic diseases. *Transfusion*, **19**, 32.
Evatt, B. L., Stein, S. F., Francis, D. P. *et al.* (1983) Antibodies to human T cell

leukaemia virus-associated membrane antigens in haemophiliacs: Evidence for infection before 1980. *Lancet*, **i**, 698–701.

Evatt, B. L., Gomperts, E. D., McDougal, J. S. *et al.* (1985) Coincidental appearance of LAV/HTLV-III antibodies in hemophiliacs and the onset of the AIDS epidemic. *N. Engl. J. Med.* **312**, 483–6.

FDA (1985) Drug Bulletin. *Progress on AIDS*, **15**, 27–32.

Felding, P., Nilsson, I. M., Hansson, B. G. and Biberfield, G. (1985) Absence of antibodies to LAV/HTLV-III in haemophiliacs treated with heat-treated factor VIII concentrate of American origin. *Lancet*, **ii**, 832–3.

Feorino, P. M., Kalyanaraman, V. S., Haverkos, H. W. *et al.* (1984) Lymphadenopathy associated virus infection of a blood donor–recipient pair with acquired immunodeficiency syndrome. *Science*, **225**, 69–72.

Feorino, P. M., Jaffe, H. W., Palmer, E. *et al.* (1985) Transfusion-associated acquired immunodeficiency syndrome: Evidence for persistent infection in blood donors. *N. Engl. J. Med.*, **312**, 1293–6.

Gallo, R. C., Robert-Guroff, M. Kalyanaraman, V. S. *et al.* (1982) Human T-cell retrovirus and adult T-cell lymphoma and leukemia: possible factors on viral incidence, in *Biochemical and Biological Markers of Neoplastic Transformation* (ed. P. Chandra), Plenum Press, New York, pp. 503–13.

Gitschier, J., Wood, W. I., Goralka, T. M. *et al.* (1984) Characterization of the human factor VIII gene. *Nature, Lond.*, **312**, 326.

Groopman, J. E., Salahuddin, S. Z., Sarngadharan, M. G. *et al.* (1984) Virologic studies in a case of transfusion-associated AIDS. *N. Engl. J. Med.*, **311**, 1419–22.

Hay, C. R. M., Preston, F. E., Triger, D. R. and Underwood, J. C. E. (1985) Progressive liver disease in haemophilia: An understated problem? *Lancet*, **i**, 1495–8.

Heldebrant, C. M., Gomperts, E. D., Kasper, C. K. *et al.* (1985) Evaluation of two viral inactivation methods for the preparation of safer factor VIII and factor IX concentrates. *Transfusion*. 25:510–15.

HIE (1986) Hemophilia Information Exchange. Factor VIII product return recommended. Medical Bulletin no. 40.

Jaffe, H. W., Francis, D. P., McLane, M. F. *et al.* (1984) Transfusion-associated AIDS: Serologic evidence of human T-cell leukemia virus infection of donors. *Science*, **223**, 1309–12.

Jaffe, H. W., Sarngadharan, M. G., DeVico, A. L. *et al.* (1985a) Infection with HTLV-III/LAV and transfusion-associated acquired immunodeficiency syndrome. *JAMA*, **254**, 770–3.

Jaffe, H. W., Feorino, P. M., Darrow, W. W. *et al.* (1985b) Persistent infection with human T-lymphotropic virus type III lymphadenopathy-associated virus in apparently healthy homosexual men. *Ann. Intern. Med.*, **102**, 627–30.

Jaye, M., De la Salle, H., Schamber, F. *et al.* (1983) Isolation of a human anti-haemophilic factor IX cDNA using a unique 52-base synthetic oligonucleotide probe deduced from the amino acid sequence of bovine factor IX. *Nucl. Acids Res.*, **11**, 2325.

Koeper, M. A., Kammsley, L. S. and Levy, J. A. (1985) Differential prevalence of antibody to AIDS-associated retrovirus in hemophiliacs treated with factor VIII concentrate versus cryoprecipitate: Recovery of infectious virus. *Lancet*, **i**, 275.

Kurachi, K. and Davie, E. W. (1982) Isolation and characterization of a cDNA coding for human factor IX. *Proc. Natl Acad. Sci. USA*, **79**, 6461.

Kuritsky, J. (1985) Results of human T-lymphotropic virus type-III test kits reported from blood collection centers – United States: April 22–June 16, 1985. Proceedings of Workshop on Experience with HTLV-III Antibody Testing, sponsored by FDA, NIH and CDC, July 31.

Levine, P. (1985) AIDS in individuals with hemophilia. *Ann. Intern. Med.* **103**, 723–6.

Lui, K. J., Lawrence, D. N., Morgan, W. M. *et al.* (1986) A model-based approach for estimating the mean incubation period of transfusion-associated acquired immunodeficiency syndrome. *Proc. Soc. Natl Sci.*, **83**, 3051–5.

McDougal, J. S., Jaffe, H. W., Cabradilla, C. D. *et al.* (1985a) Screening tests for blood donors presumed to have transmitted the acquired immunodeficiency syndrome. *Blood*, **65**, 772–5.

McDougal, J. S., Martin, L. S., Cort, S. P. *et al.* (1985b) Thermal inactivation of the AIDS virus, HTLV-III/LAV, with special reference to antihemophilic factor. *J. Clin. Invest.*, **76**, 875–7.

Mosseler, J., Schimpf, K., Auerswald, G. *et al.* (1985) Inability of pasteurised factor VIII preparations to induce antibodies to HTLV-III after long-term treatment. *Lancet*, **i**, 1111.

Okochi, K., Sato, H. and Hinuma, Y. (1984) A retrospective study on transmission of adult T cell leukemia virus by blood transfusion: seroconversion in recipients. *Vox Sang.*, **46**, 245–53.

Oncley, J. L., Melin, M., Richert, D. A. *et al.* (1949) The separation of the antibodies isoagglutinins, prothrombin, plasminogen and beta-lipoprotein into subfractions of human plasma. *J. Am. Chem. Soc.*, **71**, 541–50.

Palmer, E., Sporborg, C., Harrison, A. *et al.* (1985) Morphology and immunoelectron microscopy of AIDS virus. *Arch. Virol.*, **85**, 189–96.

Prince, A. M., Horowitz, B. and Brotman, B. (1986) Sterilisation of hepatitis and HTLV-3 viruses by exposure to tri (n-butyl) phosphate and sodium cholate. *Lancet*, **i**, 706–10.

Ramsey, R. B., Palmer, E. L., McDougal, J. S. *et al.* (1984) Antibody to lymphadenopathy-associated virus in haemophiliacs with and without AIDS. *Lancet*, **i**, 397–8.

Rouzioux, C., Chamaret, S., Montagnier, L. *et al.* (1985) Absence of antibodies to AIDS virus in haemophiliacs treated with heat-treated factor VIII concentrates. *Lancet*, **ii**, 271–2.

Schorr, J. B., Berkowitz, A., Cumming, P. O. *et al.* (1985) Prevalence of HTLV-III antibody in American blood donors. *N. Engl. J. Med.*, **313**, 384.

Soulier, J. P. (1984) Diseases transmitted by blood transfusion. *Vox Sang*, **47**, 1–6.

Tedder, R. S., Uttley, A. and Cheingsong-Popov, R. (1985) Safety of immunoglobulin preparation containing anti-HTLV-III (letter). *Lancet*, **i**, 815.

Toole, J. J., Knopf, J. L., Wozney, J. M. *et al.* (1984) Molecular cloning of a cDNA encoding human antihaemophilic factor. *Nature, Lond.*, **312**, 342.

van den Berg, W., ten Cate, J. W., Breederveld, C. and Goudsmit, J. (1986) Seroconversion to HTLV-III in haemophiliac given heat-treated factor VIII concentrate. *Lancet*, **i**, 803–4.

Vehar, G. A., Keyt, B., Eaton, D. *et al.* (1984) Structure of human factor VIII. *Nature, Lond.*, **312**, 337.

Wells, M. A., Wittek, A., Marcus-Sekura, C. *et al.* (1986) Chemical and physical inactivation of human T lymphotropic virus, type III (HTLV-III). *Transfusion*, **26**, 110–30.

White, G. C., Matthews, T. J., Weinhold, K. J. *et al.* (1986) HTLV-III seroconversion associated with heat-treated factor VIII concentrate. *Lancet*, **i**, 611–12.

Wood, W. I., Capon, D. J., Simonsen, C. C. *et al.* (1984) Expression of active human factor VIII from recombinant DNA clones. *Nature, Lond.*, **312,** 330.

Wormser, G. P., Krupp, L. B., Hanrahan, J. P. *et al.* (1983) Acquired immunodeficiency syndrome in male prisoners. New insights into an emergency syndrome. *Ann. Intern. Med.*, **98,** 297–303.

3

The human retroviruses causing AIDS

— Ulrich Desselberger —

3.1 INTRODUCTION

An infectious agent, in particular a virus, was strongly suspected in the aetiology of the acquired immune deficiency syndrome (AIDS) from the onset of the epidemic (Curran *et al.*, 1985). Retroviruses in particular were considered to be prime candidates because an animal retrovirus, feline leukaemia virus (FLV), was known to cause (besides leukaemia) a disease similar to AIDS in cats (Hardy *et al.*, 1976, Trainin *et al.*, 1983). In addition the mode of transmission, the spread of the disease and the selective T-cell tropism and depletion were reminiscent of the patterns previously seen with the then known human T-lymphotropic retroviruses (Wong-Staal and Gallo, 1985).

It has now been well established that the human T cell lymphotropic virus III/lymphadenopathy associated virus (HTLV III/LAV) is the causal agent of AIDS (Wong-Staal and Gallo, 1985; Sarngadharan, Markham and Gallo, 1985). Subsequent to its first description different names have been given to the virus: human T-cell lymphotropic virus III (HTLV-III, Gallo), lymphadenopathy associated virus (LAV, Montagnier), AIDS associated retrovirus (ARV, Levy *et al.*, 1985) and more recently human immunodeficiency virus (HIV, Varmus) has been proposed (Brown, 1986; Coffin *et al.*, 1986). In this chapter the virus will be referred to as the human immunodeficiency virus (HIV).

The earliest report of a retrovirus as the possible cause of AIDS is from Barré-Sinoussi *et al.* (1983). They described retrovirus particles in T-lymphocytes from a patient with generalized lymphadenopathy. These particles were identified in the peripheral lymph node cells after stimulation with phytohaemagglutinin and cultivation *in vitro* in the presence of interleukin 2, the human T cell growth factor (Morgan *et al.*, 1976), and antibody to human alpha-interferon. The subsequent availability of permanent T-cell lines (H9, H4; Molt 3; MT-2, MT-4) allowed growth and recovery of high titres of virus (Popovic *et al.*, 1984a, b; Montagnier *et al.*, 1984; Harada *et al.*, 1985; Folks *et al.*, 1985). Virus isolation could be achieved from over 80% of pre-AIDS and 30–50% of AIDS patients (Gallo *et al.*, 1984; Salahuddin *et al.*, 1985). Virus growth *in vitro* also allowed the production of test reagents for epidemiological surveys. The high prevalence of HIV antibody in patients with overt disease and in subpopulations at high risk (homosexuals, intravenous drug abusers, haemophiliacs and recipients of blood transfusions; Sarngadharan *et al.*, 1984; Cheingsong-Popov *et al.*, 1984; Mortimer *et al.*, 1985) with subsequent virus isolation established the final link between HIV infection and AIDS. Prospective studies have shown that 15–50% of HIV infected persons in high risk groups have developed AIDS or AIDS-related symptoms after a period of 3–4 years (Goedert *et al.*, 1986; Weber *et al.*, 1986) and over longer observation periods not many HIV-infected people may remain without symptoms.

3.2 RETROVIRUS STRUCTURE

Retrovirus particles are 80–130 nm in diameter and consist of an electron-dense core containing the capsid proteins and 2 copies of the positive-sense single-stranded RNA genome. This is surrounded by an envelope comprising a lipid bilayer (contributed by the plasma membrane of the host cell) into which virus-specific glycoprotein projections are inserted (Gelderblom *et al.*, 1987). Associated with the core is the virus-encoded RNA-dependent DNA polymerase (reverse transcriptase). Although originally regarded as C-type particles (Barré–Sinoussi *et al.*, 1983), HIV virions are now grouped as D-type particles, and their morphogenesis is closely related to that of visna virus, a member of the lentivirinae subfamily (Gonda *et al.*, 1985). The genomes of replication-competent retroviruses are similar in organization, but distinct in detail. They all possess the three genes:

1. *gag* coding for the group specific antigen proteins, which are found in the core (p18 and p24 in HIV).
2. *pol* coding for the reverse transcriptase (*pol*ymerase), an RNAse H activity, an endonuclease and a protease.
3. *env* coding for viral *env*elope proteins (the transmembrane protein gp41 and the major surface protein gp120 in HIV).

The order of these genes is always *gag-pol-env* in the direction from the 5′ to the 3′ end of the genomic RNA (Fig. 3.1). In the virion RNA of HIV these genes are flanked by long terminal repeat (LTR) sequences (Starcich *et al.*,

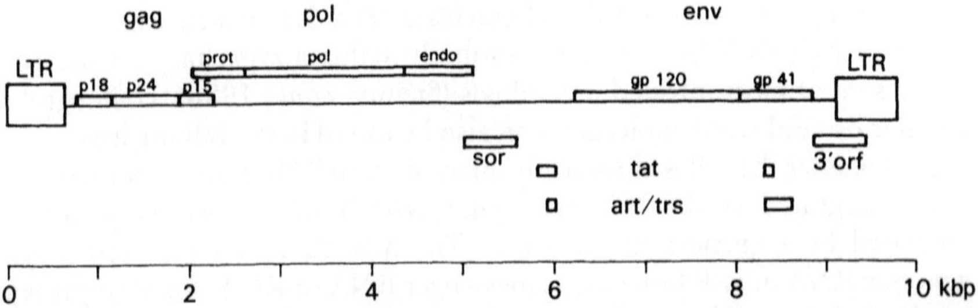

Figure 3.1 Genome organization of HIV-I in the proviral dsDNA form (modified after Rabson and Martin, 1985; Wong-Staal and Gallo, 1985; Arya *et al.*, 1985; Seigel *et al.*, 1986; Sodroski *et al.*, 1986a; Chen, 1986). The size in kilobase pairs (kbp) is indicated at the bottom of the diagram. Coding regions of genes are indicated (for abbreviations see text) as well as protein products obtained by postranslational cleavage (p, protein; gp, glycoprotein; the numbers after p and gp indicate the apparent molecular weight in kilodaltons); prot, protease; pol, polymerase (reverse transcriptase); endo, endonuclease. LTR, long terminal repeat. The tat and art/trs gene products each arise from two coding exons.

1985), and interspersed by sequences with open reading frames (ORF) of at least four other genes called *sor*, *3'orf*, *tat* and *art/trs* (Fig 3.1).

3.3 RETROVIRUS REPLICATION

The replication of retroviruses is unique and will be briefly described with specific relevance to HIV. It begins with adsorption of the virus to a specific receptor on a susceptible cell. For HIV there is strong evidence that part of the T helper (OKT4$^+$; CD4) cell antigen is involved in this process (Dalgleish *et al.*, 1984; Klatzmann *et al.*, 1984a, b; Maddon *et al.*, 1986). Binding of the virus is mediated by its main envelope glycoprotein, gp120 (McDougal *et al.*, 1986). Although HIV infects mainly the CD4 subset of T lymphocytes it can also infect macrophages (Gartner *et al.*, 1986; Koenig *et al.*, 1986), B lymphocytes (Montagnier *et al.*, 1984; Salahuddin *et al.*, 1985) and brain cells (Shaw *et al.*, 1985; Maddon *et al.*, 1986). Adsorption is followed by penetration (receptor-mediated endocytosis) (Maddon *et al.*, 1986) and uncoating (possibly in lysosomes) of the viral genome.

Subsequently, the single-stranded genomic RNA is converted into a double-stranded DNA molecule, a multistep reaction catalysed by reverse transcriptase in which part of the LTRs are duplicated, the RNA template in the initial RNA:DNA hybrid is digested by RNAse H and replaced by a second complementary DNA to form linear double-stranded (ds) DNAs with LTRs at both ends (details of these reactions can be obtained from Lowy, 1985). The dsDNA is then circularized in the cell nucleus and integrated into various non-predilected sites of the host cell chromosomes. This step is catalysed by a virus-encoded endonuclease (Fig. 3.1) which causes single-strand nicks in dsDNA molecules. Antibody to this enzyme has been detected in the sera of most infected individuals (Steimer *et al.*, 1986). Unintegrated circular ds viral DNA molecules can also be found in the cell nucleus.

At this stage the cell is chronically infected; viral RNA transcription occurs from integrated viral DNA by cellular type II RNA polymerase and is regulated by sequences in the LTRs. The new RNA is either full length genomic RNA or will function as messenger RNA (mRNA) for viral protein synthesis. Some of the mRNAs are spliced (Arya *et al.*, 1985; Sodroski *et al.*, 1985a; Sodroski *et al.*, 1986a). Most mRNAs are translated into protein precursors which are cleaved (probably by the virus coded protease; Kramer *et al.*, 1986) (Fig. 3.1) and in part processed by glycosylation (Starcich *et al.*, 1986).

The *env* gene product precursor gp160 is cleaved into the major exterior glycoprotein gp120 and the membrane bound gp41 which anchors the glycoprotein gp120 in the envelope (Di Marzo-Veronese *et al.*, 1985). Both the *sor* and the *3'orf* genes are expressed during replication and antibody against their products have been found (*sor*: Lee *et al.*, 1986; Kan *et al.*, 1986; *3'orf*: Allan *et al.*, 1985; Ratner *et al.*, 1985) but functions have not yet been assigned to either of these proteins. However, some *sor* and *3'orf* deletion mutants have been found to grow more poorly (Sodroski *et al.*, 1986b; Terwilliger *et al.*, 1986). The ORF sequence between the *sor* and the *env* genes (Fig. 3.1) codes for a protein which *t*rans-*a*ctivates *t*ranscription directed by the HIV LTR (Sodroski *et al.*, 1985a, b, 1986b; Seigel *et al.*, 1986) and was therefore named *tat*. Transactivation genes and mechanisms have also been observed in HTLVs I and II (Sodroski, Rosen and Haseltine, 1984) and in visna virus (Hess, Clements and Narayan, 1985) and play a crucial role in determining the biological activity of these viruses (Sodroski, Rosen and Haseltine, 1984; Sodroski *et al.*, 1985b; Wong-Staal and Gallo, 1985). A second transactivator gene was recently described by two research groups and named *art* (*a*nti-*r*epression *t*ransactivator; Sodroski *et al.*, 1986a) or *trs* (*t*ransacting *r*egulator of *s*plicing; Feinberg *et al.*, 1986). The products of both the *tat* and the *art* genes have been found to be essential for virus replication (Fisher *et al.*, 1986; Dayton *et al.*, 1986; Sodroski *et al.*, 1986a; Feinberg *et al.*, 1986) in contrast to the products of the *sor* and *3'orf* genes (Sodroski *et al.*, 1986b). As discussed by Chen (1986), the mechanisms of action of the transactivating genes *tat* and *art/trs* are not fully elucidated yet. The core comprising the *gag* proteins, viral RNA and reverse transcriptase is formed near the plasma membrane, and is surrounded by a plasma membrane-derived envelope containing the virus specific envelope proteins. Details of the packaging process remain to be investigated. A very rapid loss of gp120 molecules seems to occur *in vitro* during maturation of HIV particles (Gelderblom *et al.*, 1987). A small number of infected T cells may harbour the virus in latent form (Folks *et al.*, 1986). Specific antibody responses towards the internal proteins (*gag*; Kalyanaraman *et al.*, 1984; Sarin *et al.*, 1986) and against the functional proteins (reverse transcriptase, Di Marzo-Veronese *et al.*, 1986; endonuclease, Steimer *et al.*, 1986; *tat* protein, Goh *et al.*, 1986; product of the *sor* gene, Kan *et al.*, 1986; and product of the *3′orf* gene, Allan *et al.*, 1985) have been found but the significance of these observations is not fully understood at present.

Molecular clones of several HIV isolates have been obtained (Shaw *et al.*, 1984; Alizon *et al.*, 1984; Luciw *et al.*, 1984; Hahn *et al.*, 1984) and have been sequenced in full (Ratner *et al.*, 1985; Sanchez-Pescador *et al.*, 1985; Wain-Hobson *et al.*, 1985). Full length cDNA clones were found to be infectious when inserted into a plasmid and transfected into cord blood T cells of normal newborn infants (Fisher *et al.*, 1985) and a number of other cell lines, among them several human colon carcinoma cell lines (Adachi *et al.*, 1986; 1987).

3.4 ORIGIN OF HIV

HIV sequences have been compared with those of other HTLV viruses (types I and II) and with those of other retroviruses (Wong-Staal and Gallo, 1985; Alizon *et al.*, 1986; Starcich *et al.*, 1986). Whereas the HTLV-I genome is closely related to that of a simian T-lymphotropic virus type I (STLV-I) (Guo, Wong-Staal and Gallo, 1984) and the genome of HTLV-II to that of bovine leukaemia virus (BLV) (Wong-Staal and Gallo, 1985), the HIV virus has been found to show a closer homology to a simian virus called STLV-III (Kanki, Alroy and Essex, 1985) and to members of the lentivirus subfamily (Gonda *et al.*, 1985; Chiu *et al.*, 1985) of which the ovine virus, visna/maedi, are best characterized. The HIV genome also shows close homology to that of equine infectious anaemia virus (Stephens, Casey and Rice, 1986).

Recently, other retroviruses have been isolated from apparently healthy West African people and from West African patients with AIDS, which were named HTLV type IV (Kanki *et al.*, 1986) and LAV type II (Clavel *et al.*, 1986a) and are now called HIV-II. These viruses have been found to be more closely related to simian retroviruses, STLV-AGM and STLV-III MAC, respectively, than to the human retroviruses HTLV III/LAV I(HIV-I) (Clavel *et al.*, 1986a, b; Guyader *et al.*, 1987). The evolutionary relationship of all these viruses remains to be more fully elucidated. It has been postulated that the HIVs have been only recently introduced into the human population from endemically infected African monkeys (Kanki *et al.*, 1986), but this has also been disputed (Guyader *et al.*, 1987).

3.5 GENOMIC HETEROGENEITY

Among the different HIV-I isolates, there is a considerable degree of genomic diversity (Benn *et al.*, 1985; Wong-Staal *et al.*, 1985; Hahn *et al.*, 1985a, b;

Rabson and Martin, 1985; Hahn *et al.*, 1986; Alizon *et al.*, 1986; Starcich *et al.*, 1986). This diversity is greatest in the part of the envelope (*env*) gene coding for the external gp120, where areas of high variability are interspersed with areas of greater conservation. Computer-assisted analysis of the predicted *env* protein gp120 sequences of seven HIV isolates have located the majority of antigenic epitopes into highly variable regions (Modrow *et al.*, 1987) but it remains to be experimentally determined whether the variable domains of the *env* gene products represent major antigenic epitopes (Starcich *et al.*, 1986). The *gag* and *pol* sequences were found to be more conserved, but there was also a high degree of variability in certain functional HIV genes (*tat, 3'orf*; Alizon *et al.*, 1986; Starcich *et al.*, 1986). Hahn *et al.*, (1986) obtained sequential HIV isolates differing in genotype from the same chronically infected individuals. These isolates, although obtained successively, had apparently not evolved genetically in direct lineage. Similarly, new variants of equine infectious anaemia virus (EIAV), another lentivirus, obtained successively from chronically infected horses, showed non-cumulative changes (Payne *et al.*, 1987). A high mutation rate of both HIV and EIAV could mask a direct lineage between sequential isolates (Payne *et al.*, 1987). Isolates HIV-I and HIV-II are only distantly related (Guyader *et al.*, 1987).

3.6 VIRUS–HOST RELATIONSHIP

It has been shown that antigenic variation of EIAV during persistent infection is largely directed by the emergence of strong neutralizing antibody which selects for new non-neutralizable variants (Montelaro *et al.*, 1984; Salinovich *et al.*, 1986; Payne *et al.*, 1987). Similar observations have been made among consecutive isolates of visna virus (Scott *et al.*, 1979; Clements *et al.*, 1980).

The virus–host relationship in HIV infection is not clear: HIV antibody which is reactive with *env* gene products in Western blot, radioimmunoprecipitation and ELISA assays was often found to be of only weak or no neutralizing and cross-neutralizing activity (Weiss *et al.*, 1985; Clavel, Klatzmann and Montagnier, 1985). Similar findings have been reported with antibody directed against a recombinant *env* protein (Lasky *et al.*, 1986; Weiss *et al.*, 1986). Viral antigen can occasionally be found in serum and cerebrospinal fluid of patients after seroconversion (Goudsmit *et al.*, 1986). In accordance with the diversity of HIV genomes there is considerable antigenic diversity among different HIV isolates (Weiss *et al.*, 1986; Matthews *et al.*, 1986).

In contrast to HTLV-I and HTLV-II which transform T lymphocytes *in vitro* and *in vivo*, and cause adult T cell leukaemias (Yamamoto and Hinuma, 1985; Wong-Staal and Gallo, 1985), HIV is cytopathic. An activated state of the infected cells seems to be a prerequisite of HIV gene expression and replication (McDougal *et al.*, 1985; Zagury *et al.*, 1986; Nabel and Baltimore, 1987) suggesting that multiple antigenic stimulation by various micro-organisms promotes virus replication, cell death and further spread of the virus (Zagury *et al.*, 1986; Weber *et al.*, 1986; Wachter *et al.*, 1986). Depletion of the T-helper subpopulation results in the clinical manifestations of AIDS. However, the central nervous system manifestations are in part a direct result of infection with HIV (Shaw *et al.*, 1985).

HIV initiates a chronic infection, a specific antibody response does occur but is not fully neutralizing and does not affect the course of infection: the virus can be isolated from infected humans in 80% of cases during early infection and in 50% of AIDS patients, several years after the initial infection (Salahuddin *et al.*, 1985). Measurement of the presence of antibody alone thus does not indicate the stage or extent of infection (Robert-Guroff, Brown and Gallo, 1985; Bolognesi *et al.*, 1986); but recent studies reported a close association of high titres of anti-p24 (*gag*) antibody with lack of progression of AIDS (Weber *et al.*, 1987; Frösner *et al.*, 1987). Infection can be monitored in more detail: (1) by isolating virus from lymphocytes (Salahuddin *et al.*, 1985) or from cell-free plasma (Salahuddin *et al.*, 1985; Zagury *et al.*, 1985) and by checking the supernatant of cultured lymphocytes for the presence of the viral enzyme reverse transcriptase (Poiecz *et al.*, 1980); (2) by checking for the presence of the HIV genome through hybridization of sequence-specific radiolabelled DNA or RNA probes on Southern blots of cellular DNA fragments (Gelmann *et al.*, 1983) or *in situ* (Harper *et al.*, 1986).

It has been suggested that the infectivity of HIV antibody positive blood can be predicted from Western blot analysis (Esteban *et al.*, 1985); at present this should be regarded with caution as false positive Western blot reactivity to HIV has been observed (Biberfeld *et al.*, 1986). In addition virus has been found in antibody-negative homosexuals, blood donors and haemophiliacs early in infection (Levy *et al.*, 1985; Raevski *et al.*, 1986; Allain *et al.*, 1986).

3.7 HIV VACCINE AND SPECIFIC TREATMENT

Despite the considerable genomic heterogeneity of HIV isolates several approaches to vaccine development are actively being pursued. One approach being considered is to pack *env* gene products (purified from virus particles or expressed from recombinant vectors) into glycoside lattices which generate multimeric compounds called immunostimulating complexes (ISCOM) (Bolognesi *et al.*, 1986; Gallo, Reitz and Streicher, 1986). The ISCOM approach using glycoproteins from feline leukaemia virus has been found to elicit protective antibody in cats (Osterhaus *et al.*, 1985). Lasky *et al.* (1986) produced a secreted form of a slightly truncated HIV envelope glycoprotein from mammalian cells by genetic engineering techniques; anti-serum raised against this protein bound to HIV and neutralized the virus *in vitro* in low dilutions. Similar results were obtained with recombinant proteins produced in *E.coli* and containing portions of the HIV gp120 protein (Putney *et al.*, 1987). Recombinant vaccinia virus containing and expressing the *env* gene of HIV (Chakrabarti *et al.*, 1986; Hu *et al.*, 1986) is also under trial (Zagury *et al.*, 1987); however, caution has been recommended when using this approach (Redfield *et al.*, 1987). Synthetic peptides which elicit antibody reactive with the native glycoprotein are also being tested as potential vaccines (Kennedy *et al.*, 1986), but the protective efficacy of oligopeptide antibodies specific for HIV proteins remains to be demonstrated. An octapeptide which is part of a neuropeptide receptor-like portion of the T4 protein blocked HIV infection of human T lymphocytes *in vitro* at very low concentrations (0.1nM; Pert *et al.*, 1986); this finding may provide another possibility to inhibit spreading of or to prevent infection with HIV. The success of the oligopeptide approach will have to be assessed by the ability to elicit antibody of broad neutralizing activity, a task of considerable difficulty given the high degree of antigenic variation in HIV isolates. An antibody against a *gag* protein could also prove to be neutralizing (Sarin *et al.*, 1986). An alternative approach is the search for a suitable anti-idiotype antibody as immunogen (Bolognesi *et al.*, 1986; Gallo, Reitz and Streicher, 1986).

At present, there is no specific treatment for AIDS or of early HIV infection. Therapeutic options under consideration (Mitsuya and Broder, 1987) include:

1. Treatment with compounds which specifically inhibit viral reverse transcriptase (Mitsuya *et al.*, 1984; Rozenbaum *et al.*, 1985); so far promising *in vitro* compounds (Mitsuya *et al.*, 1984) have been clinically disappointing (Busch *et al.*, 1985; Rozenbaum *et al.*, 1985).
2. Clinical use has begun of a thymidine analogue, 3'azido-3-deoxythymidine (AZT), which is phosphorylated in cells, is preferentially utilized by retroviral reverse transcriptase (Furman *et al.*, 1986) and acts to terminate DNA chain synthesis (Yarchoan *et al.*, 1986, 1987). The effects of long term treatment need further investigation.
3. Finally, one suggested novel approach is to inhibit expression of the transactivating (*tat*) gene(s) (Dayton *et al.*, 1986; Fisher *et al.*, 1986) by introducing a gene transcribing *tat* anti-sense RNA into infected cells and thus blocking translation (Mariman, 1985; Chang and Stoltzfus, 1987).

REFERENCES

Adachi, A., Gendelman, H. E., Koenig, S., Folks, T., Willey, R., Rabson, A. and Martin, M. A. (1986) Production of acquired immunodeficiency syndrome-associated retrovirus in human and non-human cells transfected with an infectious molecular clone. *J. Virol.*, 59, 284–91.

Adachi, A., Koenig, S., Gendelman, H. E., Daugherty, D., Gattoni-Celli, G., Fauci, A. S. and Martin, M. A. (1987). Productive, persistent infection of human colorectal cell lines with human immunodeficiency virus. *J. Virol.* **61**, 209–213.

Alizon, M., Sonigo, P., Barre-Sinoussi, F., Chermann, J. C., Tiollais, P., Montagnier, L. and Wain-Hobson, S. (1984) Molecular cloning of lymphadenopathy associated virus. *Nature, Lond.*, **312**, 757–60.

Alizon, M., Wain-Hobson, S., Montagnier, L. and Sonigo, P. (1986) Genetic variability of the AIDS virus. Nucleotide sequence analysis of two isolates from African patients. *Cell*, **46**, 63–74.

Allain, J. P., Laurian, Y., Paul, D. A. and Senn, D. (1986). Serological markers in early stages of human immunodeficiency virus infection in haemophiliacs. *Lancet* **ii**, 1233–6.

Allan, J. S., Coligan, J. E., Lee, T. H., McLance, M. F., Kanki, P. J., Groopman, J. E. and Essex, M. (1985) A new HTLVIII/LAV encoded antigen detected by antibodies from AIDS patients. *Science*, **230**, 810–13.

Arya, S. K., Guo, C., Josephs, S. F. and Wong-Staal, F. (1985). *Trans*-activator gene of human T-lymphotropic virus type III (HTLVIII). *Science*, **229**, 69–73.

Barré-Sinoussi, F., Chermann, J. C., Rey, F., Nugeyre, M. T., Charmaret, S., Gruest, J., Dauguet, C., Axler-Blin, L., Brun-Vezinet, F., Rouzioux, C., Rozenbaum, W. and Montagnier, L. (1983) Isolation of a T-lymphotropic retrovirus from a patient at risk for acquired immune deficiency syndrome (AIDS). *Science*, **220**, 868–71.

Benn, S., Rutledge, R., Folks, T., Gold, J., Baker, L., McCormick, J., Feorionon, P., Piot, P., Quinn, T. and Martin, M. (1985) Genomic heterogeneity of AIDS retroviral isolates from North America and Zaire. *Science*, **230**, 949–51.

Biberfeld, G., Bredberg-Raden, U., Böttiger, B., Putkonen, P. O., Blomberg, J., Juto, P. and Wadell, G. (1986). Blood donor sera with false-positive Western blot reactions to human immuno-deficiency virus. *Lancet*, **ii**, 289–90.

Bolognesi, D. P., Langlois, A. J., Matthews, T. J., Fischinger, F. J. and Gallo, R. C. (1986) Prospects for development of a vaccine against human lymphotropic virus type III disease, in *New Approaches to Immunization* (ed. F. Brown, R. M. Chanock and R. A. Lerner), Cold Spring Harbor Laboratory, Cold Spring Harbor, New York, pp. 311–21.

Brown, F. (1986) Human immunodeficiency virus. *Science*, **232**, 1486.

Busch, W., Brodt, R., Ganser, A., Helm, E. B. and Stille, W. (1985). Suramin treatment for AIDS. *Lancet*, **ii**, 1247.

Chakrabarti, S., Robert-Guroff, M., Wong-Staal, F., Gallo, R. C. and Moss, B. (1986). Expression of the HTLV-III envelope gene by a recombinant vaccinia virus. *Nature, Lond.* **320**, 535–7.

Chang, L. J. and Stoltzfus, C. M. (1987). Inhibition of Rons sarcoma virus replication by antisense RNA. *J. of Virol.* **61**, 921–924.

Cheingsong-Popov, R., Weiss, R. A., Dalgleish, A., Tedder, R. S., Shanson, D. C., Jeffries, D. J., Ferns, R. B., Briggs, E. M., Weller, I. V. D., Mitton, S., Adler, M. W., Farthing, C., Lawrence, A. G., Gazzard, B. G., Weber, J., Harris, J. R. W., Pinching, A. J., Craske, J. and Barbara, J. A. J. (1984) Prevalence of antibody to human T-lymphotropic virus type III in AIDS and AIDS-risk patients in Britain. *Lancet*, **ii**, 477–80.

Chen, I. S. Y. (1986). Regulation of AIDS virus expression. *Cell*, **47**, 1–2.

Chiu, I.-M., Yaniv, A., Dalberg, J. E., Gazit, A., Skuntz, S. F., Tronick, S. R. and Aaronson, S. A. (1985) Nucleotide sequence evidence for relationship of AIDS retrovirus to lentiviruses. *Nature, Lond.*, **317**, 366–8.

Clavel, F., Guétard, D., Brun-Vezinet, F., Chamaret, S., Rey, M. A., Santos-Ferreira,

M. O., Laurent, A. G., Dauguet, C., Katlama, C., Rouzioux, C., Klatzmann, D., Champalimaud, J. L. and Montagnier, L. (1986a) Isolation of a new human retrovirus from West African patients with AIDS. *Science*, **233**, 343–6.

Clavel, F., Guyader, M., Guétard, D., Salle, M., Montagnier, L. and Alizon, M. (1986b). Molecular cloning and polymorphism of the human immunodeficiency virus type 2. *Nature Lond.*, **324**, 691–5.

Clavel, F., Klatzmann, D. and Montagnier, L. (1985) Deficient LAV1 neutralizing capacity of sera from patients with AIDS or related syndromes. *Lancet*, i, 879–80.

Clements, J., Pedersen, F., Narayan, O. and Haseltine, W. (1980). Genome changes associated with antigenic variation of visna virus during persistent infection. *Proc. Natl Acad. Sci. USA*, **77**, 4454–8.

Coffin, J., Haase, A., Levy, J. A., Montagnier, L., Oroszlan, S., Teich, N., Temin, H., Toyoshima, K., Varmus, H. E., Vogt, P. K. and Weiss, R. A. (1986). What to call the AIDS virus. *Nature, Lond.*, **321**, 10.

Curran, J. W., Morgan, W. M., Hardy, A. M., Jaffe, H. W., Darrow, W. W. and Dowdle, W. R. (1985) The epidemiology of AIDS: Current status and future prospects. *Science*, **229**, 1352–7.

Dalgleish, A. G., Beverly, P. C. L., Clapham, P. R., Crawford, D. H., Greaves, M. F. and Weiss, R. A. (1984) The CD4 (T4) antigen is an essential component of the receptor for the AIDS retrovirus. *Nature, Lond.*, **312**, 763–7.

Dayton, A. I., Sodroski, J. G., Rosen, C. A., Goh, W. C. and Haseltine, W. A. (1986) The *trans*-activator gene of the human T-cell lymphotropic virus type III is required for replication. *Cell*, **44**, 941–7.

Di Marzo-Veronese, F., Copeland, T. D., Devico, A. L., Rahman, R., Oroszlan, S., Gallo, R. C. and Sarngadharan, M. G. (1986) Characterization of highly immunogenic p66/p51 as the reverse transcriptase of HTLVIII/LAV. *Science*, **231**, 1289–91.

Di Marzo-Veronese, F., DeVico, A. L., Copeland, T. D., Orozlan, S., Gallo, R. C. and Sarngadharan, M. G. (1985) Characterization of gp41 as the transmembrane protein coded by the HTLVIII/LAV envelope gene. *Science*, **229**, 1402–5.

Esteban, J. I., Shih, J. W.-K., Tai, C.-C., Bodner, A. J., Kay, J. W. D. and Alter, H. J. (1985) Importance of Western blot analysis in predicting infectivity of anti-HTLV-III/LAV positive blood. *Lancet*, ii, 1083–6.

Feinberg, M. B., Jarrett, R. F., Aldovini, A., Gallo, R. C. & Wong-Staal, F. (1986). HTLV-III expression and production involve complex regulation at the levels of splicing and translation of viral RNA. *Cell*, **46**, 807–17.

Fisher, A. G., Collalti, E., Ratner, L., Gallo, R. C. and Wong-Staal, F. (1985) A molecular clone of HTLV-III with biological activity. *Nature, Lond.*, **316**, 262–5.

Fisher, A. G., Feinberg, M. B., Josephs, S. F., Harper, M. E., Marselle, L. M., Reyes, G., Gonda, M. A., Aldovini, A. and Debouk, C. (1986) The *trans*-activator gene of HTLVIII is essential for virus replication. *Nature, Lond.*, **320**, 367–71.

Folks, T., Benn, S., Robson, A., Theodore, T., Hoggan, M. D., Martin, M., Lightfoote, M. and Sell, K. (1985) Characterization of a continuous T-cell line susceptible to the cytopathic effects of the acquired immunodeficiency syndrome (AIDS)-associated retrovirus. *Proc. Natl Acad. Sci. USA*, **82**, 4539–43.

Folks, T., Powell, D. M., Lightfoote, M. M., Benn, S., Martin, M. A. and Fauci, A. S. (1986) Induction of HTLVIII/LAV from a nonvirus-producing T-cell line: Implications for latency. *Science*, **231**, 600–2.

Frösner, G. G. Erfle, V., Mellert, W. and Hehlmann, R. (1987). Diagnostic significance of quantitative determination of HIV antibody specific for envelope and core proteins. *Lancet*, i, 159–60.

Furman, P. A., Fyfe, J. A., St Clair, M. H., Weinhold, K. Rideout, J. L., Freeman, G. A., Nusinoff Lehrman, S., Bolognesi, D. P., Broder, S., Mitsuya, H. and Barry, D. W. (1986). Phosphorylation of 3′-azido-3′-deoxythymidine and selective interaction of the 5′-triphosphate with human immunodeficiency virus reverse transcriptase. *Proc. Natl Acad. Sci. USA* **83**, 8333–7.

Gallo, R. C., Salahuddin, S. Z., Popovic, M., Shearer, G. M., Kaplan, M., Haynes, B. F., Palker, T. J., Redfield, R., Oleske, J., Safai, B., White, G., Foster, P. and Markham, P. D. (1984) Frequent detection and isolation of cytopathic retroviruses (HTLVIII) from patients with AIDS and at risk for AIDS. *Science*, **224**, 500–3.

Gallo, R. C., Reitz, M. and Streicher, H. Z. (1986) Human T-lymphotropic virus type III (HTLVIII/LAV): Approaches to the development of a vaccine for a human retrovirus, in *New Approaches to Immunization* (ed. F. Brown, R. M. Chanock and R. A. Lerner), Cold Spring Harbor Laboratory, Cold Spring Harbor, New York, pp. 327–34.

Gartner, S., Markovits, P., Markovitz, D. M., Kaplan, M. H., Gallo, R. C. and Popovic, M. (1986) The role of mononuclear phagocytes in HTLVIII/LAV infection. *Science*, **233**, 215–9.

Gelderblom, H. R., Hausmann, H. S., Ozel, M., Pauli, G. and Koch, M. A., (1987). Fine structure of human immunodeficiency virus (HIV) and immunolocalization of structural proteins. *Virology*, **156**, 171–6.

Gelmann, E. P., Popovic, M., Blayney, D., Masur, H., Sidhu, G., Stahl, R. E. and Gallo, R. C. (1983) Proviral DNA of a retrovirus, human T-cell leukemia virus, in two patients with AIDS. *Science*, **220**, 862–5.

Goedert, J. J., Biffer, R. J., Weiss, S. H., Eyster, M. E., Melby, M., Wilson, S., Ginzburg, H. M., Grossman, R. J., DiGioia, R. A., Sanchez, W. C., Giron, J. A., Erbesen, P., Gallo, R. C. and Blattner, W. A. (1986). Three-year incidence of AIDS in five cohorts of HTLV-III-infected risk group members. *Science*, **231**, 992–5.

Goh, W. C., Rosen, C., Sodroski, J., Ho, D. D. and Haseltine, W. A. (1986) Identification of a protein encoded by the *trans* activator gene *tat* III of human T-cell lymphotropic retrovirus type III. *J. Virol.*, **59**, 181–4.

Gonda, M. A., Wong-Staal, F., Gallo, R. C., Clements, J. E., Narayan, O. and Gilden, R. V. (1985) Sequence homology and morphologic similarity of HTLV-III and Visna virus, a pathogenic lentivirus. *Science*, **227**, 173–7.

Goudsmit, J., deWolf, F., Paul, D. A., Epstein, L. G., Lange, J. M. A., Krone, W. J. A., Speelman, H., Wolters, E. C., van der Noorda, J., Oleske, J. M., van der Helm, H. J. and Coutinho, R. A. (1986) Expression of human immunodeficiency virus antigen (HIV-Ag) in serum and cerebrospinal fluid during acute and chronic infection. *Lancet*, **ii**, 177–80.

Guo, H. G., Wong-Staal, F. and Gallo, R. C. (1984) Novel viral sequences related to a human T-cell leukemia virus in T-cells of a seropositive baboon. *Science*, **223**, 1195–7.

Guyader, M., Emerman, M., Sonigo, P., Clavel, F., Montagnier, L. and Alizon, M. (1987). Genome organization and transactivation of the human immunodeficiency virus type 2. *Nature, Lond.*, **326**, 662–9.

Hahn, B. H., Shaw, G. M., Taylor, M. E., Redfield, R. R., Markham, P. D., Salahuddin, S. Z., Wong-Staal, F., Gallo, R. C., Parks, E. S. and Parks, W. P. (1986) Genetic variation in HTLV-III/LAV over time in patients with AIDS or at risk for AIDS. *Science*, **232**, 1548–53.

Hahn, B. H., Gonda, M. A., Shaw, G. M., Popovic, M., Hoxie, J. A., Gallo, R. C. and Wong-Staal, F. (1985a) Genomic diversity of the acquired immune deficiency syndrome virus HTLV III: Different viruses exhibit greatest divergence in their envelope genes. *Proc. Natl Acad. Sci. USA*, **82**, 4813–17.

Hahn, B. H., Shaw, G. M., Arya, S. K., Popovic, M., Gallo, R. C. and Wong-Staal, F. (1984) Molecular cloning and characterization of the HTLVIII virus associated with AIDS. *Nature, Lond.*, **312**, 166–9.

Hahn, B. H., Shaw, G. M., Wong-Staal, F. and Gallo, R. C. (1985b). Genomic variation of HTLVIII/LAV, the retrovirus of AIDS, in *Genetically Altered Viruses and the Environment* (ed. B. Fields, M. A. Martin and D. Kamely), Banbury Report 22, Cold Spring Harbor Laboratory, Cold Spring Harbor, New York, pp. 235–49.

Harada, S., Koyanagi, Y. and Yamamoto, N. (1985) Infection of HTLV-III/LAV in HTLV-I-carrying cells MT-2 and MT-4 and application in a plaque assay. *Science*, **229**, 563–6.

Hardy, W. D. Jr, Hess, P. W., McEwan, E. G., McClelland, A. J., Zuckerman, E. E., Essex, M., Colter, S. M. and Jarrett, O. (1976) Biology of feline leukemia virus in the natural environment. *Cancer Res.*, **36**, 582–8.

Harper, M. E., Marselle, L. M., Gallo, R. C. and Wong-Staal, F. (1986) Detection of lymphocytes expressing human T-lymphotropic virus type III in lymph nodes and peripheral blood from infected individuals by in situ hybridization. *Proc. Natl Acad. Sci. USA*, **83**, 772–6.

Hess, J. L., Clements, J. E. and Narayan, O. (1985) *Cis*- and *trans*-acting transcriptional regulation of Visna virus. *Science*, **229**, 482–5.

Hu, S. L., Kosowski, S. G. and Dalrymple, J. M. (1986). Expression of AIDS virus envelope gene in recombinant vaccinia viruses. *Nature, Lond.*, **320**, 537–40.

Kalyanaraman, V. S., Cabradilla, C. D., Getchell, J. P., Narayanan, R., Braff, E. H., Chermann, J. C., Barré-Sinoussi, F., Montagnier, L., Spira, T. J., Kaplan, J., Fishbein, D., Jaffe, H. W., Curran, J. W. and Francis, D. P. (1984) Antibodies to the core protein of lymphadenopathy associated virus (LAV) in patients with AIDS. *Science*, **225**, 321–3.

Kan, N. C., Franchini, G., Wong-Staal, F., Dubois, G. C., Robey, W. G., Lautenberger, J. A. and Papas, T. S. (1986) Identification of HTLV-III/LAV *sor* gene products and detection of antibodies in human sera. *Science*, **231**, 1553–5.

Kanki, P. J., Alroy, J. and Essex, M. (1985) Isolation of T-lymphotropic retrovirus related to HTLVIII/LAV from wild-caught African green monkeys. *Science*, **230**, 951–4.

Kanki, P. J., Barin, F., M'Boup, S., Allan, J. S., Romet-Lemonne, J. L., Marlink, R., McLane, M. F., Lee, T. H., Arbeille, B., Denis, F. and Essex, M. (1986) New human T-lymphotropic retrovirus related to simian L-lymphotropic virus type III (STLV-III AGM). *Science*, **232**, 238–43.

Kennedy, R. C., Henkel, R. D., Pauletti, D., Allan, J. S., Lee, T. H., Essex, M. and Dreesman, G. R. (1986) Antiserum to a synthetic peptide recognizes the HTLV-III envelope glycoprotein. *Science*, **231**, 1556–9.

Klatzmann, D., Barré-Sinoussi, F., Nugeyre, M. T., Dauguet, C., Vilment, E., Griscelu, C., Brun-Vezinet, F., Rouzioux, C., Gluckman, J. C., Chermann, J. C. and Montagnier, L. (1984a) Selective tropism of lymphadenopathy associated virus (LAV) for helper-inducer T lymphocytes. *Science*, **225**, 59–62.

Klatzmann, D., Champagne, E., Chamaret, S., Gruest, J., Guétard, D., Hercend, T., Gluckman, J.-C. and Montagnier, L. (1984b) T-lymphocyte T4 molecule behaves as the receptor for human retrovirus LAV. *Nature Lond.*, **312**, 767–8.

Koenig, S., Gendelman, H. E., Orenstein, J. M., Dal Canto, M. C., Pezeshkpour,

G. H., Yungbluth, M., Janotta, F., Aksamit, A., Martin, M. A. and Fauci, A. S. (1986). Detection of AIDS virus in macrophages in brain tissue from AIDS patients with encephalopathy. *Science*, **233**, 1089–93.

Kramer, R. A., Schaber, M. D., Skalka, A. M., Ganguly, K., Wong-Staal, F. and Reddy, E. P. (1986) HTLV-III gag protein is processed in yeast cells by the virus pol-protease. *Science*, **231**, 1580–4.

Lasky, L. A., Groopman, J. E., Fennic, C. W., Benz, P. M., Capon, D. J., Dowbenco, D. J., Nakamura, G. R., Nunes, W. M., Renz, M. E. and Berman, P. W. (1986) Neutralization of the AIDS retrovirus by antibodies to a recombinant envelope glycoprotein. *Science*, **233**, 209–12.

Lee, T. H., Coligan, J. E., Allan, J. S., McLane, M. F., Groopman, J. E. and Essex, M. (1986) A new HTLV-III/LAV protein encoded by a gene found in cytopathic retroviruses. *Science*, **231**, 1546–7.

Levy, J. A., Kaminski, L. S., Morrow, W. J. W., Steimer, K., Luciw, P., Dina, D., Hoxie, J. and Oshiro, L. (1985) Infection by the retrovirus associated with the acquired immuno-deficiency syndrome. Clinical, biological, and molecular features. *Ann. Intern. Med.*, **103**, 694–9.

Lowy, D. R. (1985) Transformation and oncogenesis: Retroviruses, in *Virology* (ed. B. N. Fields *et al.*), Raven Press, New York, pp. 235–63.

Luciw, P. A., Potter, S. J., Steimer, K. and Dina, D. (1984) Molecular cloning of AIDS-associated retrovirus. *Nature, Lond.*, **312**, 760–3.

Maddon, P. J., Dalgleish, A. G., McDougal, J. S., Clapham, P., Weiss, R. A. and Axel, R. (1986). The T4 gene encodes the AIDS virus receptor and is expressed in the immune system and the brain. *Cell*, **47**, 333–48.

Mariman, E. C. M. (1985) New strategies for AIDS therapy and prophylaxis. *Nature, Lond.*, **318**, 414.

Matthews, T. J., Langlois, A. J., Robey, W. G., Chang, N. T., Gallo, R. C., Fischinger, P. J. and Bolognesi, D. P. (1986). Restricted neutralization of divergent human T-lymphotropic virus type III isolates by antibodies to the major envelope glycoprotein. *Proc. Natl Acad. Sci.* USA **83**, 9709–13.

McDougal, J. S., Kennedy, M. S., Sligh, J. M., Cort, S. P., Mawle, A. and Nicholson, J. K. A. (1986) Binding of HTLVIII/LAV to $T4^{+}$T cells by a complex of the 110K viral protein and the T4 molecule. *Science*, **231**, 382–5.

McDougal, J. S., Mawle, A., Cort, S. P., Nicholson, J. K. A., Cross, G. D., Scheppler-Campbell, J. A., Hicks, D. and Sligh, J. (1985) Cellular tropism of the human retrovirus HTLVIII/LAV. I. Role of T cell activation and expression of the T4 antigen. *J. Immunol.*, **135**, 3151–62.

Mitsuya, H. and Broder, S. (1987). Strategies for antiviral therapy in AIDS. *Nature, Lond.*, **325**, 773–8.

Mitsuya, H., Popovic, R., Yarchoan, R., Matsushita, S., Gallo, R. C. and Broder, S. (1984) Suramin protection of T cells in vitro against infectivity and cytopathic effect of HTLV-III. *Science*, **226**, 172–4.

Modrow, S., Hahn, B. H., Shaw, G. M., Gallo, R. C., Wong-Staal, F. and Wolf, H. (1987). Computer-assisted analysis of envelope protein sequences of seven human immunodeficiency virus isolates: prediction of antigenic epitopes in conserved and variable regions. *J. Virol.*, **61**, 570–8.

Montagnier, L., Gruest, J., Chamaret, S., Dauguet, C., Axler, C., Guétard, D., Nugeyre, M. T., Barré-Sinoussi, F. and Chermann, J.-C. (1984) Adaptation of lymphadenopathy associated virus (LAV) to replication in EBV-transformed B lymphoblastoid cell lines. *Science*, **225**, 63–6.

Montelaro, R. C., Parekh, B., Orrego, A. and Issel, C. J. (1984) Antigenic variation during persistent infection by equine infectious anemia virus, a retrovirus. *J. Biol. Chem.*, **259**, 10539–44.

Morgan, D. A., Ruscetti, F. W. and Gallo, R. C. (1976) Selective *in vitro* growth of T-lymphocytes from normal human bone marrow. *Science*, **193**, 1007–8.

Mortimer, P. P., Vandervelde, E. M., Jesson, W. J., Pereira, M. S. and Burkhardt, F. (1985) HTLVIII antibody in Swiss and English intravenous drug abusers. *Lancet*, **ii**, 449–50.

Nabel, G. and Baltimore, D. (1987) An inducible transcription factor activates expression of human immunodeficiency virus in T cells. *Nature, Lond.*, **326**, 711–3.

Osterhaus, A., Weijer, K., Uytdehaag, F., Jarrett, O., Sundquist, B. and Morein, B. (1985) Induction of protective immune response in cats by vaccination with feline leukemia virus iscom. *J. Immunol.*, **135**, 591–6.

Payne, S. L., Salinovich, O., Nauman, S. M., Issel, C. J. and Montelaro, R. C. (1987). Course and extent of variation of equine infectious anemia virus during parallel persistent infections. *J. Virol.*, **61**, 1266–70.

Pert, C. B., Hill, J. M., Ruff, M. R., Berman, R. M., Robey, W. G., Arthur, L. O., Ruscetti, F. W. and Farrar, W. L. (1986). Octapeptides deduced from the neuropeptide receptor-like pattern of antigen T4 in brain potently inhibit human immunodeficiency virus receptor binding and T-Cell infectivity. *Proc. Natl Acad. Sci.* USA **83**, 9254–8.

Poiecz, B. J., Ruscetti, F. W., Gazdar, A. F., Bunn, P. A., Minna, J. D. and Gallo, R. D. (1980) Detection and isolation of type C retrovirus particles from fresh and cultured lymphocytes of a patient with cutaneous T cell lymphoma. *Proc. Natl Acad. Sci. USA*, **77**, 7415–19.

Popovic, M., Read-Cannole, E. and Gallo, R. C. (1984a) T4 positive human neoplastic cell lines susceptible to and permissive for HTLV III. *Lancet*, **ii**, 1472–3.

Popovic, M., Sarngadharan, M. G., Read, E. and Gallo, R. C. (1984b) Detection, isolation and continuous production of cytopathic retroviruses (HTLVIII) from patients with AIDS and pre-AIDS. *Science*, **224**, 497–500.

Putney, S. D., Matthews, T. J., Robey, W. G., Lynn, D. L., Robert-Guroff, M., Mueller, W. T., Langlois, A. J., Ghrayeb, J., Petteway, Jr, S. R., Weinhold, W. J., Fischinger, P. J., Wong-Staal, F., Gallo R. C. and Bolognesi. D. P. (1987). HTLV-III/LAV-neutralizing antibodies to an E.coli-produced fragment of the virus envelope. *Science*, **234**:1392–5.

Rabson, A. B. and Martin, M. A. (1985) Molecular organization of the AIDS retrovirus. *Cell*, **40**, 477–80.

Raevski, L. A., Cohn, D. L., Wolf, F. C., Judson, F. N., Ferguson, W. S. and Vernon, T. M. (1986). Transfusion-associated human T-lymphotropic virus type III/ lymphadenopathy associated virus infection from a seronegative donor. *Morbidity and Mortality Weekly Report* **35**, 389–91.

Ratner, L., Haseltine, W., Patarca, R., Livak, K. J., Starcich, B., Josephs, S. F., Doran, E. R., Rafalski, J. A., Whitehorn, E. A., Baumeister, K., Ivanoff, L., Petteway, S. R. Jr, Pearson, M. L., Lautenberger, J. A., Papas, T. S., Ghrayeb, J., Chang, N. T., Gallo, R. C. and Wong-Staal, F. (1985) Complete nucleotide sequence of the AIDS virus, HTLV-III. *Nature, Lond.*, **313**, 277–84.

Redfield, R. R., Wright, D. C., James, W. D., Jones, T. S., Brown, C. and Burke, D. S. (1987). Disseminated vaccinia in military recruit with human immunodeficiency virus (HIV) disease. *New Eng. J. Med.*, **316**, 673–6.

Robert-Guroff, M., Brown, M. and Gallo, R. C. (1985) HTLV III neutralizing antibodies in patients with AIDS and AIDS-related complex. *Nature, Lond.*, **316**, 72–4.

Rozenbaum, W., Dormont, D., Spire, B., Vilmer, E., Gentilini, M., Griscelli, C., Montagnier, L., Barré-Sinoussi, F. and Chermann, J. C. (1985) Antimoniotungstate (HPA23) treatment of three patients with AIDS and one with prodrome. *Lancet*, i, 450–1.

Salahuddin, S. Z., Markham, P. D., Popovic, M., Sarngadharan, M. G., Orndorff, S., Flagadar, A., Patel, A., Gold, J. and Gallo, R. C. (1985) Isolation of infectious human T-cell leukemia/lymphotropic virus type III (HTLV-III) from patients with acquired immunodeficiency syndrome (AIDS) or AIDS-related complex (ARC) and from healthy carriers: A study of risk groups and tissue sources. *Proc. Natl Acad. Sci. USA*, **82**, 5530–4.

Salinovich, O., Payne, S. L., Montelaro, R. C., Hussain, K. A., Issel, C. J. and Schnorr, K. L. (1986). Rapid emergence of novel antigenic and genetic variants of equine infectious anemia virus during persistent infection. *J. Virol.*, **57**, 71–80.

Sanchez-Pescador, R., Power, M. D., Barr, P. J., Steimer, K. S., Stempien, M. M., Brown-Shimer, S. L., Gee, W. W., Renard, A. and Randolph, A. (1985) Nucleotide sequence and expression of an AIDS-associated retrovirus (ARV-2). *Science*, **227**, 484–92.

Sarin, P. S., Sun, D. K., Thornton, A. H., Naylor, P. H. and Goldstein, A. L. (1986) Neutralization of HTLVIII/LAV replication by antiserum to thymosin α_1. *Science*, **232**, 1135–7.

Sarngadharan, M. G., Popovic, M., Bruch, L., Schüpbach, J. and Gallo, R. C. (1984) Antibodies reactive with human T-lymphotropic retroviruses (HTLVIII) in the serum of patients with AIDS. *Science*, **224**, 506–8.

Sarngadharan, M. G., Markham, P. D. and Gallo, R. C. (1985) Human T-cell leukemia viruses, in *Virology* (ed. B. N. Fields *et al.*), Raven Press, New York, pp. 1345–71.

Scott, J., Stowring, L., Haase, A., Narayan, O. and Vigne, R. (1979). Antigenic variation in visna virus. *Cell*, **18**, 321–7.

Seigel, L. J., Ratner, L., Josephs, S. F., Derse, D., Feinberg, M. B., Reyes, G. R., O'Brien, S. J. and Wong-Staal, F. (1986) Transactivation induced by human T-lymphotropic virus type III (HTLV III) maps to a viral sequence encoding 58 amino acids and lacks tissue specificity. *Virology*, **148**, 226–31.

Shaw, G. M., Harper, M. E., Hahn, B. H., Epstein, L. G., Gajdusek, D. C., Price, R. W., Navia, B. A., Patito, C. K., O'Hara, C. J., Groopman, J. E., Cho, E. S., Oleske, J. M., Wong-Staal, F. and Gallo, R. C. (1985) HTLV-III infection in brains of children and adults with AIDS encephalopathy. *Science*, **227**, 177–82.

Shaw, G. M., Hahn, B. H., Arya, S. K., Groopman, J. E., Gallo, R. C. and Wong-Staal, F. (1984) Molecular characterization of human T-cell leukemia (lymphotropic) virus type III in the acquired immune deficiency syndrome. *Science*, **226**, 1165–71.

Sodroski, J., Goh, W. C., Rosen, C., Dayton, A., Terwilliger, E. and Haseltine, W. (1986a). A second post-transcriptional *trans*-activator gene required for HTLV-III replication. *Nature Lond.*, **321**, 412–7.

Sodroski, J., Goh, W. C., Rosen, L., Tartar, A., Portetelle, D., Burny, A. and Haseltine, W. (1986b) Replicative and cytopathic potential of HTLV-III/LAV with *sor* gene deletions. *Science*, **231**, 1549–53.

Sodroski, J., Patarca, R., Rosen, C., Wong-Staal, F. and Haseltine, W. (1985a) Location of the *trans*-activating region on the genome of human T-cell lymphotropic virus type III. *Science* **229**, 74–7.

Sodroski, J., Rosen, C., Wong-Staal, F., Salahuddin, S. Z., Popovic, M., Arya, S., Gallo, R. C. and Haseltine, W. A. (1985b) *Trans*-acting transcriptional regulation of human T-cell leukemia virus type III long terminal repeats. *Science*, **227**, 171–3.

Sodroski, J. G., Rosen, C. A. and Haseltine, W. A. (1984) *Trans*-acting transcriptional activation of the long terminal repeat of human T-lymphotropic viruses in infected cells. *Science*, **225**, 381–5.

Starcich, B. R., Hahn, B. H., Shaw, G. M., McNeely, P. D., Modrow, S., Wolf, H., Parks, E. S., Parks, W. P., Josephs, S. F., Gallo, R. C. and Wong-Staal, F. (1986) Identification and characterization of conserved and variable regions in the envelope gene of HTLV-III/LAV, the retrovirus of AIDS. *Cell*, **45**, 637–48.

Starcich, B., Ratner, L., Josephs, S. F., Okamoto, T., Gallo, R. C. and Wong-Staal, F. (1985) Characterization of long terminal repeat sequences of HTLV-III. *Science*, **227**, 538–40.

Steimer, K. S., Higgins, K. W., Powers, M. A., *et. al.* (1986) Recombinant polypeptide from the endonuclear region of the acquired immune deficiency syndrome retrovirus polymerase (*pol*)gene detects serum antibodies in most infected individuals. *J. Virol.*, **58**, 9–16.

Stephens, R. M., Casey, J. W. and Rice, N. R. (1986) Equine infectious anemia virus gag and pol genes: Relatedness to Visna and AIDS virus. *Science*, **231**, 589–94.

Terwilliger, E., Sodroski, J. G., Rosen, C. A. and Haseltine, W. A. (1986). Effects of mutations within the 3′ *orf* open reading frame region of human T-cell lymphotropic virus type III (HTLVIII/LAV) on replication and cytopathogenicity. *J. Virol.*, **60**, 754–60.

Trainin, Z., Wernicke, D., Ungar-Waron, H. and Essex, M. (1983) Suppression of the humoral antibody response in natural retrovirus infections. *Science*, **220**, 858–9.

Wachter, H., Fuchs, D., Hausen, A., Reibnegger, G., Werner, E. R. and Dierich, M. P. (1986). Who will get AIDS? *Lancet*, ii, 1216–7.

Wain-Hobson, S., Sonigo, P., Danos, O., Cole, S. and Alizon, M. (1985) Nucleotide sequence of the AIDS virus, LAV. *Cell*, **40**, 9–17.

Weber, J. N., Clapham, P. R., Weiss, R. A., Parer, D., Roberts, C., Duncan, J., Weller, I., Carne, C., Tedder, R. S., Pinching A. J. and Cheingsong-Popov, R. (1987). Human immunodeficiency virus infection in two cohorts of homosexual men: neutralizing sera and association of anti-gag antibody with prognosis. *Lancet*, i, 119–22.

Weber, J. N., Wadsworth, J., Rogers, L. A., Moshtael, O., Scott, K., McManus, T., Berrie, E., Jeffries, D. J., Harris, J. R. W. and Pinching, A. J. (1986) Three-year prospective study of HTLV-III/LAV infection in homosexual men. *Lancet*, i, 1179–82.

Weiss, R. A., Clapham, P. R., Cheingsong-Popov, R., Dalgleish, A. G., Carne, C. A., Weller, I. V. D. and Tedder, R. S. (1985) Neutralization of human T-lymphotropic virus type III by sera of AIDS and AIDS-risk patients. *Nature, Lond.*, **316**, 69–72.

Weiss, R. A., Clapham, P. R., Weber, J. N., Dalgleish, A. G., Lasky, L. A. and Berman, P. W. (1986). Variable and conserved neutralization antigens of human immunodeficiency virus. *Nature Lond.*, **324**, 572–5.

Wong-Staal, F. and Gallo, R. C. (1985) Human T-lymphotropic retroviruses. *Nature, Lond.*, **317**, 395–403.

Wong-Staal, F., Shaw, G. M., Hahn, B. H., Salahuddin, S. Z., Popovic, M., Markham, P., Redfield, R. and Gallo, R. C. (1985) Genomic diversity of human T-lymphotropic virus type III (HTLVIII). *Science*, **229**, 759–62.

Yamamoto, N. and Hinuma, J. (1985) Viral aetiology of adult T-cell leukaemia. *J. Gen. Virol.*, **66**, 1641–60.

Yarchoan, R., Berg, G., Brouwers, P., Fischl, M. A., Spitzer, A. R., Wichman, A., Grafman, J., Thomas, R. V., Safai, B., Brunetti, A., Perno, C. R., Schmidt, P. J., Larson, S. M., Myers, C. E. and Broder, S. (1987). Response of human-immunodeficiency-virus-associated neurological disease to 3′-azido-3′-deoxythymidine. *Lancet*, i, 132–5.

Yarchoan, R., Klecker, R. W., Weinhold, K. J., Markham, P. D., Lyerly, H. K., Durack, D. T., Gelmann, E., Nusinoff-Lehrman, S., Blum, R. M., Barry, D. W., Shearer, G. M., Fischl, M. A., Mitsuya, H., Gallo, R. C., Collins, J. M., Bolognesi, D. P., Myers, C. E. and Broder, S. (1986) Administration of 3′-azido-3′-deoxythymidine, an inhibitor of HTLV-III/LAV replication to patients with AIDS or AIDS-related complex. *Lancet*, i, 575–80.

Zagury, D., Bernard, J., Leonard, R., Cheymier, R., Feldman, M., Sarin, P. S. and Gallo, R. C. (1986) Long-term cultures of HTLVIII-infected T cells: A model of cytopathology of T-cell depletion in AIDS. *Science*, **231**, 850–3.

Zagury, D., Fouchard, M., Vol., J. C., Cattan, A., Leibowitch, J., Feldman, M., Sarin, P. S. and Gallo, R. C. (1985) Detection of infectious HTLVIII/LAV virus in cell-free plasma from AIDS patients. *Lancet*, ii, 505–6.

Zagury, D., Leonard, R., Fouchard, M., Reveil, B., Bernard, J., Ittele, D., Cattan, A., Zirimwabagabo, L., Kalumbu, M., Justin, W., Salaun, J.-J. and Goussard, B. (1987). Immunization against AIDS in humans. *Nature Lond.*, **326**, 249–50.

4

Effects of HIV infection on the immune system

J. Steven McDougal, Janet K. A. Nicholson and Alison Mawle

4.1 INTRODUCTION

The acquired immune deficiency syndrome (AIDS) is characterized by progressive lymphopenia, predominantly of T helper/inducer cells, which renders the patient susceptible to a variety of opportunistic infections and malignancies. AIDS itself remains a clinical diagnosis and is but one manifestation of a spectrum of clinical and subclinical immunologic disorders caused by the human immunodeficiency virus (HIV), also known as HTLV-III, LAV, or ARV (Barré-Sinoussi *et al.*, 1983; Gallo *et al.*, 1984; Levy *et al.*, 1984; Coffin *et al.*, 1986).

This virus fulfils as many of Koch's postulates for cause and effect as can ethically be demonstrated in humans. It is frequently isolated from AIDS patients (Gallo *et al.*, 1984). Studies of transfusion donor–recipient pairs can reasonably be interpreted as transmission of disease by inoculation of virus (Feorino *et al.*, 1984; Groopman *et al.*, 1984; Feorino *et al.*, 1985). Virtually all AIDS patients and patients with AIDS-related syndromes show serologic evidence (antibody) of exposure to the virus; seroprevalence is lower in groups at risk for AIDS and even lower in groups at no or low risk (Sarngadharan *et al.*, 1984; Safai *et al.*, 1984). Infection occurs before (rather than as a consequence of) the development of AIDS, and seroprevalance has antedated and risen in parallel with the AIDS epidemic (Safai *et al.*, 1984; Landesman, Ginzburg and Weiss, 1985). The epidemiology of AIDS is consistent with transmission by a blood-borne agent (Curran, 1983). Finally, the biology and immunology of the virus provide compelling reasons for cause and effect. It is the latter with which this review is concerned.

From the immunologic standpoint, the AIDS phenomenon is best viewed as an HIV infectious process affecting T cells. The result is a graded severity of immunologic deficiency that, in turn, is distributed on a continuum of time and/or clinical severity. One problem with studying immunologic function in AIDS patients is that many of the opportunistic infections and malignancies that complicate the clinical course may also affect the immune system, making a distinction between primary versus secondary effects difficult. For this reason, many investigators interested in the proximate effects of HIV infection have focused on infected subjects who have not yet developed the severe immunodeficiency and clinical complications of AIDS. A second problem relates to material used for study of immunologic function. Usually, lymphocytes obtained from peripheral blood have been used, and there can be no assurance that changes in lymphocyte subpopulations detected are also reflected in lymphoid organs or represent loss/gain rather than redistribution. For the most part, however, changes found in peripheral blood have also been found in tissue such as lymph node (Modlin *et al.*, 1983; Chan *et al.*, 1985; Wood *et al.*, 1986). With these caveats in mind, we will try to distinguish primary from secondary immunologic effects of HIV infection and within the secondary effects, we will try to distinguish effects that represent an immune response to HIV from those that are a consequence of HIV cytopathology.

4.2 ORGANIZATION OF THE IMMUNE SYSTEM

The sole purpose of the immune system is to discriminate that which is foreign from that which is self, and as a consequence of this recognition, to induce immune and other cells to perform their respective immunologic functions. These immune functions can be viewed teleologically as a collective set of mechanisms geared toward the eventual destruction, inactivation, or elimination of foreign substances (Fig. 4.1). The initial discrimination of self from non-self is performed by a distinct set of thymus-derived T cells known as T helper/inducer cells. This cell set recognizes antigen that has been processed (by accessory or antigen-presenting cells such as macrophages) and is presented in the context of self-components known as class II structures, coded for by the major histocompatibility complex (MHC). Class I MHC structures are found on all nucleated cells, whereas class II structures are found only on monocytes, monocyte-derived cells, B cells, activated T cells, and haematopoietic precursors. The preponderance of evidence indicates that T helper/inducer cells recognize antigen and class II structures via a single T cell receptor-complex on the cell surface. They are at least as specific for antigen as are antibody-producing precursors, the B cells; probably have a repertoire similar in size to that of B cells; have characteristic primary and secondary responses that differ in timing and magnitude; have a bias toward recognizing denatured or processed rather than native or conformationally

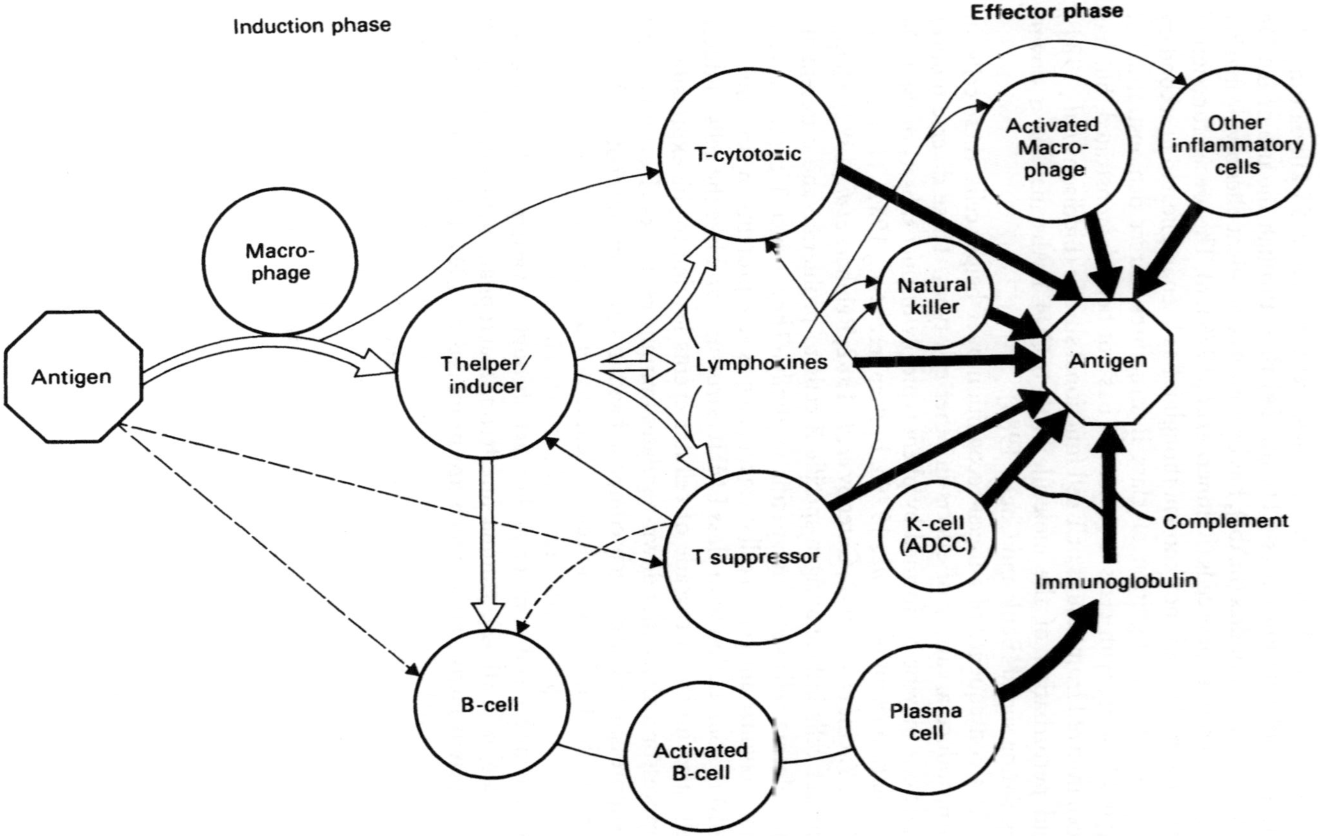

Figure 4.1 Organization of the immune system.

intact antigenic determinants; and have the additional constraint (restriction element) of class II recognition. These cells express a 55-kilodalton cell-surface molecule known as CD4 (or T4) that, through the use of α-CD4 monoclonal antibodies (mAbs), has become a convenient phenotypic marker for enumerating these cells (Reinherz *et al.*, 1979a, b). The precise function of the CD4 molecule is not known, though it has been implicated in secondary or associative recognition of class II structures (direct demonstration of ligand binding with class II structures has not been demonstrated, but has been inferred from results of T cell functional studies (Biddison *et al.*, 1984)) and perturbation of the molecule with α-CD4 mAbs may be a down-regulating signal (Bank and Chess, 1985).

As a consequence of antigen-recognition by T helper cells, these cells, in turn, induce a variety of effects in other cell types. These diverse inducer functions may be performed by phenotypically distinct subsets of the CD4 population (Reinherz *et al.*, 1979a, b; Reinherz *et al.*, 1981; Thomas *et al.*, 1982; Yachie *et al.*, 1982; Gatenby *et al.*, 1982; Reinherz *et al.*, 1982). Helper inducer cells induce antigen-specific B cells to proliferate and differentiate into plasma cells secreting specific antibody. They induce T cytotoxic cells that recognize antigen on cell surfaces (such as viral proteins on virus-infected cells) in conjunction with class I MHC structures and lyse the cells. Inducer cells also initiate a cascade of cellular events leading to the expression of suppressor activity that down-regulates immune responses. T cytotoxic and T suppressor cells are largely comprised within a phenotypic set of T cells that express the CD8 (T8) molecule (Reinherz *et al.*, 1979a, b; Reinherz and Schlossman, 1980; Ledbetter *et al.*, 1981). The inductive mechanisms may involve direct cell contact and/or act through a variety of lymphokines (interleukin 2 (IL–2), gamma interferon, macrophage-activating factor, B cell growth factor, etc.), which are produced by CD4 T cells. These lymphokines also have potent effects on other cells such as natural killer cells and macrophages. Division of T cells into mutually exclusive populations expressing either the CD4 or CD8 phenotype accounts for greater than 95% of the mature T cell pool. The association of these subpopulations with helper or cytotoxic/suppressor function, however, may not be totally appropriate. Rather, a more stringent association may be in the mode of antigen recognition. CD4 cells recognize antigen in the context of class II MHC structures, whereas CD8 T cells recognize antigen in the context of class I MHC structures (Meuer, Schlossman and Reinherz, 1982). For instance, $CD4^+$ T cytotoxic cell function has been described (in which case the cytotoxicity is class II rather than class I restricted) (Meuer, Schlossman and Reinherz, 1982). Class-I-restricted helper function by CD8 T cells has not been described.

4.3 ASSOCIATION OF SPECIFIC IMMUNE DEFECTS WITH SUSCEPTIBILITY TO CERTAIN TYPES OF INFECTIONS

Well before the AIDS epidemic, clinical studies of acquired and congenital immunodeficiency syndromes had established that certain types of immunologic defects tend to be associated with certain types of infections or malignancies. Thus, viral, fungal, or protozoal infections tend to occur in patients with T cell defects, whereas Gram-positive (and Gram-negative) infections are more of a problem in patients with B cell, antibody, or complement deficiencies (Rosen, Cooper and Wedgewood, 1984). Some infections, such as *Pneumocystis carinii* pneumonia and progressive multifocal leukoencephalopathy, are truly opportunistic in that they are virtually unheard of in subjects with intact immune systems. Other infections (herpes, cytomegalovirus (CMV), Epstein–Barr virus (EBV), toxoplasmosis) as well as certain malignancies (Kaposi's sarcoma) occur in both normal and immunodeficient subjects. Here, the distinction is in the severity, dissemination, epidemiologic restriction or life threatening nature of the infection. These associations have been garnered through accumulated clinical observations and are not absolute. Nevertheless they have been clinically useful in diagnostic prediction and clinical management, e.g. when characteristic infections occur, one considers a certain type of defect, and, conversely, when certain types of defects are present, one can be prepared for characteristic types of infection.

4.4 CELLULAR TROPISM OF HIV INFECTION *IN VITRO*

HIV is grown in activated T cells or in $CD4^+$ T cell lines. In cultures of normal human lymphocytes (stimulated with phytohaemagglutinin and cultured in the presence of IL–2), detectable cytoplasmic virus appears and then disappears in a proportion (1% to 10%) of cells (many of which form syncytia), followed by release of virus detected by particulate reverse transcriptase (RT) activity, viral antigen assay, and infectivity (Fig. 4.2). Virus infection is associated with loss of the CD4 antigen from infected cells and, ultimately, complete loss of $CD4^+$ T cells from the culture (Fig. 4.2). Residual non-$CD4^+$ cells are not susceptible to a second infection with HIV (Klatzmann *et al.*, 1985; McDougal *et al.*, 1985b). Thus, the essential immunologic feature of AIDS can be reproduced *in vitro* over a relatively short period of culture (1–2 weeks) (Klatzmann *et al.*, 1984; Fauci *et al.*, 1985; McDougal *et al.*, 1985a). A selective or preferential $CD4^+$ T cell tropism has also been demonstrated when separated cell populations (Klatzmann *et al.*, 1984; Klatzmann *et al.*, 1985; McDougal *et al.*, 1985b) or continuous cell lines are examined (Fauci *et al.*, 1985; Gallo *et al.*, 1984; Dalgleish *et al.*, 1985; Popovic, Read-Connole

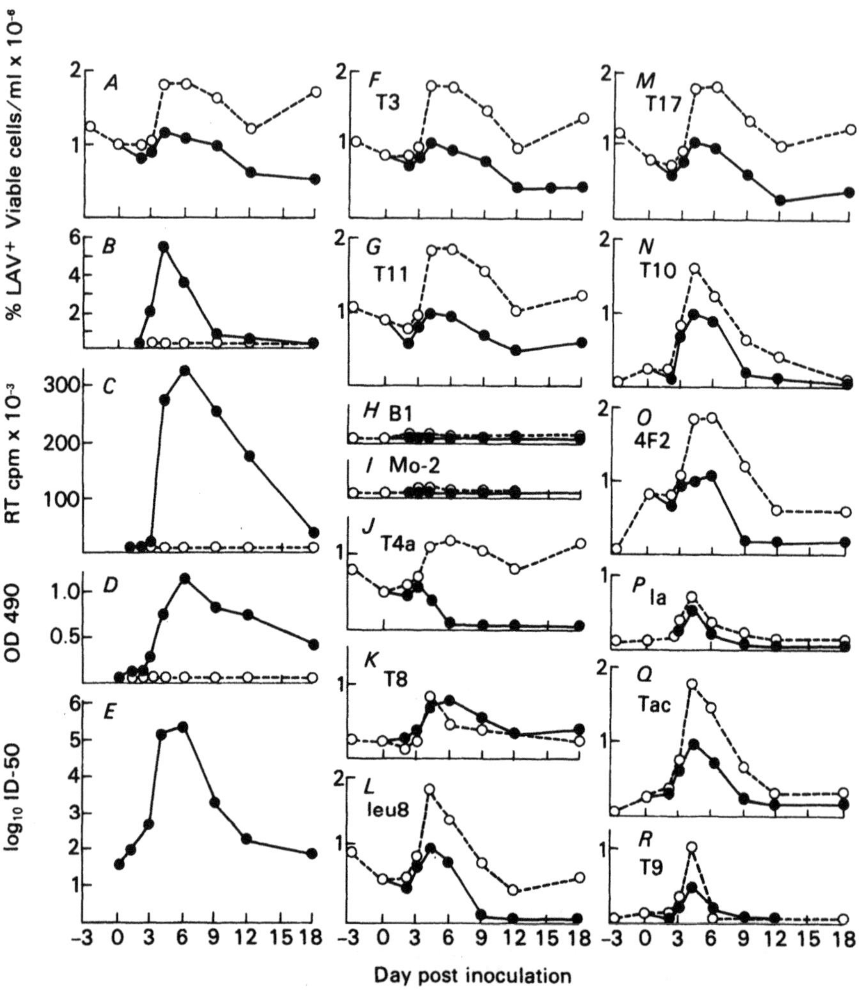

Figure 4.2 HIV infection of normal human lymphocytes. Phytohaemagglutinin-stimulated lymphocytes were divided, and half were inoculated with HIV (●——●); the other half served as control (○——○). Viable cell counts (A), cytoplasmic virus (B), supernatant RT activity (C), supernatant viral antigen (D), and infectivity titre of supernatant (E) were monitored over time as were cell surface phenotypes (F–R). (From McDougal *et al.*, 1985b reproduced with permission, American Association of Immunologists.)

and Gallo, 1984; Levy *et al.*, 1985b), although infectivity for some non-T cells has been reported (see below).

A prime determinant of cellular susceptibility to HIV infection is the presence of a cell-surface molecule with binding avidity for the virus, namely the CD4 molecule itself, which binds the gp110 envelope glycoprotein of the virus. Evidence that the CD4 molecule functions as a receptor for the virus is four-fold. First, certain CD4 monoclonal antibodies will prevent or limit the infectivity and replication of HIV in T cells (Popovic, Gallo and Mann, 1984; Dalgleish and Clapham, 1985; Klatzmann *et al.*, 1985; McDougal *et al.*, 1985b). Second, virus preferentially binds to the surface of $CD4^+$ T cells, with reciprocal inhibition of virus and CD4 mAb binding by each other (McDougal *et al.*, 1985b). Similarly, virus-infected cells bind and fuse with uninfected $CD4^+$ T cells (but not $CD4^-$ cells), resulting in syncytia formation that can be inhibited by α-CD4 mAbs (Dalgleish *et al.*, 1985; Lifson *et al.*, 1986). Third, direct demonstration of a bimolecular complex of the CD4 molecule and viral gp110 has been obtained in radioimmunoprecipitation experiments (McDougal *et al.*, 1986a). Fourth, when human cell lines that ordinarily do not express the CD4 molecule and that cannot be productively infected with native HIV are rendered CD4-positive by transfection with the human CD4 gene, virus binds and the cells are permissive for viral replication (Maddon *et al.*, 1986).

Despite suggestions to the contrary (Klatzmann *et al.*, 1984; Dalgleish *et al.*, 1985) and observations in patient groups that indicate a preferential loss of certain $CD4^+$ subsets (Nicholson *et al.*, 1984a; Fauci, 1984a; Nicholson, McDougal and Spira, 1985), there is no indication that HIV preferentially replicates in or depletes any particular $CD4^+$ T cell subset *in vitro*. The requirement for T cell activation appears to be a quantitative rather than qualitative difference. $CD4^+$ T cells that are activated or proliferating are depleted more quickly and replicate more virus than 'resting' $CD4^+$ T cells, but virus infection is cytopathic for non-activated $CD4^+$ T cells as well (McDougal *et al.*, 1985b). Thus, infection is inexorable in $CD4^+$ T cells regardless of subset or activation state, and the activation/proliferative state of the cells is not so much a determinant of infectivity, but rather, determines the amount of replication that will ensue. These distinctions may be clinically relevant. Activation/proliferation may not be an important determinant of susceptibility to infection, but it may be an important cofactor or determinant of the balance between $CD4^+$ T cell destruction and regeneration and the pace at which progressive $CD4^+$ T cell depletion and immunodeficiency occur – a cofactor of potential importance in risk groups whose life style or therapy may result in repeated antigenic stimulation of T cells.

Though cell surface expression of CD4 appears to be a necessary determinant of natural infectivity by HIV, it may not be sufficient to render all mammalian cells permissive for viral replication. All human cell lines tested that have been transfected with the human CD4 gene and express cell surface CD4 will replicate virus. CD4-transfected murine cell lines will not, though they do bind HIV (Maddon *et al.*, 1986). A panel of human–murine somatic cell hybrids, all of which expressed CD4 (coded for by chromosome 12), were tested for HIV infectivity and none replicated virus – including hybrids containing all 46 human chromosomes (Tersmette *et al.*, 1986). Thus, the apparent host range difference between $CD4^+$ cells may be related to a dominant inhibitory property (resistance trait) of mouse cells rather than a permissive property (susceptibility trait) unique to human cells. Presumably all mammalian cells will replicate virus from cloned and integrated proviral DNA introduced into the cell by transfection (Rosen, Sodroski and Haseltine, 1985; Fisher *et al.*, 1985; Levy *et al.*, 1986). If so, the difference between $CD4^+$ human and mouse cells must lie in events that occur after surface binding and before proviral transcription: penetration, endocytosis, uncoating, reverse transcription, and integration. If additional factors are identified (besides CD4 expression) that are important determinants of tropism, they are likely to act at these steps of viral replication as well.

While infection and depletion of $CD4^+$ T helper/inducer cells is probably the major contributor to quantitative viral replication and pathogenesis of immunodeficiency in the human host, infection of other cell types has also been demonstrated. Particles compatible with HIV have been observed in monocyte-derived cells such as macrophages, dendritic cells, and Langerhans' cells by electron microscopic examination of tissue specimens (Gyorkey *et al.*, 1985; Armstrong and Horne, 1985; Kolata, 1986). Monocytes express low levels of CD4 (Wood, Warner and Warke, 1983), will bind HIV, and binding is inhibited by α-CD4 mAb (Nicholson *et al.*, 1986a). Monocytes and the monocytic cell line U–937 retain infectious HIV for long periods in culture and will transmit productive viral infection to T cells (Levy *et al.*, 1985a; Levy *et al.*, 1985b; Dalgleish *et al.*, 1985; Ho, Rota and Hirsch, 1986; Nicholson *et al.*, 1986b). They also replicate virus, albeit at much lower levels and more slowly than T cells (Levy *et al.*, 1985a; Ho *et al.*, 1986a; Nicholson *et al.*, 1986a). Montagnier *et al.* (1984) first reported HIV replication in B cell lines, which were later found positive for CD4 expression (Dalgleish *et al.*, 1985). We have found two (of 10 examined) EBV-transformed B cell lines permissive for viral infection. Both lines express low levels of CD4. Neuropsychiatric symptoms may be a prominent clinical feature of HIV infection, and HIV has been identified in brain tissue by *in situ* hybridization and by culture (Shaw *et al.*, 1985; Ho *et al.*, 1985a; Levy *et al.*, 1985c). The precise cell type that is infected has not been identified. It may be as trivial as blood lymphocytes that pass through the brain; microglia, which are monocyte-derived cells, may be the source; or some brain cells may share structures homologous with the CD4 molecule (neural and thymic sharing of antigens has been reported in both mice and man). Lastly, infection of the brain may be due to mechanisms of natural infection that are independent of the CD4-virus interaction and that have yet to be described.

Taken together, the evidence supports the notion that the CD4 molecule functions as a receptor for HIV, that receptor binding is a major determinant of cell tropism (adsorption, penetration, infectivity, and eventual death), that all human CD4$^+$ T cells are susceptible to infection regardless of subset or state of activation, and that the metabolic (activation) state of the cell is a major determinant of how much and how fast virus replication will ensue. It remains unclear how cell surface binding translates to cell penetration, whether there are additional intracellular and metabolic features unique to human cells that allow or are permissive for virus replication, and why this retrovirus is cytopathic rather than transforming. In comparison to transforming retroviruses, HIV infection produces abundant viral RNA and non-integrated DNA (Wong-Staal and Gallo, 1985; Sodroski *et al.*, 1985; Rabson *et al.*, 1985). Unique genetic regions of the virus involved in transcriptional and translational control are probably responsible for its lytic potential. Two such regions, *sor* and *3'orf*, have recently been discounted for such a role (Sodroski *et al.*, 1986a, b), but further studies of deletion and site-directed mutants will likely unravel the lytic phenomenon as well. Finally, most studies of cell tropism measure replication, phenotypic depletion, and release of virus. It can be difficult to ascertain whether virus exists in a low-level, replicative form or truly latent state (proviral DNA only without transcription products) in some cell types or even in a proportion of T cells that are genetically programmed CD4 T cells that, as a result of HIV infection, do not express CD4 on their cell surface. Infection at low cell density or continued propagation of CD4$^+$ outgrowths from a predominantly lytic infection of CD4$^+$ T cells has yielded long term cultures containing cells that will transmit productive infection to fresh CD4$^+$ T cells or that can be induced to replicate virus with inducing agents such as iododeoxyuridine or allogeneic stimulation (Hoxie *et al.*, 1985; Folks *et al.*, 1985; Zagury *et al.*, 1986). In addition, infected monocytes may be a more stable reservoir for virus than the relatively short-lived, infected CD4 T cells. The relevance of these observations to viral persistence in the human host remains to be determined.

4.5 ABNORMALITIES OF CD4 T CELLS AND CD4/CD8 (T4/T8) RATIO

From the earliest reports of AIDS and well before HIV was identified as the cause, it was known that a reversal in the ratio of helper to suppressor T cells was characteristic (Gottlieb *et al.*, 1981; Masur *et al.*, 1981; Siegal *et al.*, 1981). Inverted ratios in AIDS are due to a marked decrease in the absolute number of helper/inducer T cells and a variable number (increased, normal, or decreased) of suppressor/cytotoxic T cells (Schroff *et al.*, 1983; Ammann *et al.*, 1983; Fahey *et al.*, 1984; Fauci *et al.*, 1984b). The *in vitro* biology of the virus predicts that numerical depletion of CD4 cells would reflect the primary lesion more accurately than would the CD4/CD8 ratio, and clinical studies tend to support this. However, determinations of absolute T helper cell number and T helper/suppressor ratio both have their place in clinical evaluation of HIV-infected subjects (see Chapter 5). From a technical standpoint, ratio may be a more accurate determination since intrinsic test variation is a function of a single technology, phenotyping, whereas absolute T helper count is calculated from results of three technologies: phenotyping, white cell count, and differential. Further, ratio is more sensitive to reciprocal changes in CD4 and CD8 cell counts that may occur early in infection (Melbye *et al.*, 1984; Nicholson *et al.*, 1985; Schwartz *et al.*, 1985; Eyster *et al.*, 1985; Melbye *et al.*, 1986). Absolute number of CD4 T cells is a more specific marker for severe immunodeficiency as defined by the CDC surveillance definition of AIDS (Fauci *et al.*, 1984b). From 65 to 95% of AIDS patients will manifest low numbers of CD4 T cells at diagnosis, and virtually all AIDS patients who survive long enough will ultimately develop this abnormality. However an abnormally low number of CD4 T cells is unusual in so-called pre-AIDS or AIDS-related complex (ARC), and in asymptomatic, infected individuals (Table 4.1). However, such a count is not as sensitive for AIDS or HIV infection as is determination of ratio. Low ratios occur in almost all AIDS patients at diagnosis and in a substantial proportion of HIV-infected subjects (Table 4.1).

The relationship of altered T cell subsets to the course of HIV infection continues to be defined. In cross-sectional studies, there is a spectrum of immunologic abnormalities that correlates with clinical severity. Within groups defined as having AIDS, absolute numbers of CD4 cells or CD4/CD8 ratio abnormalities are independent of risk group but are related to disease manifestation and duration of AIDS diagnosis. Patients with Kaposi's sarcoma as the sole manifestation of disease have less severe abnormalities than those with opportunistic infections (Fig. 4.3, Table 4.1). Those who recover from opportunistic infections generally have more CD4 T cells than those who do not and, once the diagnosis of AIDS is made, progressive

Table 4.1 Frequency of abnormal CD4/CD8 T cell ratio and CD4 T cells in homosexual men. Compiled from Rogers *et al.*, 1983; Nicholson, McDougal and Spira, 1985a; Nicholson *et al.*, 1985; Fishbein *et al.*, 1985; and CDC unpublished data

		% with abnormal	
Clinical Status of Homosexual Men	*Number*	*CD4/CD8 ratio (<1.00)*	*Number of CD4 cells ($<408 mm^{-3}$)*
AIDS (total meeting case definition)	130	94	81
AIDS (opportunistic infection)	99	98	96
AIDS (Kaposi's sarcoma only)	31	81	65
Lymphadenopathy syndrome	123	63	25
Asymptomatic HIV-seropositive	106	67	5
Asymptomatic HIV-seronegative	111	8	0

depletion of CD4 T cells with time is the rule (Friedman-Kein *et al.*, 1982; Mildvan *et al.*, 1982; Ammann *et al.*, 1983; Fahey *et al.*, 1984; Schroff *et al.*, 1983; Fauci *et al.*, 1984b; Lane *et al.*, 1985a). Subjects with so-called AIDS-related complex, lesser AIDS, or lymphadenopathy syndrome have abnormalities intermediate between those of AIDS patients and asymptomatic risk group members (Figs 4.3 and 4.4).

Probably the ideal group for studying the early effects of HIV infection is subjects pre- and post-exposure (as assessed by antibody). A self-limited infectious mononucleosis-like syndrome has been described in association with HIV seroconversion. Immunologic profiles consist of a low-normal or normal number of CD4 cells, a normal or elevated number of CD8 cells, and a low-normal or low CD4/CD8 ratio (Cooper *et al.*, 1985). Only a few subjects have been studied, and the logistics of identifying such patients require large-scale prospective surveillance of seronegative risk group members. These types of studies are underway in a number of centres. The next-best approach is cross-sectional and subsequent longitudinal studies of asymptomatic risk group members, and a number of these have been reported. To date, such studies in several risk groups have confirmed the following findings. Exposure to HIV is highly associated with T cell abnormalities. Of multiple immunologic tests performed, a depressed helper/suppressor ratio (reflecting a low normal count of CD4 and high-normal count of CD8 cells) has been most highly associated with exposure (Melbye *et al.*, 1984; Nicholson *et al.*, 1985; Eyster *et al.*, 1985; Lederman *et al.*, 1985; Jason *et al.*, 1985; Stein *et al.*, 1985; Goedert *et al.*, 1986), although a low number of CD4 cells rather than ratio was the best correlate in one study (Goedert *et al.*, 1984). There is also a rough correlation between degree of T cell abnormality and duration of seropositivity (Eyster *et al.*, 1985; Jaffe *et al.*, 1985; Schwartz *et al.*, 1985; Goedert *et al.*, 1986; Melbye *et al.*, 1986). Seronegative risk group members are either immunologically normal or, as a group, have milder abnormalities of borderline statistical significance (Melbye *et al.*, 1984; Goedert *et al.*, 1984; Tsoukas *et al.*, 1984; Eyster *et al.*, 1985; Nicholson *et al.*, 1986b; Jason *et al.*, 1985; Stein *et al.*, 1985; Schwartz *et al.*, 1985).

In longitudinal studies, it has generally been found that the onset of non-specific systemic symptoms and abnormally low numbers of CD4 T cells is a poor prognostic sign in exposed asymptomatic subjects as well as in subjects with AIDS-related conditions such as lymphadenopathy (Fahey *et al.*, 1984; Metroka *et al.*, 1983; Goedert *et al.*, 1984; Abrams *et al.*, 1984; Mathur-Wagh *et al.*, 1984; Schwartz *et al.*, 1985; Eyster *et al.*, 1985; Lane *et al.*, 1985a; Fishbein *et al.*, 1985; Melbye *et al.*, 1986). The occurrence of thrush or *Candida* oesophagitis is a clinical sign associated with more severe CD4 depression and may herald full-blown AIDS manifestations (Redfield, Wright and Tramont, 1986). Thus, clinical and immunologic markers for (or predictors of) more severe disease do exist. It is not at all clear, however,

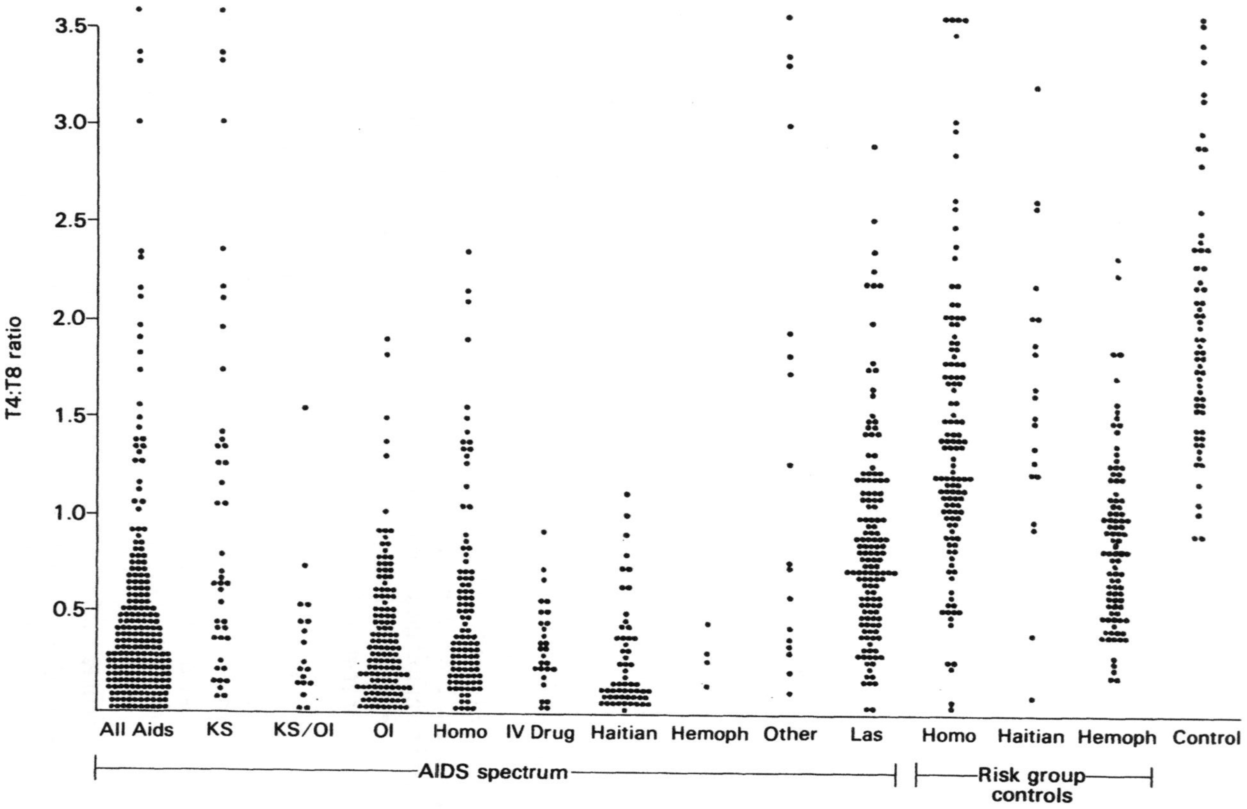

Figure 4.3 CD4/CD8 (T4/T8) T cell ratios in AIDS patients and controls. Abbreviations: KS, Kaposi's sarcoma; OI, opportunistic infection; IV Drug, intravenous drug abusers; Haemoph, haemophilia; LAS, lymphadenopathy syndrome. Compiled from consecutive specimens tested by Immunology Branch, CDC in 1982.

whether the converse exists. Not all exposed asymptomatic subjects are immunologically abnormal, and it remains to be determined whether there is a characteristic immunologic profile in exposed subjects that is independent of duration of exposure and predictive of a favourable outcome. Furthermore, it is not clear whether cofactors such as chronic antigenic stimulation, other infections, elements of life style, or therapy contribute to the pace at which progressive CD4 T cell depletion, immunodeficiency, and the onset of opportunistic infections occur. In studies of asymptomatic subjects, it has

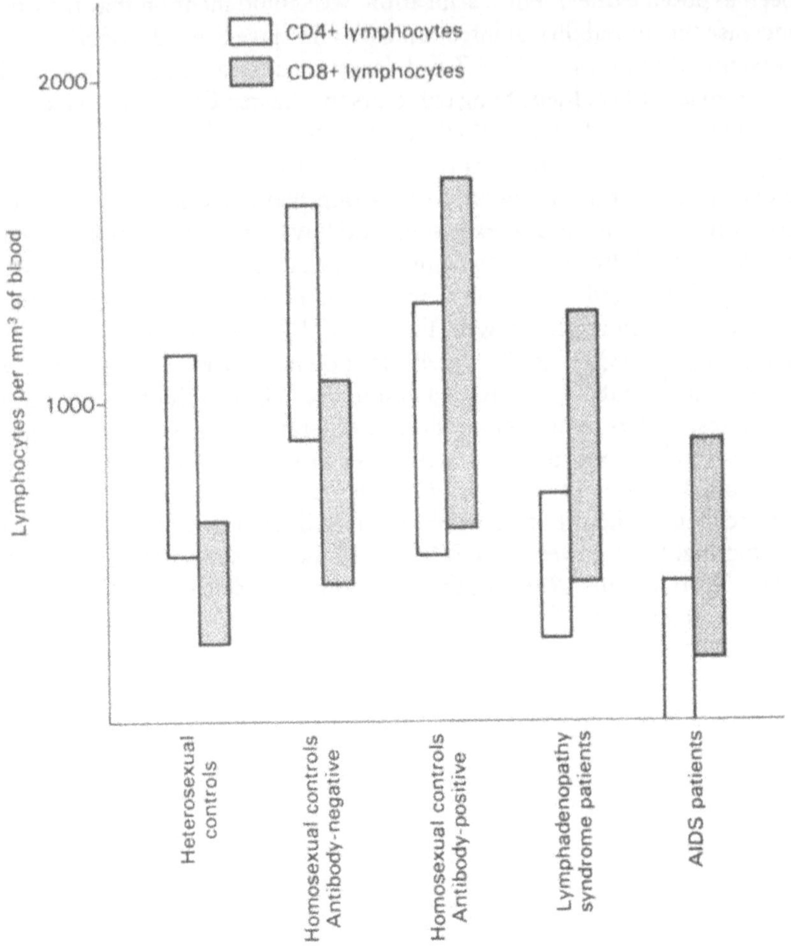

Figure 4.4 Absolute number of T helper/inducer (CD4) cells and T suppressor/cytotoxic (CD8) cells in HIV-infected subjects. Compiled from Rogers *et al.*, 1983; Nicholson, McDougal and Spira, 1985; Nicholson *et al.*, 1985; Fishbein *et al.*, 1985, and CDC, unpublished data.

generally not been possible to identify cofactors (other than duration of exposure) that act additively or synergistically with HIV exposure in predicting the degree of T cell abnormalities (Goedert *et al.*, 1984; Eyster *et al.*, 1985; Nicholson *et al.*, 1985; Melbye *et al.*, 1986; Goedert *et al.*, 1986). However, there are indications that seropositive intravenous drug abusers who continue to abuse drugs develop a greater degree of CD4 T cell depression than those who curtail their abuse (Friedman *et al.*, 1986), but it is not clear whether this reflects a real difference in natural history or other factors (e.g. subjects less likely to curb their abuse may be more likely to have been exposed earlier). For clarification, we should mention that factors that increase the probability of infection with HIV have been identified; however, cofactors that promote CD4 T cell depletion after a person is infected have not been identified. Identifying cofactors that hasten CD4 T cell depletion, on the one hand, and immunologic profiles that signify an effective immune response to this virus, on the other, is obviously relevant to disease management. Studies of asymptomatic risk group members that are longitudinal, controlled for duration of exposure, and have a reasonable followup duration will hopefully answer some of these questions.

The CD4 T cell set is functionally heterogeneous and can be further subdivided phenotypically with the use of TQ1 or Leu8 monoclonal antibodies. $CD4^+$ $TQ1^-$ $Leu8^-$ T cells are potent helpers for B cell responses. $CD4^+$ $TQ1^+$ $Leu8^+$ T cells have a minor role in B cell responses; they are the prime responders in antigen-induced proliferative assays and in the autologous mixed lymphocyte reaction; and they may induce CD8 T cell suppressor function (Reinherz *et al.*, 1982; Gatenby *et al.*, 1982). In infected subjects studied before the onset of AIDS, the initial drop in CD4 T cell numbers predominantly involves the $CD4^+$ $TQ1^+$ $Leu8^+$ subset (Nicholson *et al.*, 1984; Wood *et al.*, 1986). In the severe immunodeficiency found in AIDS patients, both CD4 T cell subsets are depleted (Nicholson, McDougal and Spira, 1985). As mentioned, there is no preferential infectivity of HIV for CD4 T cell subsets *in vitro*, and therefore the imbalance observed in patients probably reflects differences in redistribution, interconversion, or regeneration kinetics *in vivo*.

The evolution of CD4 T cell subset depletion is consistent with results of *in vitro* tests for T-cell function. When tested as isolated T cells with normal B cells in a pokeweed mitogen-driven assay for immunoglobulin production, T helper cell function is normal or depressed depending on the severity of T cell depletion in the patients selected for study (Mildvan *et al.*, 1982; Lane *et al.*, 1983; Benveniste *et al.*, 1983; Nicholson *et al.*, 1984; Pahwa *et al.*, 1984; Ammann *et al.*, 1984; Lane and Fauci, 1985). It is rarely totally abrogated except in AIDS patients with severe T cell depletion. On the other hand, proliferative responses to soluble antigen and the autologous mixed lymphocyte response are more consistently depressed or even abrogated; these may be the earliest qualitative defects in the immune system of HIV-infected subjects (Gupta and Safai, 1983; Smolen *et al.*, 1985; Lane *et al.*, 1985b). Responses to pan-T cell mitogens tend to be depressed when assayed on unseparated lymphocyte cultures but are generally normal when separated T cells, CD4 T cells, or CD8 T cells are assayed in numbers equivalent to that of controls (Lane *et al.*, 1983, 1985b; Fauci *et al.*, 1985). Proliferative responses to soluble antigen, however, are abnormal whether assayed as unseparated cells or purified T cells, leading Lane *et al.*, (1985b) to postulate an intrinsic defect in the capacity of surviving T cells to recognize soluble antigen. Antigen-driven proliferation is itself a multicellular phenomenon, and the observed defect may be due to a functional impairment of the individual responding T cell, an imbalance of TQ1/Leu8 cells within the T cell compartment, a defect in monocyte presentation of soluble antigen, or an effect of viral products that are not cytopathic but may be immunosuppressive as recently reported by Pahwa *et al.* (1985). In any event, antigen-specific proliferative responses are felt to be an *in vitro* correlate of delayed type hypersensitivity (DTH), and skin test reactivity is impaired in HIV-infected subjects. Again, total energy is more likely to be manifest in those subjects with severe T cell depletion (Gottlieb *et al.*, 1981; Masur *et al.*, 1981; Siegal *et al.*, 1981; Mildvan *et al.*, 1982; Lane and Fauci, 1985).

4.6 ABNORMALITIES OF SUPPRESSOR/CYTOTOXIC CELLS

The number of cells bearing the CD8 phenotype may be normal, elevated, or depressed (Fig. 4.4). Elevations are more frequent early in infection and in asymptomatic subjects. In full-blown, end-stage disease, severe CD4 T cell depletion may be associated with panlymphopenia including the CD8 T cell set (Stahl *et al.*, 1982; Ammann *et al.*, 1983; Fahey *et al.*, 1984; Schroff *et al.*, 1983; Lane and Fauci, 1985). This suggests that the relationship of CD8 T cell numbers to CD4 T cell numbers in HIV infection is bidirectional (that is, an early reciprocal (perhaps reactive) elevation of CD8 cells may be followed at some point by a decline that occurs in parallel with CD4 T cell depletion). However, bidirectional correlations cannot be obtained in cross-sectional studies without some arbitrary division of the data, nor have enough data from serial studies accumulated to make this distinction. In any event, there is as yet no clear or consistent association of CD8 T cell numbers with clinical course, complications, or degree of CD4 T cell depletion.

There is no evidence that normal CD8 T cells are susceptible to natural infection with HIV, and the observed perturbations are most likely secondary. CD8 T cells depend on CD4 T cells for induction of effector function and possibly for maintenance of precursor numbers as well. The extent to which changes in this population represent a secondary consequence of HIV infection or perhaps an immune response to HIV is unlikely to be determined by studies that rely on CD8 enumeration data only. Studies of phenotypic or functional subsets of the CD8 population, however, may reveal changes or responses that are clinically and therapeutically relevant.

The CD8 population can be divided into phenotypic subsets that are associated with suppressor versus cytotoxic function by using two-colour immunofluorescence analysis (Clement, Grossi and Gartland, 1984, Clement, Dagg and Landay, 1984). Asymptomatic HIV-infected subjects have higher levels of CD8 cells (and lower numbers of CD4 cells) than unifected risk group controls. This elevation is due to $CD8^+$ T cells that do not express the Leu15 antigen (Nicholson *et al.*, 1986b), a phenotypic subset associated with cytotoxic precursor and effector function (Clement, Dagg and Landay, 1984). The monoclonal antibody Leu7 marks a subpopulation of CD8 cells as well as a proportion of cells with natural killer (NK) cell function. This marker may occur on all cytotoxic cells at some point in differentiation. An increase in the $CD8^+$ $Leu7^+$ population has been described in asymptomatic HIV-infected homosexual men, in haemophiliacs, and in patients with AIDS (Lewis *et al.*, 1985; Prince *et al.*, 1985a; Ziegler-Heitbrock *et al.*, 1985; Nicholson *et al.*, 1986b; Stites *et al.*, 1986). As discussed below, HIV-infected subjects mount poor cytotoxic effector responses *in vitro* but presumably have relatively normal precursors. However, the specificity and function of the increased number of CD8 cells identified phenotypically as cytotoxic cells and their relevance to clinical course or prognosis remains to be determined.

Several studies have reported elevated numbers of T cells bearing the T10 or Ia antigen that are markers for activated or immature T cells. These increases are found within the CD8 population (Salazar-Gonzales *et al.*, 1985; Nicholson *et al.*, 1984; Schroff *et al.*, 1983). On the basis of T10/CD8 phenotype data and ecto-5′-nucleotidase activity of CD8 T cells, Salazar-Gonzales *et al.* (1985) concluded that there is an increase in the number of immature CD8 T cells. However, other markers that are more specific for immaturity (T6) or for activation/proliferation (Tac, 4F2, T9) are not elevated and, thus, not helpful in making this distinction (Nicholson *et al.*, 1984; Salazar-Gonzales *et al.*, 1985). Purified CD8 T cells from HIV-infected subjects have higher than normal rates of spontaneous proliferation (as do purified CD4 T cells and B cells) (Lane and Fauci, 1985). This finding does not distinguish activation of mature T cells from the presence of immature cells in peripheral blood. If these markers do reflect activation, it certainly does not result in heightened or fully differentiated suppressor or cytotoxic effector function – at least in those systems that have been examined (with one possible exception – described below (Laurence, Gottlieb and Kunkel, 1983)).

Because a poorly responsive immune system can result from a loss of helper induction or an excess of suppressor influences, much work has focused on the possibility that an excess of abnormal suppressor phenomena occurs in patients with AIDS. *In vitro*, lymphocytes or purified CD8 cells have been added to a variety of *in vitro* systems including mitogen assays, antigen-specific proliferation assays, autologous and allogeneic mixed lymphocyte response assays, and pokeweed mitogen-induced Ig production assays without evidence of excessive suppressor activity (Lane *et al.*, 1983; Benveniste *et al.*, 1983; Nicholson *et al.*, 1984; Smolen *et al.*, 1985; Lane and Fauci, 1985). Insofar as the induction of CD8 suppressor activity in normal lymphocytes is dependent on CD4 induction, one might predict abnormalities of suppressor cell induction, but these models have technical and interpretive difficulties and have not been reported. Though there is little evidence for excessive suppression by cells, suppressor factors have been described. Laurence, Gottlieb and Kunkel (1983) have described the spontaneous production *in vitro* of a suppressor factor dependent on T cell–monocyte interaction. This factor is similar in many respects to factors produced by suppressor T cell hybridomas and is induced in normal cells by concanavalin A stimulation (Greene *et al.*, 1982; Laurence and Mayer, 1984). Other factors present in the sera of AIDS patients have been described with suppressive or immunomodulating activity (Cunningham-Rundles, Michelis and Masur, 1983; Siegel *et al.*, 1984). They are most consistently found in patients who have severe immunodeficiency with clinical complications and quite possibly are secondary phenomena. Retrovirus products may themselves be immunosuppressive without being cytopathic, and a report bearing on this possibility has appeared (Pahwa *et al.*, 1985). A particularly appealing possibility is that the gp110 envelope glycoprotein, which is produced in excess by infected cells and binds to the CD4 molecule, may be intrinsically immunosuppressive since other reactions with the CD4 molecule (i.e. anti-CD4 monoclonal antibody) do transmit a negative signal (Bank and Chess, 1985). The role, relationship, and relative contribution of suppressor influences in the pathogenesis of AIDS remains to be defined. On balance, however, the prominent features of functional and phenotypic immunodeficiency are quite adequately explained by CD4 T cell depletion without the need to invoke excess suppression.

Functional studies of antigen-specific MHC-restricted cytotoxicity have shown that it is severely impaired in patients with AIDS or AIDS-related symptoms. Immunologically normal individuals with CMV infections have detectable CMV-specific cytotoxic T cells in their peripheral blood. Most homosexual men have been infected with CMV, and many patients with AIDS have active CMV infections. However, in testing over 80 AIDS patients for specific killing of CMV-infected MHC-matched fibroblasts, specific cytotoxicity was found in only two patients, both of whom had Kaposi's sarcoma, but no apparent opportunistic infections (Rook *et al.*, 1985b). Incubation of AIDS patients' cells in IL–2 for 72 h restored the ability of those cells to kill both MHC-matched and mismatched targets (Rook *et al.*, 1983).

Studies of the response of HIV-infected individuals to EBV have been evaluated using a regression assay. Lymphocytes from EBV-seropositive individuals, when infected with EBV and placed in culture, undergo an initial transformation of B cells that then regress as the culture continues. Regression is due to the activation of cytotoxic T cells specific for autologous EBV-infected B cells (Wallace *et al.*, 1981). When this assay was used, asymptomatic HIV-infected homosexual men showed regression comparable to that of uninfected homosexual men and heterosexual controls whereas, only 36% of patients with AIDS-related lymphadenopathy and no patients with AIDS showed regression (Mawle, Scheppler-Campbell and McDougal, 1985). Similar results were reported by Birx, Redfield and Tosato (1986). This suggests that in the EBV system, secondary T cytotoxic cell responses remain intact, at least in the early stages of HIV infection. As the clinical course progresses, however, the ability to mount such a response is lost. Cytotoxic T cells are believed to be important in regulating persistent EBV infection, and the loss of this regulation may account for the appearance of some B-cell lymphomas and the polyclonal B-cell activation that occur in AIDS patients.

A two-year longitudinal study of the cytotoxic response to influenza in asymptomatic homosexual men demonstrated that these responses remained constant over time and did not correlate with HIV antibody status, which is consistent with the findings in the EBV system (Shearer *et al.*, 1985).

It is possible to generate MHC-specific cytotoxic cells *in vitro* by allogeneic coculture of lymphocytes. Unlike the virus-specific, MHC-restricted cytotoxic assays that require cells from exposed donors, a primary allogeneic cytotoxic response can be generated and tested *in vitro*. Like virus-specific responses, the generation of alloreactive cytotoxic responses is depressed in patients with AIDS or AIDS-related clinical syndromes (asymptomatic risk group members have relatively normal responses). IL–2 partially restores or potentiates the response in both normal and infected subjects (Gerstoft, Dickmeiss and Mathiesen, 1985; Sharma and Gupta, 1985).

Taken together, these data suggest that there is a functional impairment of MHC-restricted T cell cytotoxicity in patients with AIDS and AIDS-related syndrome, but not in asymptomatic infected individuals. This defect encompasses both the primary (alloreactive) and secondary (CMV, EBV, influenza) responses. T cell help is clearly required for a primary response, and the lack of $CD4^+$ cells may play a role here. The requirement for T cell help in secondary responses is less clear-cut, though these data suggest this may be an important factor. The restoration of responses with IL–2 suggests that the defect is one of induction or differentiation rather than a lack of CD8 precursors.

NK cells are cytotoxic for a wide range of tumour cell lines without the need for previous exposure to the target cell line. They reside largely but not exclusively within a population of lymphocytes known as large granular lymphocytes (LGL). A proportion of NK cells may express the CD8, Leu15, Leu7, or Leu11 markers which, when used alone or in combination, yield populations enriched for NK activity, but precise phenotypic-functional definition has been elusive (Lanier *et al.*, 1983; Lanier and Loken, 1984). Much like the results with MHC-restricted and allogeneic cytotoxic cells, cells expressing NK-associated phenotypes and NK function tend to be well preserved in asymptomatic HIV-infected subjects but decline with severe immunodeficiency and clinical complications (Lopez, Fitzgerald and Siegal, 1983; Creemers, Stalk and Boyko, 1985; Poli *et al.*, 1985a; Jothy *et al.*, 1985; Nicholson *et al.*, 1986b; Siegal *et al.*, 1986). A more detailed analysis of patients with depressed NK function has shown that NK cells make contact with target cells (conjugate formation) normally, suggesting that the functional defect is the killing process itself (Poli *et al.*, 1985a). When depressed, NK function can be enhanced *in vitro* by the addition of IL–2 (Rook *et al.*, 1983; Reddy, Pinyavat and Greico, 1984; Lifson *et al.*, 1984; Rook *et al.*, 1985a). Again, this suggests that loss of function is not due to active suppression and that effector-precursors are present, but signals required for the induction of effector function are absent.

The relationship of LGL function to HIV infection merits attention for several reasons. First, Ruscetti *et al.*, (1986) have shown that cell lines infected with HIV are rendered susceptible to lysis by NK cells from normal subjects. Second, a population of LGL distinct from NK cells, monocytes, B cells, or T cells produces interferon-alpha (IFN-α), which potentiates NK function and has an anti-viral effect on HIV replication *in vitro* (Gidlund *et al.*, 1978; Fitzgerald, von Wussow and Lopez, 1982; Ho *et al.*, 1985b). Third, there is evidence to suggest that loss of IFN-α production (concomitant with loss of NK function) is a critical factor that acts synergistically with CD4 T-cell depletion and may herald the onset of opportunistic infections (Lopez, Fitzgerald and Siegal, 1983; Siegal *et al.*, 1986). However, the extent to which IFN-α or NK function actually limit viral replication in infected humans and whether preservation of these functions would prevent progression are unknown.

4.7 ABNORMALITIES OF B CELLS

Hypergammaglobulinaemia and elevated levels of immune complexes are characteristic findings in HIV-infected subjects (Schroff *et al.*, 1983; Gottlieb *et al.*, 1983; Ammann *et al.*, 1983; Fauci *et al.*, 1984b; Lightfoote, Folks and Sell, 1984; McDougal *et al.*, 1985c). Despite the polyclonal immunoglobulin elevation, HIV-infected subjects, and particularly AIDS patients, mount a poor antigen-specific antibody response after *in vivo* immunization. Primary responses are affected to a greater degree than secondary responses (Lane *et al.*, 1983; Ammann *et al.*, 1983). Patients mount and sustain an ongoing antibody response to HIV that can be of considerable titre, waning only with end-stage disease (Sarngadharan *et al.*, 1984; Schüpbach *et al.*, 1985; Biggar *et al.*, 1985; Kaminsky *et al.*, 1985). The normal sequence of events that occurs when precursor cells (B cells) become immunoglobulin-secreting cells (plasma cells) can be dissected *in vitro* into discrete stages of activation, proliferation, and differentiation. Largely through the work of Lane, Fauci, and coworkers, B cell responses in AIDS patients have been extremely well characterized. Lymphocytes from AIDS patients produce a poor immunoglobulin response *in vitro* to pokeweed mitogen stimulation (Lane *et al.*, 1983; Mildvan *et al.*, 1982; Nicholson *et al.*, 1984; Pahwa *et al.*, 1985). This phenomenon cannot be explained entirely by immunoregulatory T cell abnormalities because purified B cells from patients are poorly responsive when mixed with normal T cells and are not stimulated by direct B-cell activators such as formalinized staphylococci or anti-human IgM (Lane *et al.*, 1983; Mildvan *et al.*, 1982; Nicholson *et al.*, 1984; Pahwa *et al.*, 1985). They do respond to late-acting B cell growth factors and exhibit a high rate of spontaneous proliferation; a substantial portion exists in peripheral blood as differentiated Ig-secreting cells, as detected in a reverse haemolytic plaque-forming cell assay (Lane *et al.*, 1983; Pahwa *et al.*, 1984; Martin *et al.*, 1986). Thus, a high degree of apparently spontaneous, polyclonal B-cell stimulation occurs in HIV-infected subjects rendering them poorly responsive to normal early-activation signals.

The reason for B cell activation has been a matter of speculation. HIV can infect B cell lines that express the CD4 molecule, but it is not clear what proportion of B cells express CD4, and we have not been able to induce spontaneous immunoglobulin production by inoculation of purified normal B cells with HIV. Thus, the phenomenon is probably a secondary rather than primary consequence of HIV infection. Immunoregulatory abnormalities within the CD4 T cell compartment are compatible with the notion that relative preservation of the more potent CD4 helper subset in concert with a preferential loss of the CD4 subset that induces CD8 T cell suppressors allows unrestrained B cell activation. However, it has not been demonstrated that loss of suppressor-inducers necessarily results in spontaneous B-cell activation, nor has it been demonstrated that CD4 suppressor-inducer function (as opposed to phenotype) is abnormal in HIV-infected subjects. A more likely explanation postulates that abnormalities of immunoregulatory T cells allow infection or reactivation of other viral infections such as EBV or CMV that, in turn, are B cell activators. Evidence of EBV and CMV exposure is a nearly universal finding in AIDS patients (Rogers *et al.*, 1983; Quinnan *et al.*, 1984), but no one has reported a definitive correlation between EBV or CMV exposure, infection, or reactivation, on the one hand, and immunoglobulin or B-cell abnormalities, on the other, in HIV infected subjects (Crawford, Weller and Iliescu, 1984). Finally, it has been proposed that HIV-infected T cells elaborate B cell stimulating factors. Elaboration of lymphokines by cell lines transformed by HTLV-I has been reported (Salahuddin *et al.*, 1984; Arya and Gallo, 1985) but has not been found with the predominantly cytopathic HIV.

4.8 ABNORMALITIES OF MONOCYTES/MACROPHAGES

Blood monocytes and their tissue counterparts, macrophages, form one of the first lines of defence against micro-organisms by migrating toward the site of entry, phagocytosing foreign material and, in most cases, degrading and inactivating the micro-organisms. Though numerically normal, monocytes from AIDS patients may display defective chemotaxis to a variety of chemotactic stimuli (Smith *et al.*, 1984, Poli *et al.*, 1985b; Pinching *et al.*, 1983). Phagocytosis and intracellular killing have been reported as normal (Washburn, Tuazon and Bennett, 1984; Murray *et al.*, 1984) or abnormal (Pinching *et al.*, 1983), and superoxide and H_2O_2 production are generally normal (Murray *et al.*, 1984). *In vitro* assessments of monocyte-mediated, antibody-dependent, cellular cytotoxicity are reportedly abnormal in AIDS patients (Bender *et al.*, 1986), but normal in lymphadenopathy patients (Poli *et al.*, 1985b). *In vivo*, Fc-mediated clearance of IgG-coated autologous erythrocytes by the mononuclear phagocytic system is abnormally prolonged (Bender *et al.*, 1984). Those abnormalities that have been reported are most consistently found in patients with severe immunodeficiency and clinical complications.

In addition to their role in non-specific defence mechanisms, monocytes function in cellular immune responses. They process and present antigen in the context of class II MHC structures and act as accessory cells in a variety of T cell responses. Monocytes from AIDS patients express lower density class II MHC structures than normals, and class II expression is increased in both AIDS patients and normals by adding gamma-interferon *in vitro* (Heagy *et al.*, 1984). As mentioned, the qualitative defect in T cell proliferative responses to soluble antigen may relate more to a defect in antigen presentation than to the responding capacity of surviving T cells. Poor responses by lymphocytes from HIV-infected subjects to anti-CD3-induced proliferation can be partially restored with normal monocytes (Prince *et al.*, 1985b). (Anti-CD3 reacts with the CD3-T cell receptor complex and is thought to be a polyclonal correlate of antigen-specific T cell proliferation.) However, detailed examination of the antigen-presenting capacity of monocytes from HIV-infected subjects or normal monocytes infected with HIV has not been reported.

It has not been determined whether monocyte defects result from direct infection with HIV or from immunoregulatory T cell abnormalities. Defects in non-specific monocyte defence mechanisms tend to occur late in the course of infection and may well be secondary phenomena. If a defect in antigen-presentation by monocytes is shown to contribute to poor proliferative responses to soluble antigens, this defect may turn out to be a direct and early effect of HIV infection. And as mentioned before, HIV infection of monocytes may also contribute to viral persistence and be an especially troublesome problem in therapeutic strategies for eliminating virus.

4.9 ABNORMALITIES OF LYMPHOKINES AND OTHER SOLUBLE SERUM SUBSTANCES

There is a deficiency of IL–2 production in response to mitogens when whole cell populations are examined (Hauser *et al.*, 1984; Ciobanu *et al.*, 1983; Murray *et al.*, 1985; Alocer-Varela, Alarcon-Segovia and Abud-Mendoza, 1985). This deficiency is proportionate to the amount of T cell depletion in the cell preparation (Gluckman *et al.*, 1985; Prince, Kermani-Arab and Fahey, 1984). However, surviving T cells respond normally to the addition of exogenous IL–2 (proliferation, IL–2 receptor expression, enhancement of cytotoxicity and NK activity) (Gluckman *et al.*, 1985; Reddy, Pingavat and Greico, 1984; Murray *et al.*, 1985; Hauser *et al.*, 1984). Similarly, decreased production of immune or gamma interferon, a T cell-derived protein with potent antiviral and immunopotentiating effects, reflects a quantitative depletion of T cell subset numbers rather than a qualitative defect in production or responsiveness (Murray *et al.*, 1984, 1985; Fauci *et al.*, 1985).

Both IL–2 and gamma interferon are being used in therapeutic trials with the rationale of replacing or circumventing the lack of CD4 induction of cytotoxic and other immune effector mechanisms. The theoretical disadvantage is that agents which activate T cells may actually heighten viral replication and depletion of CD4 cells. The reverse pro and con exists with cyclosporin A therapy. Here, the rationale is to inhibit T cell activation in the hope of reducing viral replication, but the agent is itself immunosuppressive. To date, none of these regimens has shown clinical efficacy (Fauci *et al.*, 1985).

A unique form of alpha interferon that is acid labile has been described in both systemic lupus erythematosus (SLE) and in AIDS patients. Levels are higher in subjects with more severe immunodeficiency (Eyster *et al.*, 1983). Its role in both diseases is unknown. Since polyclonal B cell activation is found in both AIDS and SLE, it is conceivable that, in AIDS, alpha interferon is produced by B cells, perhaps as a direct (or indirect) consequence of HIV infection (Boumpas *et al.*, 1984).

Anti-lymphocyte antibodies are present in a substantial proportion of HIV-infected subjects. These antibodies are heterogeneous with respect to specificity for CD4, CD8 or B cells, and no correlation with clinical or immunologic features of the disease has been ascertained (Williams, Masur and Spira, 1984; Tomar *et al.*, 1985). They are probably a consequence of intense polyclonal B cell stimulation.

Elevated levels of immune complexes are consistently found in AIDS patients and in a high proportion of infected subjects at risk for AIDS (Gottlieb *et al.*, 1983; Lightfoote, Folks and Sell, 1984; Gupta and Licorish, 1984; McDougal *et al.*, 1985c). Levels are related to the severity of immunoregulatory T cell abnormality, hypergammaglobulinaemia, and infectious complications (McDougal *et al.*, 1985c). Immune complexes are probably responsible for decreased Fc-receptor mediated clearance by the mononuclear phagocytic system, and for idiopathic thrombocytopenic purpura or renal disease that may complicate the clinical course of HIV-infected subjects (Bender *et al.*, 1984; Morris *et al.*, 1982; Rao *et al.*, 1984).

Serum levels of the thymic hormone, alpha-l-thymosin, are elevated in AIDS patients (Biggar *et al.*, 1983; Hersch *et al.*, 1983). Its elevation is somewhat surprising since severe involution of the thymus compatible with autoimmune or viral destruction is found at autopsy (Elie *et al.*, 1983; Joshi and Oleske, 1985). The histology is similar to that found in T cell congenital immunodeficiencies which are usually associated with low rather than high levels of hormone (Incefy *et al.*, 1977). Recently a serologic cross-reaction between alpha-l-thymosin and the HIV core protein, p17, has been described, and it is possible that the competitive radioimmunoassay used for measuring alpha-l-thymosin is being affected by anti-p17 antibody or p17 antigen rather than measuring true hormone (Sarin *et al.*, 1986).

Beta-2-microglobulin is a low-molecular-weight protein associated with class I MHC structures found on the surface of all nucleated cells. Neopterin is a cellular purine metabolite. Elevated serum and urine levels of these substances correlate with degree of cell destruction or turnover in a number of diseases, and levels are elevated in AIDS patients as well (Grieco *et al.*, 1984; Wachter *et al.*, 1983).

4.10 THE IMMUNE RESPONSE TO HIV INFECTION

HIV-infected subjects mount and sustain a vigorous antibody response to HIV (Sarngadharan *et al.*, 1984; Schüpbach *et al.*, 1985; Biggar *et al.*, 1985; Kaminsky *et al.*, 1985). Antibody titres in humans, particularly to envelope glycoproteins, are often higher than those obtained after immunization of non-susceptible animals such as mice or rabbits. This suggests that viral persistence and replication is a potent antigenic stimulus, and that an ongoing immune response can be maintained in the presence of a virus that progressively depletes cells required for initiating such a response. With advanced immunodeficiency, as occurs in AIDS patients, titres do diminish with a relatively greater effect on antibodies to core proteins than to envelope glycoproteins (Schüpbach *et al.*, 1985; Biggar *et al.*, 1985). Lower ratios of core antibody to envelope antibody in AIDS patients than in asymptomatic subjects are probably a consequence of progression to severe immunodeficiency, but may be a condition that predisposes to severe immunodeficiency. In established infection, it is not clear what role antibody plays in limiting infection. It is clear that progression often occurs despite the presence of antibody. Human anti-HIV sera almost universally contain antibodies to the envelope protein, gp110 (Montagnier *et al.*, 1985; Barin *et al.*, 1985; Kitchen *et al.*, 1986), that binds to the CD4 molecule, and these sera do inhibit virus binding to $CD4^+$ T cells in reasonably high titre (McDougal *et al.*, 1986b). They also demonstrate a limited capacity to inhibit (neutralize) viral infectivity *in vitro* (McDougal *et al.*, 1985a; Weiss *et al.*, 1985; Robert-Guroff, Brown and Gallo, 1985), a phenomenon that is mediated by IgG, is independent of complement, cannot be demonstrated with all sera, is of low titre with others, and can be overcome at higher multiplicities of infectious dose. The fact that virtually all sera inhibit binding but not all sera neutralize is not necessarily a paradoxical finding and probably relates to the inherent sensitivities of the two assays. Reduction in binding of virus to a single cell by 99% may not prevent infection of the cell. Further, once infection is established *in vitro*, substantial spread may occur through cell fusion (syncytia), a process dependent on virus-CD4 interaction but which may be more resistant to inhibition by fluid-phase antibody (Dalgleish *et al.*, 1985; Lifson *et al.*, 1986). In any event, antibody may play a role in limiting the pace at which viral infectivity and CD4 depletion occurs, but it clearly is not effective in totally eliminating an established infection. It remains possible that antibody, induced by vaccination, may prevent infection from an initial exposure when virus burden and inoculum are substantially lower than in established infection.

With many viruses, antibody induced either by vaccination or as a result of primary infection protects from infection at subsequent exposure, but it is the cellular response that is primarily responsible for resolution of infection. It is disconcerting, then, that no one has reported an HIV-specific cellular response to this virus, much less demonstrated its effectiveness in limiting virus infection. This virus is unique in that the very cells that initiate a cellular response to virus are the cells destroyed by virus. It seems unlikely, however, that HIV-specific T cells involved in cellular responses (such as induction of cytotoxicity, DTH, or elaboration of lymphokines) are either rendered non-functional or killed as soon as they are produced, at a time when the antibody response to virus, which requires antigen-specific T-B collaboration, is intact. Nevertheless, a selective imbalance of functional HIV-specific T cells may exist, by mechanisms as yet unclear. Lack of documentation of a cellular response by functional assays, of course, does not mean that they do not occur. As previously discussed, several observations (e.g. elevations of cells identified phenotypically as cytotoxic cells, the susceptibility of HIV-infected cells to NK lysis, the correlation of depressed IFN-α production with poor outcome) suggest that there may be phenotypic or functional immune profiles that signify an attempt by the immune system to deal effectively with HIV infection. The challenge for the immunologist is to identify these profiles, document the mechanisms involved, establish that they correlate with favourable outcome, and hopefully manipulate them for therapeutic purposes.

4.11 CONCLUSION

From the molecular to the cellular to the clinical level, much that is known about HIV and the pathogenesis of AIDS is consistent. Given a virus that has evolved an envelope with affinity for the human CD4 molecule and a replication apparatus that is cytopathic for host cells, HIV binds to $CD4^+$ T cells, replicates in them, and destroys them. The result is numerical depletion of $CD4^+$ T cells (and possibly functional impairment of surviving or as yet uninfected $CD4^+$ T cells) occurring over a period of time. This cell set is pivotal in inducing a variety of immune responses, and decline of $CD4^+$ T cells results in progressive paralysis of immune responses, rendering the subject susceptible to opportunistic infections. The immune system, which is responsible for resolution of virus infection, is the very system attacked by HIV. Unfortunately, HIV attacks the Achilles heel of the system, and thus far the battle rages in favour of the virus. It is hoped that therapeutic or immunologic mechanisms that eliminate or control viral replication can be identified and used to tip the balance in favour of the host in this devastating disease.

REFERENCES

Abrams, D. I., Lewis, B. J., Beckstead, J. H., Casavant, C. A. and Drew, W. L. (1984) Persistent diffuse lymphadenopathy in homosexual men: endpoint or prodrome? *Ann. Intern. Med.*, **100**, 801–8.

Alocer-Varela, J., Alarcon-Segovia, D. and Abud-Mendoza, C. (1985) Immunoregulatory circuits in the acquired immune deficiency syndrome and related complex. Production of and response to interleukins 1 and 2, NK function and its enhancement by interleukin–2 and kinetics of the autologous mixed lymphocyte reactions. *Clin. Exp. Immunol.*, **60**, 31–8.

Ammann, A. J., Abrams, D., Conant, M., Chudwin, D., Cowan, M., Volberding, P., Lewis, B. and Casavant, C. (1983) Acquired immune dysfunction in homosexual men: immunologic profiles. *Clin. Immunol. Immunopath.*, **27**, 315–25.

Ammann, A. J., Schiffman, G., Abrams, D., Volberding, P., Ziegler, J. and Conant, M. (1984) B-cell immunodeficiency syndrome in acquired immune deficiency syndrome. *JAMA*, **251**, 1447–9.

Armstrong, J. A. and Horne, R. (1985) Follicular dendritic cells and virus-like particles in AIDS-related lymphadenopathy. *Lancet*, **ii**, 370–2.

Arya, S. K. and Gallo, R. C. (1985) Human T cell growth factor (interleukin 2) and α-interferon genes: expression in human T lymphotropic virus type III and type I cells. *Proc. Natl Acad. Sci.* USA, **82**, 8691–5.

Bank, I. and Chess, L. (1985) Perturbation of the T4 molecule transmits a negative signal to T cells. *J. Exp. Med.*, **162**, 1294–303.

Barin, F., McLane, M. F., Allan, J. S., Lee. T. H., Groopman, J. E. and Essex, M. (1985) Virus envelope protein of HTLV-III represents major target antigen for antibodies in AIDS patients. *Science*, **228**, 1094–6.

Barré-Sinoussi, F., Chermann, J. C., Rey, F., Nugeyre, M. T., Charmarat, S., Gruest, J., Dauguet, C., Axler-Blin, C., Vezinet-Brun, F., Rouzioux, C., Rozenbaum, W. and Montagnier, L. (1983) Isolation of a T-lymphotropic retrovirus from a patient at risk for the acquired immunodeficiency syndrome (AIDS). *Science*, **220**, 868–71.

Bender, B. S., Quinn, T. C., Lawley, T. J., Smith, W., Brickman, C. and Frank, M. M. (1984) Acquired immune deficiency syndrome: a defect in Fc-receptor specific clearance. *Clin. Res.*, **32**, 511A.

Bender, B. S., Arger, F. A., Quinn, T. C., Redfield, R., Gold, J., and Folks, T. M. (1986) Impaired antibody-dependent cell-mediated cytotoxie activity acquired immunodeficiency syndrome. *Clin. Exp. Immunol.*, **64**, 166–72.

Benveniste, E., Schroff, R., Stevens, R. H. and Gottlieb, M. S. (1983) Immunoregulatory T cells in men with a new acquired immunodeficiency syndrome. *J. Clin. Immunol.*, **3**, 359–67.

Biddison, W. E., Rao, P. E., Talle, M. A., Goldstein, G. and Shaw, S. (1984) Possible involvement of the T4 molecule in T cell recognition of class II HLA antigens. *J. Exp. Med.*, **159**, 783–97.

Biggar, R. J., Taylor, P. H., Goldstein, A. L., Melbye, M., Ebbesen, P., Mann, D. L. and Strong, D. M. (1983) Thymosin α_1 levels and helper: suppressor ratios in homosexual men. *N. Engl. J. Med.*, **309**, 49.

Biggar, R. J., Melbye, M., Ebbesen, P., Alexander, S., Nielsen, J. O., Sarin, P. and Faber, V. (1985) Variation in HTLV-III antibodies in homosexual men: decline before onset of illness related to acquired immune deficiency syndrome (AIDS). *Brit. Med. J.*, **291**, 997–8.

Birx, D. L., Redfield, R. R. and Tosato, G. (1986) Defective regulation of Epstein–Barr virus infection in patients with acquired immunodeficiency syndrome (AIDS) or AIDS-related disorders. *N. Engl. J. Med.*, **314**, 874–9.

Boumpas, D., Harris, C., Hooks, J., Popovic, M. and Mann, D. (1984) A human T cell lymphoma virus infected B lymphocyte line produces acid labile interferon alpha. *Clin. Res.*, **32**, 343A.

Chan, W. C., Brynes, R. K., Spira, T. J., Banks, P. M., Thurmond, C. C., Ewing, E. P. and Chandler, F. W. (1985) Lymphocyte subsets in lymph nodes of homosexual men with generalized lymphadenopathy correlation with morphology and blood changes. *Arch. Pathol. Lab. Med.*, **107**, 133–7.

Ciobanu, N., Welte, K., Kruger, G., Venuta, S., Gold, J., Feldman, S. P., Wang, C. Y., Koziner, B., Moore, M. A. S., Safai, B. and Mertelsmann, R. (1983) Defective T-cell response to PHA and mitogenic monoclonal antibodies in male homosexuals with acquired immunodeficiency syndrome and its *in vitro* correction by interleukin 2. *J. Clin. Immunol.*, **3**, 332–40.

Clement, L. T., Grossi, C. E. and Gartland, L. J. (1984) Morphologic and phenotypic features of the subpopulation of Leu2$^+$ cells that suppresses B cell differentiation. *J. Immunol.*, **133**, 2461–8.

Clement, L. T., Dagg, M. K. and Landay, A. (1984) Characterization of human lymphocyte subpopulations: alloreactive cytotoxic T lymphocyte precursor and effector cells are phenotypically distinct from Leu2$^+$ suppressor cells. *J. Clin. Immunol.*, **4**, 395–402.

Coffin, J., Haase, A., Levy, J. A., Montagnier, L., Oroszlan, S., Teich, N., Temin, H., Toyoshima, K., Varmus, H., Vogt, P. and Weiss, R. (1986) Human immunodeficiency viruses. *Science*, **232**, 697.

Cooper, D. A., Gold, J., Maclean, P., Donovan, B., Finlyason, R., Barnes, T. G., Michelmore, H. M., Brooke, P. and Penny, R. (1985) Acute AIDS retrovirus infection: definition of a clinical illness associated with seroconversion. *Lancet*, **i**, 537–40.

Crawford, D. H., Weller, I. and Iliescu, V. (1984) Polyclonal activation of B cells in homosexual men. *N. Engl. J. Med.*, **311**, 536–7.

Creemers, P. C., Stark, D. F. and Boyko, W. J. (1985) Evaluation of natural killer cell activity in patients with persistent generalized lymphadenopathy and acquired immune deficiency syndrome. *Clin. Immunol. Immunopathol.*, **36**, 141–50.

Cunningham-Rundles, S., Michelis, M. A. and Masur, H. (1983) Serum suppression of lymphocyte activation *in vitro* in acquired immune deficiency syndrome. *N. Engl. J. Med.*, **310**, 1279–82.

Curran, J. W. (1983) AIDS–two years later. *N. Engl. J. Med.*, **309**, 609–10.

Dalgleish, A. G., Beverely, P. C. L., Clapham, P. R., Crawford, D. H., Greaves, M. F. and Weiss, R. A. (1985) The CD4 (T4) antigen is an essential component of the receptor for the AIDS retrovirus. *Nature, Lond.*, **312**, 763–7.

Dalgleish, A. G. and Clapham, P. (1985) B cells in the pathogenesis of AIDS. *Immunol. Today*, **6**, 71.

Elie, R., Laroche, A. C., Arnous, E., Guerin, J.-M., Pierre, G. and Malebauche, R. (1983) Thymic dysplasia in acquired immunodeficiency syndrome (Haiti). *N. Engl. J. Med.*, **308**, 841–2.

Eyster, M. E., Goedert, J. J., Poon, M.-C. and Preble, O. T. (1983) Acid-labile alpha interferon. A possible preclinical marker for the acquired immunodeficiency syndrome in hemophilia. *N. Engl. J. Med.*, **309**, 583–6.

Eyster, M. E., Goedert, J. J., Sarnagadharan, M. G., Weiss, S. H., Gallo, R. C. and Blattner, W. A. (1985) Development and early natural history of HTLV-III antibodies in persons with hemophilia. *JAMA*, **253**, 2219–23.

Fahey, J. L., Prince, H., Weaver, M. M., Groopman, J., Visscher, B., Schwartz, K. and Detels, R. (1984) Quantitative changes in the Th or Ts lymphocyte subsets that distinguish AIDS syndromes from other immune subset disorders. *Am. J. Med.*, **76**, 95–100.

Fauci, A. S. (1984a) Immunologic abnormalities in the acquired immunodeficiency syndrome (AIDS). *Clin. Res.*, **32**, 491–9.

Fauci, A. S., Macher, H., Longo, D. L., Lane, H. C., Masur, M. and Gelman, E. P. (1984b) Acquired immunodeficiency syndrome: epidemiologic, clinical, immunologic, and therapeutic considerations. *Ann. Intern. Med.*, **100**, 92–106.

Fauci, A. S., Masur, H., Gelmann, E. P., Markham, P. D., Hahn, B. H. and Lane, H. C. (1985) The acquired immunodeficiency syndrome: an update. *Ann. Intern. Med.*, **102**, 800–13.

Feorino, P. M., Kalyanaraman, V. S., Haverkos, H. W., Cabradilla, C. D., Warfield, D. T., Jaffe, H. W., Harrison, A. K., Gottlieb, M. S., Goldfinger, D., Chermann, J.-C., Barre-Sinoussi, F., Spira, T. J., McDougal, J. S., Curran, J. W., Montagnier, L., Murphy, F. A. and Francis, D. P. (1984) Lymphadenopathy-associated virus (LAV) infection of a blood donor–recipient pair with acquired immunodeficiency syndrome (AIDS). *Science*, **225**, 69–72.

Feorino, P. M., Jaffe, H. W., Palmer, E., Peterman, T. A., Francis, D. P., Kalyanaraman, V. S., Weistein, R. A., Stoneburner, R. L., Alexander, W. J., Raevskey, C., Getchell, J. P., Warfield, D., Haverkos, H. W., Kilbourne, B. W., Nicholson, J. K. A. and Curran, J. W. (1985) Transfusion-associated AIDS: evidence for persistent infection in blood donors. *N. Engl. J. Med.*, **312**, 1293–6.

Fishbein, D. B., Kaplan, J. E., Spira, T. J., Miller, B., Schonberger, L. B., Pinsky, P. F., Getchell, J. P., Kalyanaraman, V. S. and Braude, J. S. (1985) Unexplained lymphadenopathy in homosexual men: a longitudinal study. *JAMA*, **254**, 930–5.

Fisher, A. G., Collalti, E., Ratner, L., Gallo, R. C. and Wong-Staal, F. (1985) A molecular clone of HTLV-III with biological activity. *Nature, Lond.*, **316**, 262–5.

Fitzgerald, P. A., von Wussow, P. and Lopez, C. (1982) Role of interferon in natural kill of HSV-1-infected fibroblasts. *J. Immunol.*, **129**, 819–23.

Folks, T., Benn, S., Rabson, A., Theodore, T., Hoggan, M. D., Martin, M., Lightfoote, M. and Sell, K. (1985) Characterization of a continuous T-cell line susceptible to the cytopathic effect of the AIDS-associated virus. *Proc. Natl Acad. Sci. USA*, **82**, 4539–43.

Friedman, S. R., Des Jarlais, D. C., Marmor, D., Yancovitz, S., Zolla-Pazner, S., El-Sadr, W., Cohen, H., Garber, J., Spira, T. J. and Beatrice, S. (1986) HTLV-III/LAV, *in vivo* immunologic stimulation, and T4 cell loss, submitted.

Friedman-Kein, A. E., Laubenstein, L., Dubin, R., Marmor, M. and Zolla-Pazner, S. (1982) Disseminated Kaposi's sarcoma in homosexual men. *Ann. Intern. Med.*, **96**, 693–700.

Gallo, R. C., Salahuddin, S. Z., Popovic, M., Shearer, A. M., Kaplan, M., Haynes, B. F., Palker, T. J., Redfield, R., Oleske, J., Safai, B., White, G., Foster, P. and Markham, P. D. (1984) Frequent detection and isolation of cytopathic retroviruses (HTLV-III) from patients with AIDS and at risk for AIDS. *Science*, **224**, 500–2.

Gatenby, P. A., Kausas, G. S., Xian, G. Y., Evans, R. L. and Engleman, E. G. (1982) Dissection of immunoregulatory subpopulations of T lymphocytes within the helper and suppressor sublineages in man. *J. Immunol.*, **129**, 1997–2000.

Gerstoft, J., Dickmeiss, E. and Mathiesen, L. (1985) Cytotoxic capabilities of lymphocytes from patients with the acquired immune deficiency syndrome. *Scand. J. Immunol.*, **22**, 463–70.

Gidlund, M., Orn, A., Wigzell, H., Senik, A. and Gresser, I. (1978) Enhanced NK cell activity in mice injected with interferon inducers. *Nature, Lond.*, **273**, 759–61.

Gluckman, J.-C., Kaltzmann, D., Cavaille-Coll, M., Brisson, E., Messiah, A., Lachiver, D. and Rozenbaum, W. (1985) Is there correlation of T cell proliferative functions and surface marker phenotypes in patients with acquired immune deficiency syndrome or lymphadenopathy syndrome? *Clin. Exp. Immunol.*, **60**, 8–16.

Goedert, J. J., Sarngadharan, M. G., Biggar, R. J., Weiss, S. H., Winn, D., Grossman, R. J., Greene, M. H., Bodner, A., Mann, D. L., Strong, D. M., Gallo, R. C. and Blattner, W. A. (1984) Determinants of retrovirus (HTLV-III) antibody and immunodeficiency conditions in homosexual men. *Lancet*, **ii**, 711–16.

Goedert, J. J., Biggar, R. J., Weiss, S. H., Eyster, M. E., Melbye, M., Wilson, S., Ginzburg, H. M., Grossman, R. J., DiGiola, R. A., Sanchez, W. C., Giron, J. A., Ebbesen, P., Gallo, R. C. and Blattner, W. A. (1986) Three year incidence of AIDS in five cohorts of HTLV-III-infected risk group members. *Science*, **231**, 992–7.

Gottlieb, M. S., Schroff, R., Schanker, H. M., Weissman, D. O., Fan, P. T., Wolf, R. A. and Saxon, A. (1981) *Pneumocystis carinii* pneumonia and mucosal candidiasis in previously healthy homosexual men: evidence for a new acquired cellular immunodeficiency. *N. Engl. J. Med.*, **305**, 1425–31.

Gottlieb, M. S., Groopman, J. E., Weinstein, W. M., Fahey, J. L. and Detels, R. (1983) The acquired immunodeficiency syndrome. *Ann. Intern. Med.*, **99**, 208–20.

Greene, W. C., Fleisher, T. A., Nelson, D. L. and Waldmann, T. A. (1982) Production of human suppressor T cell hybridomas. *J. Immunol.*, **129**, 1986–92.

Grieco, M. H., Reddy, M. M., Kothari, H. B., Lange, M., Buimovici-Klein, E. and William, D. (1984) Elevated β_2-microglobulin and lysozyme levels in patients with acquired immune deficiency syndrome. *Clin. Immunol. Immunopathol.*, **32**, 174–84.

Groopman, J. E., Salahuddin, S. Z., Sarngadharan, M. B., Mullins, M. G., Sullivan, J. L., Mulder, C., O'Hara, C. J., Cheeseman, S. H., Haverkos, H., Forgacs, P., Riedel, N., McLane, M. F., Essex, M. and Gallo, R. C. (1984) Virologic studies in a case of transfusion-associated AIDS. *N. Engl. J. Med.*, **311**, 1419–22.

Gupta, S. and Safai, B. (1983) Deficient autologous mixed lymphocyte reaction in Kaposi's sarcoma associated with deficiency of $Leu3^+$ responder cells. *J. Clin. Invest.*, **71**, 296–300.

Gupta, S. and Licorish, K. (1984) Circulating immune complexes in AIDS. *N. Engl. J. Med.*, **311**, 1530–1.

Gyorkey, F., Melnich, J. L., Sinkovics, J. G. and Gyorkey, P. (1985) Retrovirus resembling HTLV in macrophages of patients with AIDS. *Lancet*, i, 106.

Hauser, G. J., Bino, T., Rosenberg, H., Zakuth, V., Geller, E. and Spirer, Z. (1984) Interleukin–2 production and response to exogenous interleukin–2 in a patient with the acquired immune deficiency syndrome (AIDS). *Clin. Exp. Immunol.*, **56**, 14–17.

Heagy, W., Kelley, V. E., Strom, T. B., Mayer, K., Shapiro, H. M., Mandel, R. and Finberg, R. (1984) Decreased expression of human Class II antigens on monocytes from patients with acquired immune deficiency syndrome. Increased expression with interferon-γ. *J. Clin. Invest.*, **74**, 2089–96.

Hersch, E. M., Reuben, J. M., Rios, A., Mansell, W. A., Newell, G. R., McClure, J. E. and Goldstein, A. L. (1983) Elevated serum thymosin α_1 levels associated with evidence of immune dysregulation in male homosexuals with a history of infectious diseases or Kaposi's sarcoma. *N. Engl. J. Med.*, **308**, 45–6.

Ho, D. D., Rota, T. R., Schooley, R. T., Kaplan, J. C., Allan, J. D., Groopman, J. E., Resnich, L., Felsenstein, D., Andrews, C. A. and Hirsch, M. S. (1985a) Isolation of HTLV-III from cerebrospinal fluid and neural tissues of patients with neurologic syndromes related to the acquired immunodeficiency syndrome. *N. Engl. J. Med.*, **313**, 1493–7.

Ho, D. D., Hartshorn, K. L., Rota, T. R., Andrews, C. A., Kaplan, J. C., Schooley, R. T. and Hirsch, M. S. (1985b) Recombinant human interferon alpha-A suppresses HTLV-III replication *in vitro*. *Lancet*, i, 602–4.

Ho, D. D., Rota, T. R. and Hirsch, M. S. (1986) Infection of monocyte/macrophages by human T lymphotropic virus type III. *J. Clin. Invest.*, **77**, 1712–15.

Hoxie, J. A., Haggarty, B. S., Rackowski, J. L., Pillsbury, N. and Levy, J. A. (1985) Persistent noncytopathic infection of normal human lymphocytes with AIDS-associated retrovirus. *Science*, **229**, 1400–2.

Incefy, G. S., Dardenne, M., Pahwa, S., Grimmes, E., Pahwa, R. N., Smithwich, E., O'Reilly, R. and Good, R. A. (1977) Thymic activity in severe combined immunodeficiency diseases. *Proc. Natl Acad. Sci.*, **74**, 1250–3.

Isobe, M., Huecner, K., Maddon, P. J., Littman, D. R., Axel, R., Crobe, C. M. (1986) *Proc. Natl Acad. Sci.* USA, **83**, 4399–402.

Jaffe, H. W., Feorino, P. M., Darrow, W. W., O'Malley, P. M., Getchell, J. P., Warfield, D. T., Jones, B. M., Echenberg, D. F., Francis, D. P. and Curran, J. W.

(1985) Persistent infection with HTLV-III/LAV in apparently healthy homosexual men. *Ann. Intern. Med.*, **102**, 627–8.

Jason, J., McDougal, J. S., Holman, R. C., Stein, S. F., Lawrence, D. N., Nicholson, J. K. A., Dixon, G., Doxey, M. and Evatt, B. L. (1985) HTLV-III/LAV-associated antibody: association with hemophiliacs immune status and blood component usage. *JAMA*, **753**, 3409–15.

Joshi, V. V. and Oleske, J. M. (1985) Pathologic appraisal of the thymus gland in acquired immunodeficiency syndrome in children. *Arch. Pathol. Lab. Med.*, **109**, 142–6.

Jothy, S., Gilmore, N., El'Gabalaway, H. and Purchal, J. (1985) Decreased population of $Leu7^+$ natural killer cells in lymph nodes of homosexual men with AIDS-related persistent lymphadenopathy. *Can. Med. Assoc. J.*, **132**, 141–4.

Kaminsky, L. S., McHugh, T., Stites, D., Volberding, P., Henle, G., Henle, W. and Levy, J. A. (1985) High prevalence of antibodies to acquired immune deficiency syndrome (AIDS)-associated retrovirus (ARV) in AIDS and related conditions but not in other disease states. *Proc. Natl Acad. Sci. USA*, **82**, 5535–9.

Kitchen, L., Malone, G., Orgad, S., Barin, F., Zaizov, R., Ramot, B., Gazit, E., Kreiss, J., Leal, M., Wichmann, I., Martinowitz, U. and Essex, M. (1986) Viral envelope protein of HTLV-III is the major target antigen for antibodies in hemophiliac patients. *J. Infect. Dis.*, **153**, 788–90.

Klatzmann, D., Barre-Sinoussi, F., Nugeyre, M. T., Dauguet, C., Vilmer, E., Griscelli, C., Brun-Vezinet, F., Rouzioux, C., Gluckman, J. C., Chermann, J.-C. and Montagnier, L. (1984) Selective tropism of lymphadenopathy associated virus (LAV) for helper-inducer T lymphocytes. *Science*, **225**, 59–62.

Klatzmann, D., Champagne, E., Charmarat, S., Gruest, J., Guetard, D., Hercend, T., Gluckman, J.-C. and Montagnier, L. (1985) T-lymphocyte T4 molecule behaves as the receptor for human retrovirus LAV. *Nature, Lond.*, **312**, 767–8.

Kolata, G. (1986) Where is the AIDS virus harbored?. *Science*, **232**, 1197.

Landesman, S. H., Ginzburg, H. M. and Weiss, S. H. (1985) The AIDS epidemic. *N. Engl. J. Med.*, **312**, 521–3.

Lane, H. C., Masur, H., Edgar, L. C., Whalen, G., Rook, A. H. and Fauci, A. S. (1983) Abnormalities of B cell activation and immunoregulation in patients with the acquired immunodeficiency syndrome. *N. Engl. J. Med.*, **309**, 453–8.

Lane, H. C. and Fauci, A. S. (1985) Immunologic abnormalities in the acquired immunodeficiency syndrome. *Ann. Rev. Immunol.*, **3**, 477–500.

Lane, H. C., Masur, H., Gelmann, E. P., Longo, D. L., Steis, R. G., Chused, T., Whalen, G., Edgar, L. and Fauci, A. S. (1985a) Correlation between immunologic function and clinical subpopulations of patients with the acquired immune deficiency syndrome. *Am. J. Med.*, **78**, 417–22.

Lane, H. C., Depper, J. M., Greene, W. C., Whalen, G., Waldmann, T. A. and Fauci, A. S. (1985b) Qualitative analysis of immune function in patients with the acquired immunodeficiency syndrome. *N. Engl. J. Med.*, **313**, 79–84.

Lanier, L. L., Le, A. M., Phillips, J. H., Warner, N. L. and Babcock, G. F. (1983) Subpopulations of human natural killer cells defined by expression of the Leu7 (HNK–1) and Leull (NK–15) antigens. *J. Immunol.*, **131**, 1789–96.

Lanier, L. L. and Loken, M. R. (1984) Human lymphocyte subpopulations identified by using three-color immunofluorescence and flow cytometry analysis: correlation of Leu2, Leu3, Leu7, Leu8, and Leu11 cell surface antigen expression. *J. Immunol.*, **132**, 151–6.

Laurence, J., Gottlieb, A. B. and Kunkel, H. G. (1983) Soluble suppressor factors in patients with acquired immune deficiency syndrome and its prodrome. Elaboration *in vitro* by T lymphocyte-adherent cell interactions. *J. Clin. Invest.*, 72, 2072–81.

Laurence, J. and Mayer, L. (1984) Immunoregulatory lymphokines of T hybridomas from AIDS patients: constitutive and inducible suppressor factors. *Science*, 225, 66–9.

Ledbetter, J. A., Evans, R. L., Lipinski, M., Cunningham-Rundles, C., Good, R. A. and Herzenberg, L. A. (1981) Evolutionary conservation of surface molecules that distinguish T lymphocyte helper/inducer and cytotoxic/suppressor subpopulations in mouse and man. *J. Exp. Med.*, 153, 310–23.

Lederman, M. M., Ratnoff, O. D., Evatt, B. L. and McDougal, J. S. (1985) Acquisition of antibody to lymphadenopathy-associated virus in patients with classic hemophilia (Factor VIII deficiency). 102, 753–7.

Levy, J. A., Hoffman, A. D., Kramer, S. M., Landis, J. A., Shimabukuro, J. M. and Oschiro, L. S. (1984) Isolation of lymphocytopathic retroviruses from San Francisco patients with AIDS. *Science*, 225, 840–2.

Levy, J. A., Kaminsky, L. S., Morrow, J. W., Steimer, K., Luciw, P., Dina, D., Hoxie, J. and Oshiro, L. (1985a) Infection by the retrovirus associated with the acquired immunodeficiency syndrome. *Ann. Intern. Med.*, 103, 694–9.

Levy, J. A., Shimabukuro, J., McHugh, T., Casavant, C., Stites, D. P. and Oshiro, L. S. (1985b) AIDS-associated retroviruses (ARV) can productively infect other cells besides human T helper cells. *Virology*, 147, 441–8.

Levy, J. A., Shimabukuro, J., Hollander, H., Mills, J. and Kaminsky, L. (1985c) Isolation of AIDS-associated retroviruses from cerebrospinal fluid and brain of patients with neurological symptoms. *Lancet*, ii, 586–8.

Levy, J. A., Cheng-Mayer, C., Dina, D. and Luciw, P. A. (1986) AIDS retrovirus (ARV–2) clone replicates in transfected human and animal fibroblasts. *Science*, 232, 998–1000.

Lewis, D. E., Puck, J. M., Babcock, G. F. and Rich, R. R. (1985) Disproportionate expansion of a minor T cell subset in patients with lymphadenopathy syndrome and acquired immune deficiency syndrome. *J. Infect. Dis.*, 151, 555–9.

Lifson, J. D., Mark, D. F., Benike, C. J., Koths, K. and Engleman, E. G. (1984) Human recombinant interleukin–2 partly reconstitutes deficient *in vitro* immune responses of lymphocytes from patients with AIDS. *Lancet*, i, 698–702.

Lifson, J. D., Reyes, G. R., McGrath, M. S., Stein, B. S. and Engleman, E. G. (1986) AIDS retrovirus induced cytopathology: giant cell formation and involvement of CD4 antigen. *Science*, 232, 1123–6.

Lightfoote, M. M., Folks, T. M. and Sell, K. W. (1984) Analysis of immune complex components isolated from serum of AIDS patients. *Fed. Proc.*, 43, 1921.

Lopez, C., Fitzgerald, P. A. and Siegal, F. P. (1983) Severe acquired immune deficiency syndrome in male homosexuals: diminished capacity to make interferon-α *in vitro* associated with severe opportunistic infections. *J. Infect. Dis.*, 148, 962–6.

Martin, L. S., McDougal, J. S., Spira, T. J. and Loskoski, S. L. (1986) Cell surface phenotype of the spontaneous immunoglobulin-secreting cells in peripheral blood from homosexual men with generalized lymphadenopathy. *Diag. Immunol.*, 4, 117–23.

Masur, H., Michelis, M. A., Greene, J., Onorato, I., Vande Stouwe, R. A., Holtzman, R. S., Wormser, G., Brettman, L., Lange, M., Murray, H. W. and Cunningham-Rundles, S. (1981) An outbreak of community-acquired *Pneumocystis carinii* pneumonia: initial manifestation of cellular immune dysfunction. *N. Engl. J. Med.*, 305, 1431–8.

Mathur-Wagh, U., Enlow, R. E., Spigland, I., Winchester, R. J., Sacks, H. S., Rorat, E., Yancovitz, S. R., Klein, M. J., William, D. C. and Mildvan, D. (1984)

Longitudinal study of persistent generalized lymphadenopathy in homosexual men: relation to AIDS. *Lancet*, **i**, 1033–7.

Mawle, A. C., Scheppler-Campbell, J. A. and McDougal, J. S. (1985) Regression as a measure of EBV-specific T cell cytotoxicity in AIDS, AIDS-related complex, and normal homosexual men compared with heterosexual controls. *Ann. Intern. Med.*, **103**, 777.

McDougal, J. S., Cort, S. P., Kennedy, M. S., Cabradilla, C. D., Feorino, P. M., Francis, D. P., Hicks, D., Kalyanaraman, V. S. and Martin, L. S. (1985a) Immunoassay for the detection and quantitation of infectious human retrovirus, lymphadenopathy-associated virus (LAV). *J. Immunol. Methods*, **76**, 171–83.

McDougal, J. S., Mawle, A., Cort, S. P., Nicholson, J. K. A., Cross, G. D., Scheppler-Campbell, J. A., Hicks, D. and Sligh, J. (1985b) Cellular tropism of the human retrovirus HTLV-III/LAV. I. Role of T cell activation and expression of the T4 molecule. *J. Immunol.*, **135**, 3151–62.

McDougal, J. S., Hubbard, M., Nicholson, J. K. A., Jones, B. M., Holman, R. C., Roberts, J., Fishbein, D. B., Jaffe, H. W., Kaplan, J. E., Spira, T. J. and Evatt, B. L. (1985c) Immune complexes in the acquired immunodeficiency syndrome (AIDS): relationship to disease manifestation, risk group, and immunologic defect. *J. Clin. Immunol.*, **5**, 130–8.

McDougal, J. S., Kennedy, M. S., Sligh, J. M., Cort, S. P., Mawle, A. and Nicholson, J. K. A. (1986a) Binding of HTLV-III/LAV to $T4^+$ T cells by a complex of the 110K viral protein and the T4 molecule. *Science*, **231**, 382–5.

McDougal, J. S., Nicholson, J. K. A., Cross, G. D., Kennedy, M. S., Cort, S. P., Rao, P., Goldstein, L., Goldstein, G. and Mawle, A. (1986b) Binding of the human retrovirus HTLV-III/LAV/ARV/HIV to the CD4 (T4) molecule: conformation dependence, epitope mapping, antibody inhibition, and potential for idiotypic mimicry. *J. Immunol.*, **137**, 2937–44.

Melbye, M., Biggar, R. J., Ebbesen, P., Sarngadharan, M. G., Weiss, S. H., Gallo, R. C. and Blattner, W. A. (1984) Seroepidemiology of HTLV-III antibody in Danish homosexual men: prevalence, transmission, and disease outcome. *Brit. Med. J.*, **289**, 573–5.

Melbye, M., Biggar, R. J., Ebbesen, P., Neuland, C., Goedert, J. J., Faber, V., Lorenzen, I., Skinhoj, P., Gallo, R. C. and Blattner, W. A. (1986) Long-term seropositivity for human T-lymphotropic virus type III in homosexual men without the acquired immunodeficiency syndrome: development of immunologic and clinical abnormalities. *Ann. Intern. Med.*, **104**, 496–500.

Metroka, C. E., Cunningham-Rundles, S., Pollack, M. S., Sonnabend, J. A., Davis, J. M., Gordon, B., Fernandez, R. D. and Mouradian, J. (1983) Generalized lymphadenopathy in homosexual men. *Ann. Intern. Med.*, **99**, 585–91.

Meuer, S. C., Schlossman, S. F. and Reinherz, E. L. (1982) Clonal analysis of human cytotoxic T lymphocytes: $T4^+$ and $T8^+$ effector T cells recognize products of different major histocompatibility complex regions. *Proc. Natl Acad. Sci. USA*, **79**, 4395–9.

Mildvan, D., Mathur, U., Enlow, R. W., Roman, P. L., Winchester, R. J., Colp, C., Singman, H., Adelsberg, B. R. and Spigland, I. (1982) Opportunistic infections and immune deficiency in homosexual men. *Ann. Intern. Med.*, **96**, 700–4.

Modlin, R. L., Meyer, P. R., Hofman, F. M., Mehlmauer, M., Levy, N. B., Lukes, R. J., Parker, J. W., Ammann, A. J., Conant, M. A., Rea, T. H. and Taylor, C. R. (1983) T-lymphocyte subsets in lymph nodes from homosexual men. *JAMA*, **250**, 1302–5.

Montagnier, L., Gruest, J., Charmaret, S., Dauguet, C., Axler, C., Guetard, D.,

Nugeyre, M. T., Barre-Sinoussi, F., Chermann, J. C., Brunet, J. B., Klatzmann, D. and Gluckman, J. C. (1984) Adaptation of lymphadenopathy associated virus (LAV) to replication in EBV-transformed B-lymphoblastoid cell lines. *Science*, **225**, 63–7.

Montagnier, L., Clavel, F., Krust, B., Charmaret, S., Rey, F., Barre-Sinoussi, F. and Chermann, J. C. (1985) Identification and antigenicity of the major envelope glycoprotein of lymphadenopathy-associated virus. *Virology*, **141**, 283–9.

Morris, L., Distenfeld, A., Amorosi, E. and Karpatkin, S. (1982) Autoimmune thrombocytopenic purpura in homosexual men. *Ann. Intern. Med.*, **96**, 714–17.

Murray, H. W., Rubin, B. Y., Masur, H. and Roberts, R. B. (1984) Impaired production of lymphokines and immune (gamma) interferon in the acquired-immunodeficiency syndrome. *N. Engl. J. Med.*, **310**, 883–9.

Murray, H. W., Welte, K., Jacobs, J. L., Rubin, B. Y., Mertelsmann, R. and Roberts, R. B. (1985) Production of and *in vitro* response to interleukin 2 in the acquired immunodeficiency syndrome. *J. Clin. Invest.*, **76**, 1959–64.

Nicholson, J. K. A., McDougal, J. S., Spira, T. J., Cross, G. D., Jones, B. M. and Reinherz, E. L. (1984) Immunoregulatory subsets of the T helper and T suppressor cell population in homosexual men with chronic unexplained lymphadenopathy. *J. Clin. Invest.*, **73**, 191–201.

Nicholson, J. K. A., McDougal, J. S. and Spira, T. J. (1985a) Alterations of functional subsets of T helper and T suppressor cell populations in acquired immunodeficiency syndrome (AIDS) and chronic unexplained lymphadenopathy. *J. Clin. Immunol.*, **5**, 269–74.

Nicholson, J. K. A., McDougal, J. S., Jaffe, H. W., Spira, T. J., Kennedy, M. S., Jones, B. M., Darrow, W. W., Morgan, M. and Hubbard, M. (1985b) Exposure to human T-lymphotropic virus type III/lymphadenopathy associated virus and immunologic abnormalities in asymptomatic homosexual men. *Ann. Intern. Med.*, **103**, 37–42.

Nicholson, J. K. A., Cross, G. D., Callaway, C. S. and McDougal, J. S. (1986a) *In vitro* infection of human monocytes with human T-lymphotropic virus type III/lymphadenopathy-associated virus (HTLV-III/LAV). *J. Immunol.*, **137**, 323–9.

Nicholson, J. K. A., Echenberg, D. F., Jones, B. M., Jaffe, H. W., Feorino, P. M. and McDougal, J. S. (1986b) T cytotoxic/suppressor cell phenotypes in a group of asymptomatic homosexual men with and without exposure to HTLV-III/LAV. *Clin. Immunol. Immunopathol*, **40**, 505–14.

Pahwa, S. G., Quilop, M. T. J., Lange, M., Pahwa, R. N. and Grieco, M. H. (1984) Defective B lymphocyte function in homosexual men in relation to the acquired immunodeficiency syndrome. *Ann. Intern. Med.*, **101**, 757–63.

Pahwa, S., Pahwa, R., Saxinger, C., Gallo, R. C. and Good, R. A. (1985) Influence of the human T-lymphotropic virus/lymphadenopathy-associated virus on functions of human lymphocytes: Evidence for immunosuppressive effects and polyclonal B cell activation by banded viral preparations. *Proc. Natl Acad. Sci. USA*, **82**, 8198–202.

Pinching, A. J., McManus, T. J., Jeffries, D. J., Moshtael, O., Donaghy, M., Parkin, J. M., Munday, P. E. and Harris, J. R. W. (1983) Studies of cellular immunity in male homosexuals in London. *Lancet*, **ii**, 126–9.

Poli, G., Introna, M., Zanaboni, F., Peri, G., Carbonari, M., Aiuti, F., Lazzarin, A., Moroni, M. and Mantovani, A. (1985a) Natural killer cells in intravenous drug abusers with lymphadenopathy syndrome. *Clin. Exp. Immunol.*, **62**, 128–35.

Poli, G., Bottazzi, B., Acero, R., Bersani, L., Ross, V., Introna, M., Lazzarin, A., Galli, M. and Mantovani, A. (1985b) Monocyte function in intravenous drug abusers with lymphadenopathy syndrome and in patients with acquired immunodeficiency syndrome: selective impairment of chemotaxis. *Clin. Exp. Immunol.*, **62**, 136–42.

Popovic, M., Gallo, R. C. and Mann, D. L. (1984) OKT4 bearing molecule is a receptor for the human retrovirus HTLV-III. *Clin. Res.*, **33**, 560A.

Popovic, M., Read-Connole, E. and Gallo, R. C. (1984) T4 positive human neoplastic cell lines susceptible to and permissive for HTLV-III. *Lancet*, ii, 1472.

Prince, H. E., Kermani-Arab, V. and Fahey, J. L. (1984) Depressed interleukin–2 receptor expression in acquired immunodeficiency and lymphadenopathy syndromes. *J. Immunol.*, **133**, 1313–17.

Prince, H. E., Kressi, J. K., Kasper, C. K., Kleinman, S., Saunders, A. M., Waldbeser, L., Manding, O. O. and Kaplan, H. S. (1985a) Distinctive lymphocyte subpopulation abnormalities in patients with congenital coagulation disorders who exhibit lymph node enlargement. *Blood*, **66**, 64–8.

Prince, H. E., Moody, D. J., Shubin, B. I. and Fahey, J. L. (1985b) Defective monocyte function in acquired immune deficiency syndrome (AIDS): evidence from a monocyte-dependent T-cell proliferative system. *J. Clin. Immunol.*, **5**, 21–5.

Quinnan, G. V., Masur, H., Rook, A. H., Armstrong, G., Frederick, W. R., Epstein, I., Manischewitz, J. F., Macher, A. M., Jackson, L., Ames, J., Smith, H. A., Parker, M., Pearson, G. R., Parillo, J., Mitchell, C. and Strauss, S. E. (1984) Herpes virus infections in the acquired immune deficiency syndromes. *JAMA*, **252**, 72–7.

Rabson, A. B., Daugherty, D. F., Venkatesan, S., Boulukos, K. E., Benn, S., Folks, T. M., Feorino, P. M. and Martin, M. A. (1985) Transfection of novel open reading frame of AIDS retrovirus during infection of lymphocytes. *Science*, **229**, 1388–90.

Rao, T. K. S., Filippone, E. J., Nicastri, A. D., Landesman, S. H., Frank, E., Chen, C. K. and Friedman, E. A. (1984) Associated focal and segmental glomerulosclerosis in the acquired immunodeficiency syndrome. *N. Engl. J. Med.*, **310**, 669–73.

Reddy, M. M., Pinyavat, N. and Greico, M. H. (1984) Interleukin 2 augmentation of natural killer cell activity in homosexual men with acquired immune deficiency syndrome. *Infect. Immun.*, **44**, 339–43.

Redfield, R. R., Wright, D. C. and Tramont, E. C. (1986) The Walter Reed staging classifications for HTLV-III/LAV infection. *N. Engl. J. Med.*, **314**, 131–2.

Reinherz, E. L., Kung, P. C., Goldstein, G. and Schlossman, S. F. (1979a) Separation of functional subsets of human T cells by a monoclonal antibody. *Proc. Natl Acad. Sci. USA*, **76**, 4061–5.

Reinherz, E. L., Kung, P. C., Pesando, J. M., Ritz, J., Goldstein, G. and Schlossman, S. F. (1979b) Ia determinants on human T cell subsets defined by monoclonal antibody: activation stimuli required for expression. *J. Exp. Med.*, **150**, 1472–82.

Reinherz, E. L. and Schlossman, S. F. (1980) The differentiation and function of human T lymphocytes. *Cell*, **19**, 821–7.

Reinherz, E. L., Morimoto, C., Penta, A. C. and Schlossman, S. F. (1981) Subpopulations of the $T4^+$ inducer T cell subset in man: evidence for an amplifier population preferentially expressing Ia antigen upon activation. *J. Immunol.*, **126**, 67–70.

Reinherz, E. L., Morimoto, C., Fitzgerald, K. A., Hussey, R. E., Daley, J. F. and Schlossman, S. F. (1982) Heterogeneity of human $T4^+$ inducer T cells defined by a monoclonal antibody that delineates two functional subpopulations. *J. Immunol.*, **128**, 463–8.

Robert-Guroff, M., Brown, M. and Gallo, R. C. (1985) HTLV-III neutralizing antibodies in patients with AIDS and AIDS-related complex. *Nature, Lond.*, **316**, 72–4.

Rogers, M. F., Morens, D. M., Stewart, J. A., Kaminski, R. M., Spira, T. J., Feorino, P. M., Larsen, S. A., Francis, D. P., Wilson, M. and Kaufman, L. (1983) National case-control study of Kaposi's sarcoma and *Pneumocystis carinii* pneumonia in homosexual men: Part 2, laboratory results. *Ann. Intern. Med.*, **99**, 151–8.

Rook, A. H., Masur, H., Lane, H. C., Frederick, W., Kasahara, T., Macher, A. M., Djeu, J. Y., Manischewitz, J. F., Jackson, L., Fauci, A. S. and Quinnan, G. V. (1983) Interleukin–2 enhances the depressed natural killer and cytomegalovirus-specific cytotoxic activities of lymphocytes from patients with the acquired immune deficiency syndrome. *J. Clin. Invest.*, **72**, 398–403.

Rook, A. H., Hooks, J. J., Quinnan, G. V., Lane, H. C., Manischewitz, J. F., Macher, A. M., Fauci, A. S. and Djeu, J. Y. (1985a) Interleukin 2 enhances the natural killer cell activity of acquired immunodeficiency syndrome patients through a α-interferon-independent mechanism. *J. Immunol.*, **134**, 1503–7.

Rook, A. H., Manischewitz, J. F., Frederick, W. R., Epstein, J. S., Jackson, L., Gelmann, E., Steis, R., Masur, H. and Quinnan, G. V. (1985b) Deficient HLA-restricted, cytomegalovirus-specific cytotoxic T cells and natural killer cells in patients with the acquired immune deficiency syndrome. *J. Infect. Dis.*, **152**, 627–30.

Rosen, C. A., Sodroski, J. G. and Haseltine, W. A. (1985) The location of cis-acting regulatory sequences in the human T cell lymphotropic virus type III (HTLV-III/LAV) long terminal repeat. *Cell*, **41**, 813–23.

Rosen, F. S., Cooper, M. D. and Wedgewood, R. J. P. (1984) The primary immunodeficiencies (parts 1 and 2). *N. Engl. J. Med.*, **311**, 235–42, 300–10.

Ruscetti, F. W., Mikouits, J. A., Kalyanaraman, V. S., Overton, R., Stevenson, H., Stromberg, K., Herberman, R. B., Farrar, W. L. and Ortaldo, J. R. (1986) Analysis of effector mechanisms against HTLV-I and HTLV-III/LAV infected lymphoid cells. *J. Immunol.*, **136**, 3619–24.

Safai, B., Sarngadharan, M. G., Groopman, J. E., Arnett, K., Popovic, M., Slinski, A., Schupbach, J. and Gallo, R. C. (1984) Seroepidemiological studies of human T-lymphotropic retrovirus type III in acquired immunodeficiency syndrome. *Lancet*, **i**, 1438–40.

Salahuddin, S. Z., Markham, P. D., Lindner, S. G., Gootenberg, J. and Popovic, M. (1984) Lymphokine production by cultured human T cells transformed by HTLV-I. *Science*, **223**, 703–7.

Salazar-Gonzales, J. F., Moody, D. J., Giorgi, J. V., Martinez-Maza, O., Mitsuyasu, R. T. and Fahey, J. L. (1985) Reduced ecto-5′-nucleotidase activity and enhanced OKTIO and HLA-DR expression on CD8 (T suppressor/cytotoxic) lymphocytes in the acquired immune deficiency syndrome: Evidence of CD8 immaturity. *J. Immunol.*, **135**, 1778–85.

Sarin, P. S., Sun, D. K., Thornton, A. H., Naylor, P. H. and Goldstein, A. L. (1986) Neutralization of HTLV-III/LAV replication by antiserum to thymosin α1. *Science*, **232**, 1135–7.

Sarngadharan, M. G., Popovic, M., Bruch, L., Schupbach, J. and Gallo, R. C. (1984) Antibodies reactive with human T-lymphotropic retroviruses (HTLV-III) in the serum of patients with AIDS. *Science*, **224**, 506–8.

Schroff, R. W., Gottlieb, M. S., Prince, H. E., Chai, L. L. and Fahey, J. L. (1983) Immunological studies of homosexual men with immunodeficiency and Kaposi's sarcoma. *Clin. Immunol. Immunopathol.*, **27**, 300–14.

Schüpbach, J., Haller, O., Vogt, M., Lathy, R., Joller, H., Oelz, O., Popovic, M., Sarngadharan, M. G. and Gallo, R. C. (1985) Antibodies to HTLV-III in Swiss patients with AIDS and pre-AIDS and in groups at risk for AIDS. *N. Engl. J. Med.*, **312**, 265–70.

Schwartz, K., Visscher, B. R., Detels, R., Taylor, J., Nisharian, P. and Fahey, J. L. (1985) Immunological changes in lymphadenopathy virus positive and negative symptomless male homosexuals: two years of observation. *Lancet*, **ii**, 831–2.

Sharma, B. and Gupta, S. (1985) Antigen-specific primary cytotoxic T lymphocyte (CTL) responses in acquired immune deficiency syndrome (AIDS) and AIDS-related complexes (ARC). *Clin. Exp. Immunol.*, **62**, 296–303.

Shaw, G. M., Harper, M. E., Hahn, B. H., Epstein, L. G., Gajdusek, D. C., Price, R. W., Navia, B. A., Petito, C. K., O'Hara, C. J., Groopman, J. E., Cho, E.-S., Oleske, J. M., Wong-Staal, F. and Gallo, R. C. (1985) HTLV-III infection in brains of children and adults with AIDS encephalopathy. *Science*, **227**, 177–82.

Shearer, G. M., Salahuddin, S. Z., Markham, P. D., Joseph, L. J., Payne, S. M., Kriebel, P., Bernstein, D. C., Biddison, W. E., Sarngadharan, M. G. and Gallo, R. C. (1985) Prospective study of cytotoxic T lymphocyte responses to influenza and antibodies to human T lymphotropic virus-III in homosexual men. *J. Clin. Invest.*, **76**, 1699–1704.

Siegal, F. P., Lopez, C., Hammer, G. S., Brown, A. E., Kornfeld, S. J., Gold, J., Hassett, J., Hirschman, S. Z., Cunningham-Rundles, C., Adelsberg, B. R., Parkham, D. M., Siegal, M., Cunningham-Rundles, S. and Armstrong, D. (1981) Severe acquired immunodeficiency in homosexual males, manifested by chronic perianal ulcerative herpes simplex lesions. *N. Engl. J. Med.*, **305**, 1439–44.

Siegal, F. P., Lopez, C., Fitzgerald, P. A., Shah, K., Baron, P., Leiderman, I. Z., Imperato, D. and Landesman, S. (1986) Opportunistic infections in acquired immune deficiency syndrome result from synergistic defects of both the natural and adaptive components of cellular immunity. *J. Clin. Invest.*, in press.

Siegel, J. P., Djeu, J. Y., Stocks, N. I., Masur, H., Fauci, A. S., Lane, H. C., Gelmann, E. P. and Quinnan, G. P. (1984) Serum from patients with the acquired immune deficiency syndrome suppresses production of interleukin–2 by normal peripheral blood lymphocytes. *Clin. Res.*, **32**, 358A.

Smith, P. D., Ohura, K., Masur, H., Lane, H. C., Fauci, A. S. and Wahl, S. M. (1984) Monocyte function in the acquired immune deficiency syndrome: defective chemotaxis. *J. Clin. Invest.*, **74**, 2121–8.

Smolen, J. S., Bettelheim, P., Koller, U., McDougal, S., Graninger, W., Luger, T. A., Knapp, W. and Lechner, K. (1985) Deficiency of the autologous mixed lymphocyte reaction in patients with classic hemophilia treated with commercial factor VIII concentrate. *J. Clin. Invest.*, **75**, 1828–34.

Sodroski, J., Patarca, R., Rosen, C., Wong-Staal, F. and Haseltine, W. (1985) Location of the transactivating region on the genome of human T-cell lymphotropic virus type III. *Science*, **229**, 74–7.

Sodroski, J., Goh, W. C., Rosen, C., Tartar, A., Portetelle, D., Burny, A. and Haseltine, W. (1986a) Replicative and cytopathic potential of HTLV-III/LAV with sor gene deletions. *Science*, **231**, 1549–53.

Sodroski, J., Goh, W. C., Rosen, C., Dayton, A., Terwilliger, E. and Haseltine, W. (1986b) A second post-transcriptional trans-activator gene required for HTLV-III replication, *Nature, Lond.*, **321**, 412–17.

Stahl, R. E., Friedman-Kein, A. E., Dubin, R., Marmor, M. and Zolla-Pazner, S. (1982) Immunologic abnormalities in homosexual men: relationship to Kaposi's sarcoma. *Am. J. Med.*, **73**, 171–8.

Stein, S. F., Evatt, B. L., McDougal, J. S., Lawrence, D. N., Holman, R. C., Ramsey, R. B. and Spira, T. J. (1985) A longitudinal study of patients with hemophilia:

immunologic correlates of infection with HTLV-III/LAV and other viruses. *Blood*, **66**, 973–9.

Stites, D. P., Casavant, C. H., McHugh, T. M., Moss, A. R., Beal, S. L., Ziegler, J. L., Saunders, A. M. and Warner, N. L. (1986) Flow cytometric analysis of lymphocyte phenotypes in AIDS using monoclonal antibodies and simultaneous dual immunofluorescence. *Clin. Immunol. Immunopathol.*, **38**, 161–77.

Tersmette, M., Van Dongen, J. J. M., De Goede, R. E. Y., Van Kessel, A. G., Huisman, H. G. and Miedema, F. (1986) $T4^+$ human-murine T cell hybrids cannot be productively infected with HTLV-III. *International AIDS Conference*, Paris, June 21–3.

Thomas, Y., Rogozinski, L., Irigoyen, O. H., Shen, H. H., Talle, M. A., Goldstein, G. and Chess, L. (1982) Functional analysis of human T cell subsets defined by monoclonal antibodies. V. Suppressor cells within the activated $OKT4^+$ population belong to a distinct subset. *J. Immunol.*, **128**, 1386–90.

Tomar, R. H., John, P. A., Hennig, A. K. and Kloster, B. (1985) Cellular targets of antilymphocyte antibodies in AIDS and LAS. *Clin. Immunol. Immunopathol.*, **37**, 37–47.

Tsoukas, C., Gervais, F., Shuster, J., Gold, P., O'Shaughnessy, M. and Robert-Guroff, M. (1984) Association of HTLV-III antibodies and cellular immune status of hemophiliacs. *N. Engl. J. Med.*, **311**, 1514–15.

Wachter, H., Fuchs, D., Hausen, A., Huber, C., Kuosp, O., Reibnegger, G. and Spira, T. J. (1983) Elevated urinary neopterin levels in patients with the acquired immunodeficiency syndrome (AIDS). *Hoppe-Seyler's Z. Physiol. Chem.*, **364**, 1345–6.

Wallace, L. E., Moss, D. J., Rickinson, A. B., McMichael, A. J. and Epstein, M. A. (1981) Cytotoxic T cell recognition of Epstein–Barr virus-infected cells. II. Blocking studies with monoclonal antibodies to HLA determinants. *Eur. J. Immunol.*, **11**, 694–9.

Washburn, R. G., Tuazon, C. U. and Bennett, J. E. (1984) Phagocytic and fungicidal activity of monocytes from patients with acquired immunodeficiency syndrome. *J. Infect. Dis.*, **151**, 565–6.

Weiss, R. A., Clapham, P. R., Cheingsong-Popov, R., Dalgleish, A. G., Carne, C. A., Weller, I. V. D. and Tedder, R. S. (1985) Neutralization of human T-lymphotropic virus type III by sera of AIDS and AIDS-risk patients. *Nature, Lond.*, **316**, 69–72.

Williams, R. C., Masur, H. and Spira, T. J. (1984) Lymphocyte-reactive antibodies in acquired immune deficiency syndrome. *J. Clin. Immunol.*, **4**, 118–23.

Wong-Staal, F. and Gallo, R. C. (1985) Human T-lymphotropic retroviruses. *Nature, Lond.*, **317**, 395–403.

Wood, G. S., Warner, N. L. and Warke, R. A. (1983) Anti-Leu3/T4 antibodies react with cells of monocyte/macrophage and Langerhans lineage. *J. Immunol.*, **131**, 212–16.

Wood, G. S., Burnes, B. F., Dorfman, R. F. and Warnke, R. A. (1986) In situ quantitation of lymph node helper, suppressor, and cytotoxic T cell subsets in AIDS. *Blood*, **67**, 596–603.

Yachie, A., Miyawaki, T., Yokoi, T., Nagaoki, T. and Taniguchi, N. (1982) Ia positive cells generated by PWM-stimulation within the $OKT4^+$ subset interact with $OKT8^+$ cells for inducing active suppression on B cell differentiation *in vitro*. *J. Immunol.*, **129**, 103–6.

Zagury, D., Bernard, J., Leonard, R., Cheynier, R., Feldman, M., Sarin, P. S. and Gallo, R. C. (1986) Long-term cultures of HTLV-III infected T cells: a model of cytopathology of T cell depletion in AIDS. *Science*, **231**, 850–3.

Ziegler-Heitbrock, H. W. L., Schramm, W., Satchel, D., Rumpold, H., Kraft, D., Wernicke, D., Von Der Helm, K., Eberle, J., Deinhardt, F., Rieber, G. P. and Rietmuller, G. (1985) Expansion of a minor subpopulation of peripheral blood lymphocytes ($T8^+/Leu7^+$) in patients with hemophilia, *Clin. Exp. Immunol.*, **61**, 633–41.

5

T cell phenotyping in the diagnosis and management of AIDS and AIDS related disease

Michael S. Gottlieb, Roger Detels
—— and John L. Fahey ——

5.1 INTRODUCTION

The topic of this chapter is the utility, if any, of T lymphocyte subset quantitation in the assessment and management of patients infected with human immunodeficiency viruses (HIV). The answer to this question cannot be definitive at this time because of the novelty of this epidemic and the nature of the data. The perceptions of practising physicians on T cell phenotyping have far-reaching consequences for the well-being of their patients, on laboratory services utilization and on health care expenditures. Additional studies are needed to address the utility of T lymphocyte testing. Clinical practitioners, faced with an incompletely resolved medical issue, must continue to critically assess the relevance of this test to decision-making in patients with HIV infection.

It is now well appreciated that AIDS and other illness due to HIV infection are frequently associated with measurable immunologic abnormalities. The central abnormalities are listed in Table 5.1.

In this chapter, cells with helper phenotype are referred to as T4, suppressor cells as T8, and helper to suppressor ratio as T4/8 (Table 5.2). The standard method for calculation of the lymphocyte count and quantitative T4 and T8 counts is defined in Table 5.3.

T cell phenotyping of the first AIDS patients at UCLA indicated major depletion of T4 helper/inducer cells (Gottlieb *et al.*, 1981; Schroff *et al.*, 1983). This abnormality stimulated the search for a T4 tropic retroviruses as the aetiologic agents of the clinical syndrome (Barre-Sinoussi *et al.*, 1983;

Popovic *et al.*, 1984). Molecular studies have confirmed that the T4 lymphocyte is one important immune cell target for infection by HIV with the virus binding to the T4 molecule (probably via the virus envelope glycoprotein) (Klatzmann *et al.*, 1984; Dalgliesh *et al.*, 1984; McDougal *et al.*, 1986). More recent information indicates infection of the cells of monocyte/macrophage lineage (Smith *et al.*, 1984) perhaps explaining macrophage functional defects. Thus T cell phenotyping has made a critical contribution to our current understanding of the aetiology and pathogenesis of AIDS.

T cell phenotyping has been controversial from the beginning in part because it was new, availability was limited, and it was and remains costly. Accurate information on its clinical utility for diagnosis, screening and patient management is very limited, contributing to overuse and inappropriate applications.

Prior to HIV antibody testing, this test was used as a non-specific indicator of immune imbalance in epidemiologic studies (Kornfeld *et al.*, 1982; Fahey, Detels and Gottlieb, 1983; Gottlieb *et al.*, 1984; Goldsmith *et al.*, 1983; Lederman *et al.*, 1983; Luban, Kelleher and Remon, 1983; Pinching, 1983) and in some clinics and blood screening programs. In this period the T cell

Table 5.1 Major immunologic abnormalities in HIV infection

Decreased absolute lymphocyte count
Decreased number of T helper/inducer cells
Decreased T helper/T suppressor ratios
Cutaneous anergy
Defective monocyte function

Table 5.2 T cell phenotyping terminology

	Surface Marker (synonyms)
T helper/inducer cells	T4, OKT-4, CD-4, Leu 3
T suppressor/cytoxic cells	T8, OKT-8, CD-8, Leu-2
T helper/suppressor ratio	T4/8 OKT-4/OKT-8, CD-4/CD-8

Table 5.3 Calculation for quantitative T cell subset enumeration

Absolute lymphocyte count	Total white blood cell count multiplied by percentage lymphocytes on Wright's-stained smear
Absolute T4 or T8	Absolute lymphocyte count multiplied by percentage T4 or T8 cells

ratio was a candidate surrogate marker for infection with the then suspected AIDS virus. In the last two years, increased use in clinical setting of the much less costly and less technically demanding HIV antibody tests has clearly proved more definitive than T cell analysis in answering the most important diagnostic question, namely whether a patient *has* or *has not* been infected with HIV. Although very useful, the antibody assay does not answer important questions which come up in clinical practice. These include: (1) the duration of HIV infection, (2) the extent of immune system damage, i.e. staging, (3) the prognosis for development of AIDS or other symptomatic HIV syndrome, and lastly, (4) the risk of incipient serious infection. A central question for patients and their health providers is whether any test beyond HIV antibody can provide information which helps to further define the overall situation and options of the patient. A reasonable possibility exists that quantitative T cell studies, particularly T4 number and ratio, when applied with appreciation of their limits, can yield clinically useful information. Until this is more thoroughly studied, these tests can provide the clinician and patient only with insights, not definitive answers.

5.2 LABORATORY TESTS

Laboratory tests have several possible purposes (Griner *et al.*, 1981). These are: in diagnosis, in screening asymptomatic populations, and in patient management. The intelligent selection of a laboratory test depends on a choice appropriate for the purpose intended. In the process of *diagnosis*, sensitive tests, *when normal*, allow the physician to confidently exclude the disease.

The primary purpose of *screening* is to detect diseases or states whose morbidity and mortality can be reduced by early diagnosis and treatment. Basic decision analysis indicates that a particular test should be done when the benefits outweigh the costs in terms of money, patient risk or discomfort. Guidelines for application of screening include: (1) the disease in question should be common enough in the population to be tested to justify the effort to detect it; (2) the disease should cause significant morbidity if not treated; (3) effective therapy should exist to alter its natural history; and finally, (4) detection and treatment of the presymptomatic state should result in benefits beyond those obtained from treatment of the early symptomatic patient. Once the criteria are met, the issue should be examined from the standpoint of laboratory test specificity and sensitivity.

The third purpose of laboratory tests is in *patient management* (Griner, 1981). Tests can, when repeated, monitor the status of a disease process, its progression, stability or resolution. They may also aid in prognosis. Optimal frequency of test performance is determined from expected rate of change of underlying disease which may influence the test result.

5.3 THE T HELPER CELL AND RATIO IN HIV INFECTION

Considerable although incomplete information on the utility, if any, of T cell studies is available from prospective epidemiologic studies in homosexual male populations and retrospective studies of symptomatic populations. Selected series from which data for this review were obtained are listed in Table 5.4. Critical points for assessment of natural history studies of AIDS are the geographic location, the number of participants, and importantly, the clinical status of the subject population, i.e. symptomatic and asymptomatic. Only studies in homosexual subjects are reviewed here because the largest amount of information has been gathered in this population. It is recognized that, because of cofactors for development of AIDS, the result in one risk group cannot necessarily be extrapolated to others.

Table 5.4 Selected series

Series	*Date*	*Location*	*Population*	*N*	*Clinical status*
Nicholson	1985	US	Homosexual	120	asym*
Goedert	1984	NY, Wash	Homosexual	66	sym† and asym
Goedert	1986	NY, Wash	Homosexual	86	sym and asym
Melbye	1986	Denmark	Homosexual	250	asym
Detels	1986	LA	Homosexual	167	asym
Detels	1986	LA (MACS)	Homosexual	1637	asym
Gottlieb	1986	LA	Homosexual	101	sym

*Asymptomatic.
†Symptomatic.

With rare exception, studies of this type have demonstrated clear relationships between the presence of HIV antibody and immunologic findings. These relationships are summarized in Table 5.5. Men with HIV antibody have lower T4 cell numbers, higher or normal T8 cell numbers and lower ratio than men without HIV antibody.

Nicholson and associates at CDC studied 120 randomly selected asymptomatic homosexual men from throughout the US who had been controls for CDC epidemiologic studies (Nicholson *et al.*, 1983). The group with HIV antibody (41%) had significantly lower T4/8 ratios, lower numbers of T4 cells, and higher numbers of T8 cells. The men without antibody were not significantly different from laboratory controls. Of the men with HIV antibody 63% had an abnormal T4/8 ratio compared to 8% with seronegatives. Conversely, 84% of men with low T4/8 ratio were seropositive. The most frequent cause for a low ratio in those with antibody was an elevation of the T8 count or the combination of a low-normal T4 cell count and high

Table 5.5 Consensus conclusions from immunologic studies of HIV seropositives and seronegatives

Presence of HIV antibodies correlates with:	
	Lower T4
	Higher T8
	Lower T4/8

normal T8 count. Lower T4/8 ratios were most strongly related to seropositivity, although T4 count was related. It is noteworthy that in these studies of asymptomatic men, the absolute lymphocyte count did not correlate with the presence or absence of antibody. This was a relatively healthy group with no progression to AIDS over a 17 month average follow-up.

Melbye and colleagues from Denmark published longitudinal immunologic studies in 250 homosexual males (Melbye *et al.*, 1986). Only 8.8% had antibody to HIV initially. After December, 1981, 6% per year seroconverted. The duration of seropositivity correlated with decreased T4 number and to a lesser extent increased T8 number.

Perhaps the most unsettling finding in Melbye's study was a significant and steady time-related decline in T cell ratio among men with antibody. This resulted from both a decline in T4 and an increase in T8. Of subjects antibody positive for greater than 29 months 60% had low absolute T4 numbers compared to only 25% of subjects antibody positive for less than 19 months. In other words, these data suggest that duration of HIV infection is a key predictor of T4 lymphopenia. If T4 lymphopenia, in turn, is a predictor of AIDS in antibody positive populations, as data from our own studies and those of Goedert and colleagues suggest, T cell analysis may provide the clinician and patient with more information than antibody testing alone. Clearly this interpretation is tentative and requires further study. While it is not firmly established and by no means uniformly accepted, it is possible that this information can lead to more informed decision-making by physician and patient.

Unpublished data from UCLA epidemiologic and clinical studies further explore the relationship of T cell status to prognosis. In an early prospective study (Detels, *et al.* in preparation), Detels and colleagues followed a cohort of 167 homosexual men in Los Angeles. These men were followed for 2 years for immune changes and for more than 3 years for the development of AIDS. Some 35 (35%) had antibody at baseline. Eight men (8%) developed AIDS.

Table 5.6 compares baseline T cell levels among HIV seronegatives, seropositives, and AIDS cases. As in other studies seropositives had significantly fewer T4 cells and significantly greater T8 cells compared to seronegatives. The mean T4 cells count of the 8 cases was lower at the first visit compared with seropositives who did not develop AIDS but only at the 0.05

Table 5.6 Comparison of baseline T cell levels among seronegatives, seropositives and cases

	No. T4 cells		No. T8 cells	
Seronegatives (N=79)	839 ± 321	$p<0.01$	676 ± 281	$p<0.006$
Seropositives (N=42)	679 ± 293	$p<0.053$	877 ± 454	p=NS
Cases (N=8)	467 ± 187		920 ± 233	

level. At the baseline visit, 4/8 showed low ratio only, 2 had reduced T4 cells, 1 had increased T8 cells, and 1 was normal.

A steady decline in the number of T4 cells but not of T8 cells preceded the development of clinical AIDS in the 8 cases as illustrated in Fig. 5.1. At the visit nearest to diagnosis all 8 cases had abnormally low T4 cell numbers. Confirmatory information from a larger group comes from the UCLA Multicenter AIDS Cohort or MACS study which is in progress in 5 US cities under the auspices of the National Institute of Allergy and Infectious Diseases. At the Los Angeles sites, 1637 homosexual males are enrolled; 55% were seropositive to HIV at the time of enrolment. Table 5.7 compares the 624 seropositive men and 609 seronegative men who have completed one year of follow-up to date. Statistically but not clinically significant differences in total white cell count and absolute lymphocyte count were observed. The presence of antibody was associated with relative leukopenia and lymphopenia. Significant differences between seropositives and seronegatives were observed for T4, T8 and ratio. In this cohort, 59 men (7% of

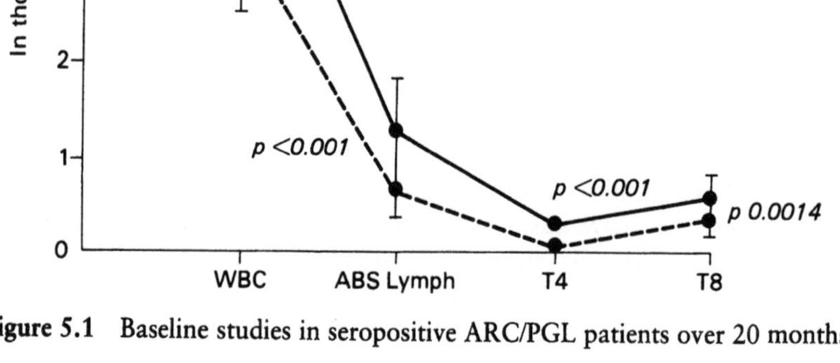

Figure 5.1 Baseline studies in seropositive ARC/PGL patients over 20 months.

Table 5.7 WBC and T cell studies in consistently seropositive and seronegative high risk individuals over 1 year (LA MACS Cohort)*

	Seropositive (N = 624)		*Seronegative* (N = 609)		*Difference between groups*
	Mean	(+ SD)	Mean	(+ SD)	*p* value
WBC	5763	(1589)	6859	(1909)	< 0.0001
ABS lymph	1722	(529)	2009	(614)	< 0.0001
T4	539	(221)	839	(324)	< 0.0001
T8	793	(335)	620	(255)	< 0.0001
Ratio	0.77	(0.40)	1.59	(0.66)	< 0.0001

*Multicentre AIDS Cohort Study supported by National Institute of Allergy and Infectious Diseases.

seropositives) developed AIDS over 18 months followup. Table 5.8 compares the baseline immunologic variables for the 59 seropositive men who developed AIDS to the 754 seropositives who did not. T4 cell number and ratio were the most powerful discriminating variables between those seropositives who did and those who did not develop AIDS. T4 number at entry among the 59 who developed AIDS were 299 ± 167 compared to 555 ± 225 among the 754 who did not develop AIDS.

The next studies to be discussed are of patient populations seeking care in tertiary clinics at UCLA. T cell and antibody studies were performed under research protocols. These studies were done in patients with non-neoplastic manifestations of HIV infection. Patients presenting with Kaposi's Sarcoma (KS) were evaluated in separate clinics.

In 101 patients referred for persistent lymphadenopathy and previously reported by Gottlieb (Gottlieb *et al.*, 1985), progression to AIDS was associated with several haematologic variables. As shown in Fig. 5.2, those with less than 200 T4 cells/mm^3 had a 60% probability of progression to

Table 5.8 Baseline WBC and T cell studies in 813 consistently seropositive high risk individuals developing AIDS over 18 months

	Did not develop AIDS (n = 754)		*Developed AIDS* (n = 59)		*Difference between groups*
	Mean	(+ SD)	Mean	(+SD)	*p* value
WBC	5863	(1616)	5361	(1477)	0.0208
ABS lymph	1747	(537)	1610	(633)	0.0627
T4	555	(225)	299	(167)	< 0.0001
T8	800	(342)	927	(376)	0.0064
T4/8	0.79	(0.42)	0.35	(0.21)	< 0.0001

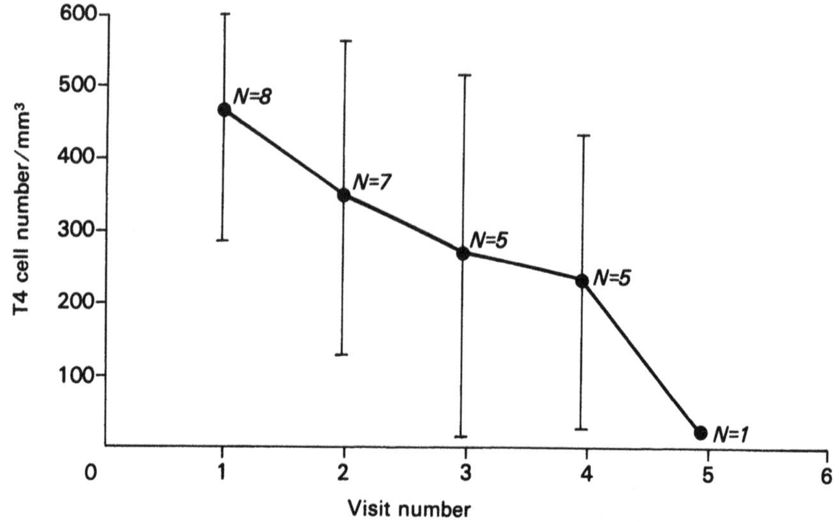

Figure 5.2 Serial T4 cell number in UCLA (study no. 1) subjects developing AIDS.

AIDS over 20 months compared to 10% progression over the same time period among patients with greater than 350 T4 cells. The 5th percentile for normals at the UCLA medical immunology laboratory was 350.

Subsequent further analysis of this series revealed that in these symptomatic patients, leukopenia and lymphopenia on a simple complete blood count were equally predictive of an AIDS outcome as seen in Table 5.9. This data is similar to that reported by Goedert *et al.* (1984, 1985, 1986) in a relatively symptomatic cohort in New York where the number of T4 cells was a strong predictor of the future development of AIDS among seropositive men with an inverse relationship between development of AIDS and T4 count. Of those with less than 400 T4 cells 46% developed AIDS compared to 9% with higher T4 counts. Absolute lymphocyte numbers were not reported.

Table 5.9 Baseline studies in seropositive ARC/PGL patients over 20 months

	Progressed to AIDS (n = 16)		*Did not progress to AIDS* (n = 52)		*Difference between groups*
	Mean	(+ SD)	Mean	(+ SD)	*p* value
WBC	3139	1056	4869	1617	< 0.0005
ABS lymph	688	289	1272	499	< 0.001
T4	50	60	313	175	< 0.001
T8	374	170	608	261	< 0.001

Published studies by Taylor and Mitsuyasu in AIDS/Kaposi's sarcoma patients indicated that survival correlated with absolute T4 count (Taylor *et al.*, 1986; Mitsuyasu *et al.*, 1986).

In summary, these studies suggest that significant changes in T4, T8 and T4/T8 ratio are associated with HIV infection. Lower T4 cell number and ratio may be early predictors of AIDS in seropositive populations. In highly symptomatic patients particularly at tertiary care clinics, total white cell count and absolute lymphocyte count may have equal predictive value.

5.4 T CELL STAGING IN HIV INFECTION

Although we have not yet formally studied T cell based clinical decision making, observations from our research studies suggest potential clinical utility. In the otherwise asymptomatic patient with HIV antibody, knowing the T4 is sometimes helpful for physician management in assessing the significance of symptomatology such as fever, weight loss or dyspnoea. For example in the febrile patient, it is our experience that T4 numbers which are normal or mildly depressed make evolving *Pneumocystis carinii* pneumonia or other serious infection less likely. This can be reassuring to the patient (Gottlieb, 1986; Gottlieb *et al.*, 1985).

In order to be useful in this setting, these studies must have been repeated at intervals. In our own clinical practice, 4 month intervals were arbitrarily selected. Clearly in serial testing, the reproducibility characteristics of the test are critical. The standard for utility of a test in early diagnosis would be that earlier detection and treatment of the presymptomatic state should result in benefits beyond those obtainable from treatment of the early symptomatic state (Griner *et al.*, 1981). Some patients with marked T4 depletion may be candidates for prophylaxis against *P. carinii* pneumonia infection (Gottlieb *et al.*, 1984). An alternative course of action for such patients would be to encourage closer medical followup in order to make early diagnosis of treatable opportunistic infections.

It must be acknowledged that early diagnosis in AIDs has not been proven to materially influence morbidity or survival. It is our anecdotal experience, and a reasonable expectation, that early diagnosis would lead to treatment and reduced morbidity from some infections. The risks and benefits of this option must be weighed by the patient and practitioner. The costs incurred and the risks of inducing inappropriate or disabling fear of full-blown AIDS must be considered.

In the era before antibody testing, screening T lymphocyte testing in asymptomatic members of groups with increased risk, the so-called 'worried well', was not recommended. Indeed even today some controversy about screening antibody testing remains. A major argument against T cell testing derives from lack of specificity and speculation on the extent of 'background' immunologic noise in populations at increased risk, particularly homosexual males (Weber *et al.*, 1986). It is furthermore argued that the finding of an abnormality does not change the basic prevention message of a health provider.

With rare exceptions, however, the large cohort studies do not support the notion of high immunologic noise levels in *antibody negative* high risk group members. Thus the linkage of T cell analysis withHIV antibody testing could increase the specificity of T cell testing for staging, as a barometer of sorts for the immunologic effects of the infection.

Prior to the antibody test, the non-specificity of T cell testing produced unrealistic psychological unrest. However, an unavoidable conclusion from the natural history studies cited earlier is that many asymptomatic homosexual males are infected with HIV. In the absence of proven treatment for AIDS or HIV, some have questioned the need for any further assessment of immunologic status. This is ironic since in most areas of medicine, early diagnosis of organ failure is a much sought after objective.

In any view, there are potential advantages to knowing more. Early clinical trials of antiviral agents (Yarchoan *et al.*, 1986) and immune modulators suggest that T4 number and other phenotypes are endpoints for efficacy and toxicity of candidate antiviral agents. Also when effective drugs are identified, it is likely that categories of patients with earlier HIV-related disease will be included if the agents are safe when administered over extended periods. It is unlikely that without long-term demonstrated safety that candidate agents will be tested in patients with antibody who do not have immune dysfunction. As trials increase in size and geographic distribution, the assessment of T cell phenotype by the practitioner may be increasingly relevant in the process of qualifying subjects for participation. If the T cell phenotyping test did not exist, based on our current concepts of the pathogenesis of AIDS, there would be major effort to develop a test that provides a quantitative assessment of T4 phenotype. T cell testing should be studied for benefits including cost-effectiveness.

5.5 CONCLUSIONS

In conclusion T4 cell injury is a central feature of HIV infection. The assessment of T cell phenotype continues to have significant potential applications in stratifying antibody positive patients for prognosis, and for patient management of AIDS and HIV related immune deficiency. The risk-to-benefit ratio and cost-effectiveness of this testing warrants further studies.

REFERENCES

Barré-Sinoussi, F., Chermann, J. C., Rey, F. *et al.* (1983) *Science*, **220**, 868–71.

Dalgliesh, A. G., Beverly, P. C., Clapham, P. R. *et al.* (1984) *Nature, Lond.*, **312**, 763–7.
Detels, R., Visscher, B. R., Fahey, J. L., Sever, J. L., Gravell, M., Madden, D. L., Schwartz, K., Dudley, J. P., English, P. A., Powers, H., Clark, V. A. and Gottlieb, M. S. *Ann. Intern. Med.*, in preparation.
Fahey, J. L., Detels, R. and Gottlieb, M. S. (1983) *N. Engl. J. Med.*, **308**, 842–3.
Fahey, J. L., Prince, H., Weaver, M., Groopman, J., Visscher, B. R., Schwartz, K. and Detels, R. (1984) *Am. J. Med.*, **76**, 95–100.
Goedert, J. J., Biggar, R. J., Weiss, S. H., Eister, M. E., Melbye, M., Wilson, S., Ginzberg, H. M., Grossman, J., DiVioia, R. A., Sanchez, W. C., Jirone, J. A., Ebbeson, P., Gallo, R. C. and Blattner, W. A. (1986) *Science*, **231**, 992–5.
Goedert, J. J., Biggar, R. J., Winn, D. M., Greene, M. H., Mann, D. L., Gallo, R. C., Sarngadharan, N. M. G., Weiss, S. H., Grossman, R. J., Bodner, A. J., Strong, D. M. and Blattner, W. A. (1984) *Lancet*, **ii**, 711–15.
Goedert, J. J., Biggar, R. J., Winn, D. M., Mann, D. L. *et al.* (1985) *Am. J. Epidemiol.*, **121**, 629–36.
Goldsmith, J. C., Moseley, P. L., Monick, M. *et al.* (1983) *Ann. Intern. Med.*, **98**, 294–6.
Gottlieb, M. S. (1986) *Clinics of North America*, W. B. Saunders, Philadelphia.
Gottlieb, M. S. *Clinical Approach to Infections in the Compromised Host* (ed. L. S. Young and R. Rubins), in press.
Gottlieb, M. S., Wolfe, P. R., Fahey, J. L., Knight, S., Hardy, D., Eppolito, L., Ashida, E., Patel, A., Beall, G. and Sun, N. (1985) *AIDS-Associated Syndromes*, Plenum Publishing Corp., New York.
Gottlieb, M. S., Knight, S., Mitsuyasu, R., Weisman, J., Roth, M. and Young, L. S. (1984) *Lancet*, **ii**, 398–9.
Gottlieb, M. S., Schroff, R., Schanker, H. M., Weisman, J. *et al.* (1981) *N. Engl. J. Med.*, **305**, 1425–31.
Griner, P. F., Mayewski, R. J., Mushlin, A. I. and Greenland, P. (1981) *Ann. Intern. Med.*, **94**, 559–63.
Klatzmann, D., Champagne, E., Chameret, S. *et al.* (1984) *Nature, Lond.*, **312**, 763–7.
Kornfeld, H., Vande-Stouwe, R. A., Lange M., Reddy, M. M. and Grieco, M. H. (1982) *N. Engl. J. Med.*, **307**, 729–31.
Lederman, M. M., Ratnoff, O., Scillian, J. J. *et al.* (1983) *N. Engl. J. Med.*, **308**, 79–83.
Luban, N. L. C., Kelleher, J. F. and Remon, G. H. (1983) *Lancet*, **i**, 503–5.
McDougal, J. S., Kennedy, M. S., Sligh, J. M., Cort, S. P., Mawle, A. and Nicholson, J. K. (1986) *Science*, **231**, 382–5.
Melbye, M., Biggar, R. J., Ebbesen, P., Neuland, C., Goedert, J. J., Faber, V., Lorenzen, I. B., Skinhog, P., Gallo, R. C. and Blattner, W. A. (1986) *Ann. Intern. Med.*, **104**, 496–500.
Mitsuyasu, R. T., Taylor, J. M. G., Glaspy, J. and Fahey, J. L. (1986) *Cancer*, **57**(8 suppl.), 1657–61.
Nicholson, J. K., McDougal, J. S., Jaffe, H. W., Spira, T. J., Kennedy, M. S., Jones, B. M., Darrow, W., Morgan, M. and Hubbard, M. (1983) *Ann. Intern. Med.*, **103**, 37–42.
Pinching, A. J., Jeffries, D. J., Donaghy, M. *et al.* (1983) *Lancet*, **ii**, 126–30.
Popovic, M., Sarngadharan M. G., Read, E., Gallo, R. C. *et al.* (1984) *Science*, **224**, 497–500.
Schroff, R. W., Gottlieb, M. S., Prince, H. *et al.* (1983) *Clin. Immunol. Immunopathol.*, **27**, 300–14.

Smith, P. D., O'Hara, K., Masur, H., Lane, H. C., Fauci, A. S. and Wahl, S. M. (1984) *J. Clin. Invest.*, **74**, 2121–8.
Taylor, J., Afrasiabi, R., Fahey, J. L., Korns, E., Weaver, M. and Mitsuyasu, R. (1986) *Blood*, **67**, 666–71.
Weber, J. N., Rogers, L. A., Scott, K., Berrie, E., Harris, J. R. W., Wadsworth, J., Moshtael, O., McManus, T., Jeffries, D. J. and Pinching, A. J. (1986) *Lancet*, **ii**, 1179–82.
Yarchoan, R., Klecker, R. W., Weinhold, K. J., Markham, P. D. *et al.* (1986) *Lancet*, **i**, 575–80.

6

The immunosuppressive effects of blood

Alison M. MacLeod, Andrew Innes and Graeme R. D. Catto

6.1 INTRODUCTION

The role of blood transfusion in the development of acquired immune deficiency syndrome (AIDS) is two-fold. Firstly, human immunodeficiency virus (HIV) may be directly transmitted by a blood transfusion and secondly, there is evidence that transfusions can suppress the immune response in several ways and may predispose the recipient to HIV infection.

6.2 TRANSFUSION AS A CAUSE OF AIDS

Even before the HIV virus was identified as the causal agent in AIDS there were indications that the disease could be transmitted by blood transfusion. In 1983 an infant was described who received blood and platelet transfusions from 18 different donors within eight weeks of his birth (Ammann *et al.*, 1983). In the 2 years until his death he suffered recurrent infections, showed raised levels of immunoglobulin and impaired cellular immunity. One of the platelet donors died 17 months later of AIDS. In addition, an adult Frenchman, who was not homosexual, a drug addict or a haemophiliac, developed AIDS four years after receiving a blood transfusion while working in Haiti (Andreani *et al.*, 1983).

It seemed likely, therefore, that an agent transmissible by blood or blood products was responsible for AIDS and that this agent had a long incubation time. Further evidence for this came firstly, when altered T cell function was noted in haemophiliacs receiving treatment with factor VIII concentrate (Luban, Kelleher and Reaman, 1983) and secondly, when eleven cases of clinical AIDS in haemophiliacs, without other risk factors, were reported to the Centers for Disease Control (Gordon, 1983).

The first analysis of data from several centres (Curran *et al.*, 1984) showed that 64 of 2157 patients notified as suffering from AIDS were not in the usual 'high-risk' groups. Eighteen of these had received multiple blood transfusions and at least one donor for each fully investigated recipient was found to be at risk of AIDS. Further confirmation of the association between blood transfusion and AIDS was obtained in the following months (Gordon, 1984).

Shortly thereafter reports from the United States and France suggested a possible role for a human T cell leukaemia retrovirus in the aetiology of AIDS; it was named HTLV-III by the American group (Gallo *et al.*, 1983) and LAV by the French (Vilmer *et al.*, 1984). Within a few months antibodies to HTLV-III were demonstrated by Western blot analysis in sera from both a high-risk blood donor and a recipient of his blood who developed AIDS in the absence of other risk factors. The virus itself was isolated from the donor's peripheral blood lymphocytes and viral sequencing showed HTLV-III related RNA sequences in her splenocytes (Groopman *et al.*, 1984). As well as providing strong evidence for the transmission of AIDS by blood transfusion this study provided confirmation that HTLV-III was the primary aetiological agent in AIDS.

A study of over 9000 cases of AIDS (Feorino *et al.*, 1985) reported that 2.2% had blood or blood product administration as their only risk factor. All recipients investigated had at least one blood donor in the 'high-risk' category for AIDS and all but four of these donors had antibodies to HTLV-III detected by an enzyme-linked immunosorbent assay (ELISA); in 90% the virus itself was recovered from peripheral blood lymphocytes. For the majority of recipients only one blood donor was found to have HTLV-III antibodies and most of these were asymptomatic. The authors therefore suggested that serological screening of all blood donors was necessary.

That the HIV can be transmitted directly by blood transfusion is not in doubt. However, it is possible also that the transfusion of uncontaminated blood may diminish immune responsiveness allowing activation of the virus. The immunosuppressive effects of blood transfusion may therefore predispose to the development of this condition.

6.3 THE IMMUNE EFFECTS OF BLOOD TRANSFUSION

Interest in the immunosuppressive effects of blood is focused principally in two areas of medical research. Firstly, those involved in the investigation of AIDS have studied these effects over the past four years. In addition, it was noted in 1973 that the administration of blood transfusions in the months and years before renal transplantion correlated with an improved allograft survival. This suggests an immunosuppressive role for blood and the past decade has seen intensive study of the possible mechanisms responsible for this beneficial effect.

6.3.1 AIDS and the immunosuppressive effects of blood

Those investigating AIDS have attempted to determine whether blood transfusions or blood products themselves produce immunodeficiency. Certain features of immunodeficiency found in AIDS have been noted in asymptomatic members of 'high-risk' groups such as homosexual men (Kornfeld *et al.*, 1982). It was unclear, however, whether these abnormalities highlighted patients who were susceptible to the AIDS agent or whether they indicated an early or mild infection with that agent.

The major immunological abnormalities found in AIDS are (a) a low ratio of helper (T_H) to suppressor (T_S) T lymphocytes and (b) a decrease in natural killer (NK) cell activity.

(a) T helper and T suppressor cell changes

Helper T lymphocytes are required to maintain antibody responses to virus infection (Burns and Allison, 1975). Suppressor T cells, in contrast, switch off effector cells taking part in an immune response when their task is complete. T_S cells along with antibodies, interferons and prostaglandins comprise a group of immunological modulators capable of immunosuppression. In AIDS the T_H/T_S ratio is low due to a decrease in the numbers of T_H cells (Seligmann *et al.*, 1984).

Several groups have noted a decreased T_H/T_S ratio in haemophiliacs receiving Factor VIII (Kessler *et al.*, 1983; Luban, Kelleher and Reaman, 1983; Gascon, Zoumbas and Young, 1984). This has also been reported by some (Kessler *et al.*, 1983) but not by others (Gascon, Zoumbas and Young, 1984) in patients who have received multiple blood transfusions for sickle cell anaemia. Kaplan and his group (1984) studied not only the T_H/T_S ratio but also the absolute numbers of these cells and showed that the T_H/T_S ratio was decreased in transfused patients compared to untransfused patients with sickle cell disease and that this was accounted for by a rise in T_S cells. The reduced ratio in haemophiliacs resulted from both a decrease in T_H cells and an increase in T_S cells compared to a normal population. A more recent study (Jason *et al.*, 1985) reported a decrease in T_H cells resulting in a low T_H/T_S ratio in haemophiliacs receiving Factor VIII and an increase in T_S cells in those receiving multiple transfusions although no change in the ratio was noted in this latter group. Thus the results are not in complete agreement but overall it appears that the T_H/T_S ratio is frequently decreased in those receiving blood or blood products and that whole blood transfusion induces a rise in T_S cells whereas treatment with Factor VIII results mainly in a fall in T_H

cells. These studies must be interpreted with care as in none of them were antibodies to HIV sought in either the recipients or donors of the blood products.

A study from Scotland (Ludlam *et al.*, 1985) performed after HIV antibody testing became available showed low levels of T_H cells in seronegative haemophiliacs receiving locally harvested factor VIII; at that time HIV antibodies were only found in sera from patients receiving commercial factor VIII. Many of these patients were subsequently exposed to one batch of contaminated Factor VIII and those who underwent seroconversion had significantly lower levels of T_H cells than those who remained seronegative; a reduced number of T_H, it was felt, might predispose to infection with HIV. Kaplan also reviewed his data in 1985 (Kaplan, Sarnack and Levy, 1985) and reported that the patients who had low T_H/T_S ratios after multiple blood transfusion, principally because of a rise in T_S cells, were all seronegative for HIV.

A diminished helper/suppressor ratio as a result of blood or blood product administration may thus predispose to the development of AIDS. Whether this results from an increase in T_S or a decrease in T_H lymphocytes may depend on whether blood or factor VIII is given. It should be noted, however, that in none of these studies was the function of T_H or T_S cells evaluated.

(b) Natural killer cell activity

Natural killer (NK) cells are directly cytotoxic to virus infected cells and are activated by interferon within one or two days of virus infection. There is also evidence, particularly from studies in the mouse (Bancroft, Shellam and Chalmer, 1981), that NK cells play an important role in the natural resistance to virus infection.

Decreased NK activity, such as is found in AIDS itself (Seligmann *et al.*, 1984), might thus predispose to virus infection. NK cell activity has therefore been assayed in patients receiving multiple blood transfusions or blood products. In haemophiliacs and transfused patients without antibodies to HIV the activity of NK cells was decreased (Kaplan *et al.*, 1984). These observations have been confirmed by others (Gascon, Zoumbas and Young, 1984) who went further and indicated that the degree of depression of NK cell activity was directly related to the amount of blood transfused. More recently it has been shown that NK cell response to certain types of interferon is impaired in haemophiliacs (this was independent of HIV antibody status) (Matheson *et al.*, 1986); this may represent a possible mechanism by which blood can impair NK cell function.

6.3.2 The induction of the immunosuppressive effects of blood

Blood transfusion and blood products clearly do suppress the immune response but the components of blood which cause this effect and the mechanisms by which it is accomplished are at present unclear. Some suggestions have been made, however, by those studying the blood transfusion effect in relation to the development of AIDS.

Those receiving multiple transfusions are repeatedly exposed to chronic stimuli from foreign cellular or soluble antigens, e.g. histocompatibility and viral antigens. Such chronic antigenic stimulation can result in an increase in T_S cells and in addition, NK cell activity may be modified by lymphocytes and their products. When human T lymphocytes are stimulated in this way they express HLA DR antigens which they normally do not. Increased HLA DR expression has been noted on T cells of patients with sickle cell anaemia who have received multiple blood transfusions (Gascon, Zoumbas and Young, 1984). Chronic antigenic stimulation may also be responsible for the down modulation of interferon receptors which could result in a decreased response of NK cells to interferon (Matheson *et al.*, 1986).

The importance of the immunosuppressive effects of blood on the development of AIDS is at present not known. Clearly the major risk of administering both blood or blood products must be the transmission of the HIV.

6.3.3 Renal transplantation and the immunosuppressive effects of blood

Blood transfusions exert a beneficial effect on renal allograft survival by actively inducing a state of immunological unresponsiveness. The mechanism for this is unclear. The two major areas which are currently under investigation are (a) the induction and activation of suppressor cells and (b) the generation of protective antibodies.

(a) Induction and activation of suppressor cells

Evidence that T suppressor cells played a part in prolonging allograft survival came before any link with the blood transfusion effect was made. It was first shown that the tolerance of an allogeneic transplant in a neonate is mediated by T_S cells (Dorsch and Roser, 1975). Later T_S cells were shown to prevent the rejection of cardiac transplants in an animal model (Hall, Roser and Dorsch, 1979). Functional assays showed that T_S cells caused the immunosuppressive effect in both studies.

Even before experimental evidence became available it was suggested that suppressor cells might be induced by transfusion and hence improve transplant survival (van Rood, Balner and Morris, 1978). Increased T_S function was later found in dialysis patients three weeks after the administration of two units of blood although this effect had disappeared by 20 weeks. No increase in suppressor cell numbers was noted in blood from these patients in contrast to those who had received multiple blood transfusions for sickle cell anaemia (Kaplan *et al.*, 1984). The increase in T_S cell function without an increase in their numbers was confirmed by others (Lenhard *et al.*, 1982).

Further animal studies showed that induction of T_S cells, detected by functional assays, improved allograft survival in animal models (Marquet *et al.*, 1982; Maki *et al.*, 1981). In these studies, however, suppressor cell activity was 'donor specific'. This means that transfusion from one inbred rat strain A to another B, differing at the major histocompatibility complex (MHC), induced T_S cells to strain B only and prolonged the survival of a transplant from strain B alone. Such classical 'donor specific immunosuppression' has been investigated extensively by those studying transplantation particularly in the animal model. If suppression could be induced to the antigens of the kidney transplant alone and not to all antigens, risks of non-specific immunosuppression, such as infection, could be avoided.

Kidney transplant survival, however, in many patients is improved by as few as one to three pre-transplant transfusions; the response is therefore unlikely to be entirely 'donor specific'. This problem has been considered in some detail by Hutchinson's group in Oxford (Hutchinson and Morris, 1986). They showed that minimal sharing of antigens induces suppression; for example activation of T_S cells by shared minor antigens can suppress rejection against MHC antigens to which there has been no previous exposure. Suppression could be specifically induced by a given blood transfusion and mediated by non-specific suppressive factors.

(b) Generation of protective antibodies

Anti-idiotypic antibodies

The immune response is regulated in many different ways. One of these is the idiotypic–anti-idiotypic network proposed by Jerne (Jerne, 1974). Antibodies which are induced in response to an antigen have a combining site for that antigen. Antigenic determinants are carried by the molecules which make up the combining sites and these define the idiotype of that antibody. An antibody response can occur to the idiotype and to the idiotypic markers of T cell receptors for the antigen. Such anti-idiotypic antibodies can therefore control the antibody response to an antigen.

In animal studies anti-idiotypic antibodies have been shown to inhibit selectively T cell mediated responses in the mixed lymphocyte culture (MLC) assay and also to prevent the rejection of allografts (Binz *et al.*, 1982). Similar antibodies have been noted in sera from transfused patients awaiting transplantation and have been found to be directed specifically to the transfusion donor (Fagnilli and Singal, 1982; Singal, Joseph and Ludwin, 1985). Subsequently serum from patients with a successful transplant obtained before and after transplant, inhibited a mixed lymphocytic culture between donor and recipient lymphocytes; no inhibitory activity was noted in sera from patients who had rejected their graft. Anti-idiotypic antibodies therefore represent one means by which transfusions induce immunosuppression in patients awaiting transplantation.

Fc receptor blocking antibodies
In the 1970s it was shown that kidney transplant survival in the animal model was enhanced when certain non-cytotoxic B lymphocyte antibodies were present in recipient serum prior to transplantation. These antibodies were capable of blocking Fc receptors and could be induced prior to transplant by injection of spleen cells (Suthanthiran *et al.*, 1979). They enhanced grafts only from animals sharing the same MHC as the donor of the spleen cells (Catto *et al.*, 1977). Such MHC linked protective antibodies were found in human sera. Patients with Fc receptor blocking activity in serum obtained prior to transplantation had significantly better graft survival than those who did not (MacLeod *et al.*, 1982a). These antibodies occurred more frequently in those who had received five or more blood transfusions and they developed in untransfused patients following blood transfusion (MacLeod *et al.*, 1982b). A further study showed that such transfusion induced antibodies were HLA linked (MacLeod *et al.*, 1985). Fc receptor blocking antibodies may represent another method of enhancement of kidney transplant survival as a result of blood transfusions.

In summary, both cellular and humoral responses have been shown to change in response to blood transfusion. How these responses integrate to cause improved allograft survival is as yet unknown.

6.4 BLOOD TRANSFUSION AND RENAL ALLOGRAFT SURVIVAL

6.4.1 Blood transfusion in the recipient of a cadaver donor transplant

(a) The blood transfusion effect and sensitization

Although the beneficial effect of transfusion on the outcome of a renal transplant was first noted in 1973 (Opelz *et al.*, 1973) it was not until 1980 that over 80% of patients received blood transfusions prior to their first cadaver donor renal transplant (Opelz and Terasaki, 1982). Physicians delayed instituting a policy of deliberate blood transfusion because of the risk of inducing lymphocytotoxic antibodies in their patients' sera and indeed most centres adopted restrictive transfusion policies to minimize the risk of such presensitization.

The evidence on which this was based came from analyses of extensive data by Paul Terasaki's group in Los Angeles. In a study of over 1000 patients they showed that transplant outcome was significantly worse when lymphocytotoxic antibodies were present in recipient sera prior to transplantation (Terasaki, Kreisler and Mickey, 1971). No mention of the number of transfusions was made and hence the effect of blood transfusion on allograft survival could not be assessed. Since the animal studies of the early 1970s suggested a beneficial effect of blood transfusion on experimental transplant outcome (Jenkins and Woodruff, 1971; Fabre and Morris, 1972) the Los Angeles group felt it imperative to evaluate the influence of the number of transfusions given prior to transplantation on human allograft survival (Opelz *et al.*, 1973). Contrary to their expectations they found a one year survival of 66% in those transfused with over 10 units of blood compared with 29% in untransfused patients. These results were confirmed by the London Transplant and the Eurotransplant groups (Festenstein *et al.*, 1976; van Hooff, Kalff and van Poelgeest, 1976). Analysis of the combined United Kingdom data, however, failed to confirm this (National Organ Matching Service, UK, 1975) and the registry of the European Dialysis and Transplantation Association showed a beneficial effect of transfusion only in recipients well matched for HLA antigens (Brunner *et al.*, 1976).

By the late 1970s no clear indication of the effect of pre-transplant blood transfusions on transplant outcome had emerged. Many centres analysed their own results and all demonstrated significantly improved allograft survival in recipients transfused prior to transplantation (Briggs *et al.*, 1978; Feduska *et al.*, 1979; Williams *et al.*, 1979; Solheim *et al.*, 1980). In 1980, after analysis of data from over 2000 patients, the Los Angeles group concluded that 'the marked beneficial effect of transfusions outweighs the risk of sensitisation' (Opelz and Terasaki, 1980). These data are supported by recent results showing that pre-transplant transfusions improve allograft survival by 20% (Opelz, 1985). The current policy of most centres is, therefore, to ensure that each patient receives between three and five units of blood prior to entering the transplant waiting list. There is some evidence however, that great care should be taken in deciding whether certain groups of patients should receive transfusions.

Previous pregnancies and failed transplants as well as blood transfusions can induce the formation of lymphocytotoxic antibodies. In particular, 10% of women who had more than three previous pregnancies but only two transfusions became sensitized to lymphocytes from over 90% of members of a normal panel (Opelz *et al.*, 1981). A similar high degree of sensitization is noted in patients with a previously failed graft when compared with untransplanted patients (Opelz, 1984). Since the presence of cytotoxic antibodies to donor lymphocytes generally precludes transplantation from that donor, less than 10% of donors would be suitable for individuals in these groups of potential recipients. Certain transplant units are therefore modifying their elective transfusion protocols, particularly for parous women (Ting, A. and Hendricks, F., personal communications).

Administering azathioprine along with a blood transfusion in an attempt to prevent sensitization has been attempted unsuccessfully (Raftery *et al.*, 1985a) but preliminary results using cyclosporin A are encouraging (Raftery *et al.*, 1985b).

(b) Nature of blood product

Elective blood transfusions are usually given in the form of packed red cells although whole blood is equally effective in producing the transfusion effect (Muller *et al.*, 1982). Blood which has been depleted of lymphocytes is ineffective (Persijn *et al.*, 1981) as are platelet transfusions (Chapman *et al.*, 1985). Lymphocytes therefore are essential to produce a beneficial effect in clinical renal transplantation.

(c) Timing of blood transfusion

It is not clear whether the time at which transfusion is given is important. Some (Werner-Favre *et al.*, 1979) but not others (Corry *et al.*, 1980) found it advantageous to transfuse patients within a particular time limit before transplantation. The effect of administering blood during the transplant operation in previously untransfused patients is also controversial; some groups claiming (Stiller *et al.*, 1978; Williams *et al.*, 1979) and others denying benefit (Persijn, Cohen and Landsbergen, 1979; Opelz and Terasaki, 1982).

(d) The effect of cyclosporin A

Cyclosporin A is now frequently used as routine immunosuppressive therapy with a marked improvement in transplant outcome reported almost universally. Some groups have claimed that the effect of cyclosporin is so strong that no further improvement in graft survival is gained by giving pre-transplant blood transfusions (Klintmalm *et al.*, 1985; Gardner *et al.*, 1985). A large multicentre trial of over 10 000 patients, however, showed that both cyclosporin A and pre-transplant blood transfusion independently improve transplant outcome (Opelz, 1985).

(e) Blood transfusion and the incidence of tumours in transplant recipients

Cancer does occur more frequently in transplant recipients than in the normal population; the relationship to pre-transplant transfusion is, however, obscure. The Australia and New Zealand Dialysis and Transplant Registry followed patients for 19 years and noted an incidence of cancer six times that expected in recipients of both living related and cadaver donor transplants (Sheil *et al.*, 1985); the transfusion histories of the patients were not mentioned. The types of cancer commonly occurring in such patients, lymphomas, Kaposi's sarcoma, cancer of the skin, lip and uterine cervix are those in which oncogenic viruses are believed to play a role (Penn, 1977). Immunosuppression, to which pre-transplant transfusions might contribute, may render the recipient vulnerable to such viruses. Any study attempting to define the effect of transfusion on the incidence of cancer in renal transplant recipients would have to take the amount and type of post-transplant immunosuppressive therapy given to the patient into account.

6.4.2 Donor specific blood transfusion in the recipient of a living related donor transplant

The one and three year transplant survival rates of a kidney from an HLA identical sibling are 90%; those of a one haplotype mismatched graft are 75% (Simmons *et al.*, 1977). In 1980 Salvatierra's group in San Francisco transfused the potential recipients of a one haplotype mismatched transplant with blood from the prospective donor and found that the one year graft survival rose to 94% (Salvatierra, Vincenti and Amend, 1980). Several other groups have confirmed these observations (Mendez *et al.*, 1982; Yamauchi *et al.*, 1983) and donor specific transfusion is now widely practised. The practical clinical problem is again the development of cytotoxic antibodies to donor lymphocytes necessitating cancellation of the planned transplant from that relative. Donor sensitization rates of between 11 and 29% have been reported (Barry *et al.*, 1985; Salvatierra, Vincenti and Amend, 1980). Whether sensitization after donor specific transfusion occurs may depend on previous sensitization by third party transfusions, pregnancies or failed grafts. In the initial report (Salvatierra, Vincenti and Amend, 1980) all but one of the 10 patients who developed sensitization to donor T lymphocytes had received previous random transfusions. Furthermore, Mendez and colleagues (1982) showed that sensitization did not occur in previously untransfused patients.

The administration of immunosuppressive drugs, including azathioprine and cyclosporin A along with donor specific transfusions has decreased the number of patients sensitized (Glass *et al.*, 1983; Hillis *et al.*, 1986). However, recent evidence suggests that azathioprine may be ineffective if the patient already has cytotoxic antibodies against lymphocytes from several members of a normal panel (Salvatierra *et al.*, 1985). Certain groups of patients only may benefit from therapy with immunosuppressive drugs given along with donor specific transfusion.

In a different approach to the problem of sensitization prospective recipients of a one haplotype mismatched transplant received third party blood transfusions only (Frisk, Brynger and Sandberg, 1982; Opelz, 1984). Transplant survival similar to that achieved with donor specific transfusion was reported and sensitization rates were lower since the patient had not been exposed to donor antigens. Donor specific transfusion may not therefore be the only method of improving survival of one haplotype mismatched living related transplants.

6.5 BLOOD TRANSFUSION AND THE INCIDENCE OF GROWTH, METASTASIS AND RECURRENCE OF TUMOURS

The beneficial effects of blood transfusion on allograft survival may, it has been postulated, be expected to reduce the immune response to other antigens, for example, those produced by a tumour. The evidence supporting such a hypothesis is not yet definitive but preliminary experimental work on animal models and studies in man is available.

Francis and Shenton (1981) found an increased rate of growth of a chemically-induced sarcoma in rats given allogeneic blood transfusion but not in those given syngeneic blood. They also noted decreased lymphocyte reactivity (to purified protein derivative of old tuberculin (PPD) and phytohaemagglutinin (PHA)) and increased plasma suppressive activity after allogeneic blood transfusion. Other workers (Jeekel *et al.*, 1982), however, found the converse with a reduction in tumour growth after allogeneic transfusion both in radiation induced basal cell carcinoma and in a chemically-induced adenocarcinoma of the duodenum.

In man, the evidence for a transfusion effect is also conflicting. It has previously been noted (Matas *et al.*, 1975; Herr, Engen and Hostetler, 1979) that patients undergoing chronic haemodialysis have an increased incidence of carcinoma of the lung, kidney, stomach and colon. Such a predisposition may be related to the non-specific immunosuppression of uraemia but frequent exposure to blood transfusion may also be a factor. The effect of blood transfusion on human malignancies has been most extensively studied in patients with carcinoma of the colon. Several studies have now reported a decreased recurrence-free survival after colectomy and blood transfusion. Burrows and Tartter (1982), in a retrospective study, found a significantly reduced recurrence-free survival in patients with adenocarcinoma of the colon and rectum who had received peri-operative blood transfusion; all patients studied had undergone potentially curative resections. This trend was observed irrespective of clinical staging (by Dukes classification) or location of the tumour; others have subsequently confirmed these results (Blumberg, Agarwal and Chuang, 1985). There was no correlation in either study between patient survival and the number of units of blood given or the timing of the transfusions. Foster and colleagues (1985) observed a significantly poorer prognosis after 'curative' resection associated with blood transfusion irrespective of staging, age, histological differentiation, location or pre-operative haemoglobin. Foster, in collaboration with others (Hyman *et al.*, 1985) studying lung cancer patients also found a similar reduction in survival rate after lung resection requiring blood transfusion. In contrast, no adverse relationship between blood transfusion and outcome after mastectomy for breast cancer was noted (Foster, Foster and Costanza, 1984).

The studies on colonic malignancy have been criticized for including patients with rectal tumours; these frequently require longer, technically more difficult operations, involving a greater degree of manipulation which may predispose to metastatic seeding. For these reasons, blood transfusions are required more frequently (Taylor, 1985). Such tumours also have a significantly poorer prognosis than intra-abdominal lesions with the same Dukes' staging. Ota *et al.* (1985) examining the effect found no evidence that survival at either 5 or 10 years was altered by pre-operative blood transfusion. In this study, survival in those transfused patients with rectal tumours was reduced but not to a significant degree. A prospective trial, with a three year follow up period, could not confirm an adverse relationship between peri-operative blood transfusion and recurrence of colorectal cancer (Frankish *et al.*, 1985). Indeed Blair and Janvrin (1985) found the converse to be true, noting a protective effect of a high haemoglobin level and blood transfusion. This, they suggested, may be due to an anticoagulant effect since anticoagulation has been shown experimentally to prevent circulating malignant cells forming metastatic lesions.

It therefore seems an attractive hypothesis that random donor blood transfusion may lead to decreased immune responsiveness of a host to a tumour, but at present the evidence in man remains to be substantiated. Furthermore it is not known whether any such association is cause or effect – it is for example possible that patients with more advanced forms of malignancy require more blood. Blood loss and the need for transfusion may relate to the degree of manipulation during surgery. The amount of blood transfused may be only an indicator of other factors involving length of surgery and anaesthesia, either or both of which may have an effect on the immune system (Riddle, 1967; Jubert *et al.*, 1973).

Although there is as yet little objective evidence for an adverse effect of blood transfusion on malignancy a variety of possible immunomodulatory mechanisms have been proposed:

1. A non-specific immunosuppression mediated by increased suppressor cell and decreased natural killer T cell activity.
2. Changes in antibody response which may be specific unresponsiveness

due to the development of (a) anti-idiotypic antibodies against certain T cell clones or (b) the development of Fc blocking antibodies.

3. T cell responsiveness in mixed lymphocyte culture is suppressed by ferritin and there is an inverse relationship between serum ferritin and the ratio of helper:suppressor T cells.

In the present state of knowledge, however, caution should be exercised in the administration of blood transfusion to patients with colonic carcinoma. Prior autodonation by patients, the correction of anaemia with haematinics and strenuous efforts to prevent surgical bleeding may all be useful. Transfusion of frozen blood has theoretical but unproven advantages – it has a markedly reduced leukocyte content and causes less histocompatibility antigen isosensitization (Huggins *et al.*, 1973).

6.6 IS THERE A LINK BETWEEN SEMEN RELATED IMMUNO-SUPPRESSION AND BLOOD TRANSFUSION?

Although spermatozoa are highly immunogenic, antibody to sperm components is not usually demonstrable in men or women. Immune tolerance to sperm surface antigens should not normally occur since sperm do not develop until puberty. In males, the lack of antibody is thought to be due to the impermeability of the reproductive tract to immunocompetent cells, the 'blood-testis' barrier. If this barrier is breached, however, by vasectomy, anatomical abnormalities or inflammation, then such antibodies may be readily produced. The alimentary tract, however, is not so privileged and homosexual males are subject to exposure to sperm both orally and rectally. It is also surprising that although all sexually active women are exposed to an extensive antigen load, very few develop humoral immunity to sperm. This may be firstly because vaginal secretions flush away spermatozoa and reduce their numbers (Lord, Sensabaugh and Stites, 1977) and secondly because certain components of seminal fluid are immunosuppressive. There is also considerable phagocytosis of sperm in the genital tract. Moreover, unlike micro-organisms, spermatozoa are incapable of replicating and therefore of perpetuating an antigenic stimulus. Agglutinating antibodies to sperm in women may often be related to a breach in the intact mucosa of the genital tract. Thus high levels are demonstrable in patients with carcinoma of the cervix (Jones, Kaye and Ing, 1973). Increased titres in prostitutes may be related to high sperm load or the high incidence of genital infections (Schwimmer, Ustay and Behrman, 1967).

In situations in which spermatozoa may act as an antigenic stimulus they may indeed induce immune suppression similar to that attributed to blood transfusion. Several sperm surface antigens have been identified which may stimulate such immunomodulation. On their surfaces, sperm display ABO blood group antigens and also both Class I and Class II HLA histocompatibility antigens (Edwards, Ferguson and Coombs, 1964; Ingerslev, 1981). There is also evidence of antigenic cross-reactivity between spermatozoa and T lymphocytes (Mathur *et al.*, 1980). Such cross-reactivity was particularly marked with immature thymocytes but was less clear when mature circulating T lymphocytes were studied. Antigenic cross-reaction may therefore be related to early T cell differentiation antigens and may explain the lower circulating total lymphocyte count in women with antisperm antibody.

Interest in AIDS has recently prompted the study of humoral and cellular immune responses to spermatozoa in homosexual men. Such individuals have repeated exposure to spermatozoa via both intact and lacerated rectal and oral mucosae and a marked increase in incidence of antisperm antibodies. An ELISA technique showed that 28.6% of homosexual males studied had demonstrable IgG or IgM antisperm antibodies (Wolff and Schill, 1985) compared with 4% of a control population of male dermatology patients of proven fertility and 9.6% of infertile men.

The extent of immune dysregulation correlates with the degree of allogeneic stimulation by sperm (Mavligit *et al.*, 1984). In a group of 30 monogamously paired homosexual males 19 of 26 anal sperm recipients showed evidence of allogeneic immunization whereas 4 of 4 exclusive sperm donors did not. In 8 sperm recipients reduced effector/suppressor T cell ratios were found (Te/Ts<1.0): five of these men had evidence of antisperm antibodies; three had a functional T cell deficiency with a diminished graft versus host reaction. Furthermore a similar reduced effector/suppressor T cell ratio was observed in the female partner of a heterosexual pair practising anal intercourse.

Similar functional T cell impairment has been found by Shearer *et al.* (1984). None of those studied had symptoms of AIDS and the percentages of T helper and suppressor cells were the same as in a control group. In the homosexual group only one-third exhibited even a weak cytotoxic response to influenza virus compared to a strong response in the entire heterosexual group studied. Significantly higher levels of IgG antisperm antibody titres were found in sera from homosexual men when compared to sera from heterosexuals (Witkin and Sonnabend, 1983). In addition high levels of circulating immune complexes (CICs) were found in 61% of the homosexuals tested. Such CICs are known to react with Fc or complement receptors on T and B lymphocytes, both *in vivo* and *in vitro*, and thus modulate cellular and humoral immune responses. The presence of the IgG antibodies and CICs may either be due to frequent rectal and oral deposition of semen or to the high incidence of venereal disease. Indeed, the initial genital infection may cause lymphocyte sensitization to spermatozoa with subsequent rectal or oral deposition leading to a secondary response.

Evidence of elevated cytotoxic T lymphocyte (CTL) activity has been found in one study (Tung *et al.*, 1985). Two of 11 homosexuals studied, however, were HIV positive. Although there was no correlation with homosexual practices, there was a significant relationship between elevated CTL activity and (a) number of lifetime partners, (b) use of recreational drugs, (c) T_H/T_S ratio and (d) antibodies to hepatitis B surface antigen, cytomegalovirus and Epstein–Barr virus. Sera from several individuals contained considerable quantities of antigen–antibody complexes suggesting extensive allogeneic stimulation. Exposure to HIV did not appear to be related to either high or normal levels of CTL activity. The basis for such activity in homosexuals is unknown. However, it may be related to one or more of the following: (a) exposure to alloantigens in passive anogenital partners, (b) viral infections cross-reacting with HLA alloantigens (though this was not detectable in autologous controls) and (c) protozoal infections possessing lectin activity.

The absorption from the gastrointestinal tract of allogeneic specificities expressed on spermatozoa may induce changes in both cellular and humoral immunity similar to those produced by blood transfusion. In homosexuals, such alterations may play some part in the increased susceptibility to infections including HIV.

6.7 PREGNANCY – ROLE OF LEUKOCYTE TRANSFUSION FOR RECURRENT ABORTION

It has been suggested that a blocking antibody response induced by the conceptus helps to maintain normal pregnancy. This may be analogous to the beneficial effect of blood transfusion on subsequent renal transplantation.

Antibodies thought to be implicated in this protective response include (a) auto-anti-idiotypic antibodies binding to maternal T cell receptors for paternal HLA specificities (Suciu-Foca *et al.*, 1983), (b) anti-TLX (cross-reacting trophoblast-lymphocyte) antibodies stimulated by exposure to the trophoblast (Faulk and McIntyre, 1983) and (c) non-cytotoxic antibodies to the Fc receptor on paternal B cells (Power *et al.*, 1983). Such Fc receptor blocking antibodies are absent from the sera of women undergoing spontaneous abortion (Power *et al.*, 1983) suggesting an immunological basis for this condition. Indeed in most cases of recurrent abortion, no anatomical, chromosomal or endocrinological cause is found. Further evidence in favour of an immunological basis for spontaneous abortion is provided by the increased sharing of HLA antigens reported between women subject to recurrent spontaneous abortions and their partners (Gerencer *et al.*, 1978). Such HLA sharing has also been associated with neural tube defects and pre-eclamptic toxaemia (PET) (Schacter *et al.*, 1979).

The concept of protective antibodies in normal pregnancy is further supported by the decreased incidence of PET in women transfused before their first pregnancy. Moreover, women who have had a normal pregnancy may have spontaneous abortion or develop PET when pregnant by another man (Mowbray and Underwood, 1985).

The increased sharing of HLA antigens between women subject to recurrent abortion and their partners suggests that HLA incompatibility between partners may convey biological advantages perhaps perpetuating genetic diversity and also preventing lethal homozygous combinations early in pregnancy. HLA antigen sharing might therefore be responsible for the lack of a 'protective' blocking antibody response.

Animal studies are difficult to perform as abortion is uncommon in small animals. However CBA/J mice demonstrated a high degree of fetal resorption when mated with DBA/2J males. When spleen cells from BALB/c males (but not DBA/2J males) were infused the resorption rate fell from 23% to 5% (Chaouat *et al.*, 1985). This study also demonstrated the appearance of a factor suppressing the mixed lymphocyte reaction to the serum of the treated mice. Immunological factors therefore appear to be important in the maintenance of at least some pregnancies.

Beer *et al.*, (1981) took three couples sharing antigens at the HLA, A, B and D/DR loci (MLR non-responders) and sensitized the women intradermally with paternal leukocytes. Two of the three couples established pregnancies into the third trimester and one couple demonstrated reactivity in MLR.

Taylor and Faulk (1981) gave third party transfusions of leukocyte-enriched plasma to three women each of whom not only had a history of three previous spontaneous abortions but who also shared several HLA antigens with their husbands. They were transfused repeatedly pre- and post-conception from at least 16 different erythrocyte compatible donors. All three women had successful pregnancies producing normal babies with normal placentae.

Unander, Lindholm and Olding (1985) demonstrated reduced activity in MLR in the sera of 20 women subject to recurrent abortion transfused with third party blood containing leukocytes and erythrocytes. In this study three transfusions were given pre-pregnancy at intervals of 4–8 weeks. Unfortunately, no details of the subsequent pregnancies were given. Other studies have used paternal peripheral blood lymphocytes given by intradermal, subcutaneous and intravenous sites to immunize women with recurrent abortion. Such patients, without either detectable suppressive antibody activity in MLR or serological evidence of cytotoxic antibody were immunized with paternal lymphocytes on a single occasion (Mowbray *et al.*, 1983). Antipaternal antibodies were then demonstrable by MLR inhibition and the lymphocytotoxicity assay in all but two women. In the small group immunized pre-pregnancy, no further abortions occurred: those immunized while pregnant completed their pregnancies successfully apart from two women treated late in pregnancy. It may be argued that immunization with paternal cells would be unlikely to provide an antigenic stimulus not present on spermatozoa but the route of administration may be important. In this study there was no evidence of excessive HLA antigen sharing by aborting couples.

A later study (Mowbray *et al.*, 1985) adopted a double blind approach giving the patient either her own or her husband's leukocytes. Seventeen of 22 women given paternal cells compared with 10 of 27 controls had successful pregnancies. Pregnancy rates in both groups were similar. It has, however, been suggested (MacLeod, Power and Catto 1985) that the presence of cytotoxic antibodies to paternal lymphocytes, while indicative of a maternal immune response, may not provide even an indirect indicator that subsequent pregnancies will be successful since they occurred as frequently in those who became successfully pregnant as in those who subsequently aborted. Other workers (Reznikoff-Etievant *et al.*, 1985) also infused paternal lymphocytes, demonstrated a greater success rate giving several leukocyte injections and observed a correlation between antipaternal antibody (detected by microlymphocytotoxicity assay) production and successful pregnancy.

Theoretical problems, however, exist with such techniques – why should a protective immunological response follow infusion of paternal leukocytes and yet not be stimulated by spermatozoa or trophoblast? What is the mechanism of action of the infusions? While graft-versus-host (GVH) disease is a theoretical problem (Grogan, Broughton and Doyle, 1975) it has not been noted in any of the trials reported to date. Fortunately in such clinical trials, there has been no evidence of anti-erythrocyte antibodies, infection or anaphylactic reactions. In the double-blind trial (Mowbray *et al.*, 1985), 2 births were below the 10th centile for weight and one baby had a ventricular septal defect. One woman immunized with paternal cells had a genetically abnormal (trisomy 15) abortion but later without further treatment had a normal pregnancy.

It would appear that leukocyte infusions have a place in the management of recurrent spontaneous abortion. However, there continue to be reservations regarding potential adverse side effects particularly on other aspects of the immune system. Also the optimum route of immunization and whether third party or paternal cells should be used have yet to be determined.

In conclusion, blood transfusion along with infusion of other allogeneic material such as spermatozoa or lymphocytes may suppress the immune response. This may result in improved renal transplant survival or increase the chance of a successful pregnancy occurring. It is possible also that malignant tumour growth may be prompted and that diminished immune responsiveness may result in increased susceptibility to infection.

REFERENCES

Ammann, A. J., Cowan, M. J., Wara, D. W., Weintrub, P., Dritz, S., Goldman, H. and Perkins, H. A. (1983) Acquired immunodeficiency in an infant: possible transmission by means of blood products. *Lancet*, i, 956–8.

Andreani, T., Modigliani, R., Le Charpentier, Y., Galian, A., Brouet, J.-C., Liance, M., Lachance, J.-R., Messing, B. and Vernisse, B. (1983) Acquired immunodeficiency with intestinal cryptosporidiosis: possible transmission by Haitian whole blood. *Lancet*, i, 1187–91.

Bancroft, G. J., Shellam, G. R. and Chalmer, J. E. (1981) Genetic influences on the augmentation of natural killer (NK) cells during murine cytomegalovirus infection: correlation with patterns of resistance. *J. Immunol.*, **126**, 988–94.

Barry, J. M., Norman, D. J., Bohanon, L. L., Wetzsteon, P. and Fischer, S. (1985) Comparison of two donor-specific transfusion protocols. *Transplantation Proceedings*, **17**, 1072–4.

Beer, A. E., Quebbeman, J. F., Ayers, J. W. T. and Hawes, R. F. (1981) Major histocompatibility complex antigens, maternal and paternal immune responses and chronic habitual abortions in humans. *Am. J. Obstet. Gynaec.*, **141**, 987–99.

Binz, H., Soots, A., Nemlander, A., Wight, E., Fenner, M., Meier, B., Hayry, P. and Wigzell, H. (1982) Induction of specific transplantation tolerance via immunisation with donor specific idiotypes. *Ann. N. Y. Acad. Sci.*, **392**, 360–74.

Blair, S. D. and Janvrin, S. B. (1985) Relationship between cancer of the colon and blood transfusion. *Brit. Med. J.*, **290**, 1516–17.

Blumberg, N., Agarwal, M. M. and Chuang, C. (1985) Relations between recurrence of cancer of the colon and blood transfusions. *Brit. Med. J.*, **290**, 1037–9.

Briggs, J. D., Canavan, J. S. F., Dick, H. M., Hamilton, D. N. H., Kyle, K. F., MacPherson, S. G., Paton, A. M. and Titterington, D. M. (1978) Influence of HLA matching and blood transfusion on renal allograft survival. *Transplantation*, **25**, 80–5.

Brunner, F. B., Giesecke, B., Gurland, H. J., Jacobs, C. J., Parsons, F. M., Scharer, K., Seyffart, G., Spies, G. and Wing W. J. (1976) Combined report on regular dialysis and transplantation in Europe V, 1974, in *Dialysis, Transplantation, Nephrology* (ed. J. Moorhead, C. Mion and R. Baillod) Pitman Medical, London, pp. 3–64.

Burns, W. H. and Allison, A. C. (1975) In *The Antigens*, Vol. 3 (ed. M. Sela), New York, Academic Press.

Burrows, L. and Tartter, P. (1982) Effect of blood transfusions on colonic malignancy recurrence rate. *Lancet*, ii, 662.

Carlson, J., Hinricks, S., Bryant, M., Levy, M., Yamamoto, J., Yee, J., Gardner, M., Higgins, J., Peterson, N. and Holland, P. (1985) HTLV-III antibody screening of blood bank donors. *Lancet*, i, 523–4.

Catto, G. R. D., Carpenter, C. B., Strom, T. B. and Williams, R. M. (1977) Passive enhancement of rat renal allograft by antibodies to a non-SD (Ag-B) locus of the MHC analogous to Ia. *Transplantation Proceedings*, **9**, 957–60.

Chaouat, G., Kolb, J.-P., Kiger, N., Stanislawski, M. and Wegmann, T. G. (1985) Immunologic consequences of vaccination against abortion in mice. *J. Immunol.*, **134**, 1594–8.

Chapman, J. R., Fisher, M., Ting, A. and Morris, P. J. (1985) Platelet transfusion before renal transplantation in humans. *Transplantation Proceedings*, **17**, 1038–40.

Corry, R. J., West, R. C., Hunsicker, L. G., Schanbacher, B. A. and Lachenbruch, P. A.

(1980) Effect of timing of administration and quantity of blood transfusion on cadaver renal transplant survival. *Transplantation*, **30**, 425–8.

Curran, J. W., Lawrence, D. N., Jaffe, H., Kaplan, J. E., Zyla, L. D., Chamberland, M., Weinstein, R., Lui, K.-J., Schonberger, L. B., Spira, T. J., Alexander, W. J., Swinger, G., Amman, A., Solomon, S., Auerbach, D., Mildvan, D., Stoneburner, R., Jason, J. M., Haverkos, H. W. and Evatt, B. L. (1984) Acquired immunodeficiency syndrome (AIDS) associated with transfusions. *N. Engl. J. Med.*, **310**, 69–75.

Dorsch, S. E. and Roser, B. (1975) T cells mediate transplantation tolerance. *Nature, Lond.*, **258**, 223–5.

Edwards, R. G., Ferguson, L. C. and Coombs, R. R. A. (1964) Blood group antigens on human spermatozoa. *J. Reprod. Fert.*, **7**, 153–61.

Fabre, J. and Morris, P. J. (1972) The mechanism of specific immunosuppression of renal allograft rejection by donor strain blood. *Transplantation*, **14**, 634–40.

Fagnilli, L. and Singal, D. P. (1982) Blood transfusions may induce anti-T cell receptor antibodies in renal patients. *Transplantation Proceedings*, **14**, 319–21.

Faulk, W. P. and McIntyre, J. A. (1983) Immunological studies of human trophoblast: markers, subsets and functions. *Immunolog. Rev.*, **75**, 139–75.

Feduska, N. J., Vincenti, F., Amend, W. J., Duca, L., Cochrum, K. and Salvatierra, O. (1979) Do blood transfusions enhance the possibility of a compatible transplant? *Transplantation*, **27**, 35–8.

Feorino, P. M., Jaffe, H. W., Palmer, E., Peterman, T. A., Francis, D. P., Kalyanaraman, V. S., Weinstein, R. A., Stoneburner, R. L., Alexander, W. J., Raevsky, C., Getchell, J. P., Warfield, D., Haverkos, H. W., Kilbourne, B. W., Nicholson, J. K. A. and Curran, J. W. (1985) Transfusion-associated acquired immunodeficiency syndrome. *N. Engl. J. Med.*, **312**, 1293–7.

Festenstein, H., Sachs, J. A., Paris, A. M. I., Pegrum, G. D. and Moorhead, J. F. (1976) Influence of HLA matching and blood transplant group renal-graft recipients. *Lancet*, **i**, 157–61.

Foster, R. S., Costanza, M. C., Foster, J. C., Wanner, M. C. and Foster, C. B. (1985) Adverse relationship between blood transfusions and survival after colectomy for colon cancer. *Cancer*, **55**, 1195–201.

Foster, R. S., Jr, Foster, J. C. and Costanza, M. C. (1984) Blood transfusions and survival after surgery for breast cancer. *Arch. Surg.*, **119**, 1138–40.

Francis, D. M. A. and Shenton, B. K. (1981) Blood transfusion and tumour growth: evidence from laboratory animals. *Lancet*, **ii**, 871.

Frankish, P. D., McNee, R. K., Alley, P. G. and Woodfield, D. G. (1985) Relation between cancer of the colon and blood transfusions. *Brit. Med. J.*, **290**, 1827.

Frisk, B., Brynger, H. and Sandberg, L. (1982) Two random transfusions before primary renal transplantation. *Transplantation Proceedings*, **14**, 386–8.

Gallo, R. C., Sarin, P., Gelman, E. P., Robert-Guroff, M., Richardson, E., Kalyanaraman, V. S., Mann, D., Sidhu, G. D., Stahl, R. E., Zola-Pazner, S., Leibowitch, J. and Popovic, M. (1983) Isolation of human T cell leukaemia virus in acquired immune deficiency syndrome (AIDS). *Science*, **220**, 865–7.

Gardner, B., Harris, K. R., Digard, N. J., Gosling, D., Campbell, M. J., Tate, D. G., Sharman, V. L. and Slapak, M. (1985) Do recipients of a cadaveric renal allograft on cyclosporine require prior transfusions? Experience in a single unit. *Transplantation Proceedings*, **17**, 1032–3.

Gascon, P., Zoumbas, N. C. and Young, N. S. (1984) Immunologic abnormalities in patients receiving multiple blood transfusions. *Ann. Intern. Med.*, **100**, 173–7.

Gerencer, M., Kastelan, A., Drazanic, A., Kerhin-Brkljacicic, V. and Madjaric, M.

(1978) The HLA antigens in women with recurrent abnormal pregnancies of unknown aetiology. *Tissue Antigens*, **12**, 223–7.

Glass, N. R., Miller, D. J., Sallinger, H. W. and Belzer, F. O. (1983) Comparative analysis of the DST and Imuran-plus-DST protocols for live donor renal transplantation. *Transplantation*, **36**, 636–41.

Gordon, R. J. (1983) Factor VIII products and disordered immune regulation. *Lancet*, **i**, 991.

Gordon, R. J. (1984) More on blood transfusion and AIDS. *N. Engl. J. Med.*, **312**, 1742.

Grogan, T. M., Broughton, D. D. and Doyle, W. F. (1975) Graft-versus-host reaction (GVHR). A case report suggesting GVHR occurred as a result of maternofetal cell transfer. *Arch. Path.*, **99**, 330–4.

Groopman, J. E., Salahuddin, S. Z., Mangalasseril, G., *et al.*, (1984) Virologic studies in a case of transfusion-associated AIDS. *N. Engl. J. Med.*, **311**, 1419–23.

Hall, B. M., Roser, B. J. and Dorsch, S. E. (1979) A model for study of the cellular mechanisms that maintain long-term enhancement of cardiac graft survival. *Transplantation Proceedings*, **11**, 958–61.

Herr, H. W., Engen, D. E. and Hostetler, J. (1979) Malignancy in uraemia: dialysis versus transplantation. *J. Urol.*, **121**, 584–5.

Hillis, A. N., Duguid, J., Evans, C. M., Bome, J. M. and Sells, R. A. (1986) Three year experience of donor specific transfusion DST and concomitant cyclosporin A (CyA). *Abstracts British Transplantation Society*, April 1986, p. 22.

van Hooff, J. P., Kalff, M. W. and van Poelgeest, A. E. (1976) Blood transfusions and kidney transplantation. *Transplantation*, **22**, 306–7.

Huggins, C. E., Russell, P. S., Winn, P. J. *et al.* (1973) Frozen blood in transplant patients: Hepatitis and HLA isosensitisation. *Transplantation Proceedings*, **5**, 809–12.

Hutchinson, I. V. and Morris, P. J. (1986) The role of major and minor histocompatibility antigens in active enhancement of rat kidney allograft survival by blood transfusion. *Transplantation*, **41**, 166–70.

Hyman, N. H., Foster, R. S. Jr., De Mueles, D. E. and Costanza, M. C. (1985) Blood transfusions and survival after lung cancer resection. *Am. J. Surg.*, **149**, 502–7.

Ingerslev, H. J. (1981) Antibodies against spermatozoal surface membrane antigens in female infertility. *Acta Obstetricia et Gynaecologica Scandinavica*, Supplement 100.

Jason, J., Hilgartner, M., Holman, R. C., Dixon, G., Spira, T. J., Aledort, L. and Evatt, B. (1985) Immune status of blood product recipients. *JAMA*, **253**, 1140–5.

Jeekel, J., Eggermont, A., Heystek, G. and Marquet, R. (1982) Inhibition of tumour growth by blood transfusions. *Europ. Surg. Res.*, **14**, 124–5.

Jenkins, A. M. and Woodruff, M. F. (1971) The effect of prior administration of donor strain blood or blood constituents on the survival of cardiac allografts in rats. *Transplantation*, **12**, 57–60.

Jerne, N. K. (1974) Towards a network theory of the immune system. *Annal. Immunolog. (Institute Pasteur)*, **125C**, 373–89.

Jones, W. R., Kaye, M. D. and Ing, R. M. Y. (1973) Sperm microagglutinating activity in the serum of patients with carcinoma of the cervix. *Am. J. Obstet. Gynec.*, **116**, 883–4.

Jubert, A. V., Lee, E. T., Hersh, E. M. and McBride, C. M. (1973) Effects of surgery, anaesthesia and intraoperative blood loss on immunocompetence. *J. Surg. Res.*, **15**, 399–403.

Kaplan, J., Sarnack, S., Gitlin, J. and Lusler, J. (1984) Diminished helper/suppressor lymphocyte ratios and natural killer activity in recipients of repeated blood transfusions. *Blood*, **64**, 308–10.

Kaplan, J., Sarnack, S. and Levy, J. (1985) Transfusion-induced immunologic abnormalities not related to AIDS virus. *N. Engl. J. Med.*, **313**, 1227.

Kessler, C. M., Schulof, R. S., Goldstein, A., Naylor, P. H., Luban, N. W. C., Kelleher, J. F. and Reaman, G. H. (1983) Abnormal T lymphocyte subpopulations associated with transfusions of blood-derived products. *Lancet*, **i**, 991–2.

Klintmalm, G., Brynger, H., Flatmark, A., Frodin, W., Husberg, B., Thorsby E. and Groth, C. G. (1985) The blood transfusion, DR matching and mixed lymphocyte culture effects are not seen in cyclosporine-treated renal transplant recipients. *Transplantation Proceedings*, **17**, 1026–31.

Kornfeld, H., Vande Stave, R. A., Lange, M., Reddy, M. and Grieco, M. H. (1982) T-lymphocyte subpopulations in homosexual men. *N. Engl. J. Med.*, **74**, 433–41.

Lenhard, J., Masen, G., Seifert, R., Johannsen, R. and Grosse-Wilde, H. (1982) Characterisation of transfusion-induced suppressor cells in prospective kidney allograft recipients. *Transplantation Proceedings*, **14**, 329–32.

Lord, E. M., Sensabaugh, G. F. and Stites, D. P. (1977) Immunosuppressive activity of human seminal plasma. *J. Immunol.*, **118**, 1704–11.

Luban, N. L. C., Kelleher, J. F. and Reaman, G. H. (1983) Altered distribution of T-lymphocyte subpopulations in children and adolescents with haemophilia. *Lancet*, **1**, 503–5.

Ludlam, C. A., Tucker, J., Steel, C. M., Tedder, R. S., Cheingsong-Popov, R., Weiss, R. A., McClelland, D. B. L., Philip, I. and Prescot, R. J. (1985) Human T-lymphotopic virus type III (HTLVIII) infection in seronegative haemophiliacs after transfusion of factor VIII. *Lancet*, **ii**, 233–6.

MacLeod, A. M., Mason, R. J., Stewart, K. N., Power, D. A., Shewan W. G., Edward, N. and Catto, G. R. D. (1982a) Association of Fc receptor-blocking antibodies and human renal transplant survival. *Transplantation*, **34**,

MacLeod, A. M., Mason, R. J., Shewan, W. G., Power, D. A., Stewart K. N., Edward, N. and Catto, G. R. D. (1982b) Possible mechanism of action of transfusion effect in renal transplantation. *Lancet*, **ii**, 468–70.

MacLeod, A. M., Catto, G. R. D., Mather, A., Mason, R., Stewart, K. N., Power, D. A., Shewan, G. and Urbaniak, S. (1985) Beneficial antibodies in renal transplantation developing after blood transfusion: evidence for HLA linkage. *Transplantation Proceedings*, **17**, 1057–8.

MacLeod, A. M., Power, D. A. and Catto, G. R. D. (1985) Pregnancy after treatment with paternal lymphocytes. *Lancet*, **ii**, 508.

Maki, T., Okazaki, H., Wood, M. L. and Monaco, A. P. (1981) Suppressor cells in mice bearing intact skin allografts after blood transfusions. *Transplantation*, **32**, 463–6.

Marquet, R. L., Heystek, G. A., Niessen, G. J. C. M. and Jeekel, J. (1982) Induction of suppressor cells by a single blood transfusion in rats. *Transplantation Proceedings*, **14**, 397–9.

Matas, A. J., Simmons, R. L., Kjellstrand, C. M., Buselmeier, T. J. and Najarian, J. S. (1975) Increased incidence of malignancy during chronic renal failure. *Lancet*, **i**, 883–6.

Matheson, D. S., Green, B. J., Poon, M. C., Fritzler, M. J., Hoar, D. I. and Bowen, T. J. (1986) Natural killer cell activity from hemophiliacs exhibits differential responses to various forms of interferon. *Blood*, **67**, 164–7.

Mathur, S., Goust, J.-M., Williamson, H. O. and Fudenberg, H. H. (1980) Antigenic cross-reactivity of sperm and T-lymphocytes. *Fertility and Sterility*, **34**, 469–76.

Mavligit, G. M., Talpaz, M., Hsia, F. T., Wong, W., Lichtiger, B., Mansel, P. W. A. and Mumford, D. M. (1984) Chronic immune stimulation by sperm alloantigens. *JAMA*, **251**, 237–41.

Mendez, R., Iwaki, T., Mendez, R. G., Bogaard, T., Volpicelli, M., Self, B. (1982) Seventeen consecutive one-haplotype matched living related transplants using donor-specific blood transfusions. *Transplantation*, **33**, 621–4.

Mowbray, J. F., Gibbings, C. R., Sidgwick, A. S., Ruskiewicz, M. and Beard, R. W. (1983) Effects of transfusion in women with recurrent spontaneous abortion. *Transplantation Proceedings*, **XV**, 896–9.

Mowbray, J. F., Gibbings, C., Liddell, H., Reginald, P. W., Underwood, J. L. and Beard, R. W. (1985) Controlled trial of treatment of recurrent spontaneous abortion by immunisation with paternal cells. *Lancet*, **i**, 9412–3.

Mowbray, J. F. and Underwood, J. L. (1985) Immunology of abortion. *Clin. Exp. Immunol.*, **60**, 1–7.

Muller, J. Y., Kaplan, C., Betuel, H., Bignan, J. D., Fauchet, R., Gluckman, J. C., Soulillou, J. P. and Thilbault, P. H. (1982) Effet des transfusions sanguines sur les greffes de rein. *Nouvelle Presse Medicale*, **11**, 3697–701.

National Organ Matching Service, United Kingdom (1975) Annual Report 1974–1975, Bristol, England.

Opelz, G. (1984) In *Kidney Transplantation: Principles and Practice* (ed. P. J. Morris), Grune and Stratton, London, Chap. 16.

Opelz, G. (1985) Effect of HLA matching, blood transfusions and presensitisation in cyclosporine-treated kidney transplant recipients. For the Collaborative Transplant Study, 1985. *Transplantation Proceedings*, **17**, 2179–83.

Opelz, G. and Terasaki, P. I. (1980) Dominant effect of transfusions on kidney graft survival. *Transplantation*, **29**, 153–8.

Opelz, G. and Terasaki, P. I. (1982) International study of histocompatibility in renal transplantation. *Transplantation*, **33**, 87–95.

Opelz, G., Mickey, M. R., Sengar, D. P. S. and Terasaki, P. I. (1973) Effect of blood transfusions on subsequent kidney transplants. *Transplantation Proceedings*, **5**, 253–9.

Opelz, G., Graner, B., Mickey, M. R. and Terasaki, P. I. (1981) Lymphocytotoxic antibody responses to transfusions in potential kidney transplant recipients. *Transplantation*, **32**, 177–83.

Ota, D., Alvarez, L., Lichtiger, B., Giacco, G. and Guinee, V. (1985) Perioperative blood transfusion in patients with colon carcinoma. *Transfusion*, **25**, 392–4.

Penn, I. (1977) Development of cancer as a complication of clinical transplantation. *Transplantation Proceedings*, **9**, 1121–7.

Persijn, G., Cohen, G. and Landsbergen, Q. (1979) Retrospective and prospective studies on the effect of transplantation in the Netherlands. *Transplantation*, **28**, 396–401.

Persijn, G. G., van Leeuwen, A., Parlevliet, J., Cohen, B., Landsbergen, Q., D'Amaro, J. and van Rood, J. J. (1981) Two major factors influencing kidney graft survival in Eurotransplant: HLA-DR matching and blood transfusion. *Transplantation Proceedings*, **13**, 150–4.

Power, D. A., Catto, G. R. D., Mason, R. J. and MacLeod, A. M. (1983) The fetus as an allograft: Evidence for protective antibodies to HLA-linked paternal antigens. *Lancet*, **ii**, 701–4.

Raftery, M. J., Lang, C. J., Schwarz, G., O'Shea, J., Varghese, Z., Sweny, P., Fernando, O. N. and Moorhead, J. F. (1985a) Failure of azathioprine to prevent sensitisation due to third party transfusion. *Transplantation Proceedings*, **17**, 1044–6.

Raftery, M. J., Lang, C. J., Schwarz, G., O'Shea, J. M., Varghese, Z., Sweny, P., Fernando, O. N. and Moorhead, J. F. (1985b) Prevention of sensitisation resulting from third party transfusion. *Transplantation Proceedings*, **17**, 2499–500.

Reznikoff-Etievant, M. F., Simonney, N., Janaud, D., Darbois, Y. and Netter, A. (1985) Treatment of recurrent spontaneous abortions by immunization with paternal leukocytes. *Lancet*, **i**, 1398.

Riddle, P. R. (1967) Disturbed immune reactions following surgery. *Brit. J. Surg.*, **54**, 882–6.

van Rood, J. J., Balner, H. and Morris, P. J. (1978) Blood transfusion and transplantation. *Transplantation*, **26**, 275–7.

Salvatierra, O., Vincenti, F. and Amend, W. (1980) Deliberate donor-specific blood transfusions prior to living related renal transplantation. *Ann. Surg.*, **192**, 543–51.

Salvatierra, O., Melzer, J., Potter, D., Garovay, M., Vincenti, F., Amend, W. J. C., Husing, R., Hopper, S. and Feduska, N. J. (1985) A seven year experience with donor-specific blood transfusions. *Transplantation*, **40**, 659–62.

Schacter, B., Gyves, A., Muir, A. and Tasin, M. (1979) HLA-A, B compatibility in parents of offspring with neural tube defects of couples experiencing involuntary fetal wastage. *Lancet*, **i**, 796–9.

Schwimmer, W. B., Ustay, K. A. and Behrman, S. J. (1967) Sperm-agglutinating antibodies and decreased fertility in prostitutes. *Obstet. Gynaec.*, **30**, 192–200.

Seidl, S. and Kuhnl, P. (1985) HTLV-III antibody screening in German blood donors. *Lancet*, **i**, 1047.

Seligmann, M., Chess, L., Fahey, J. L., Fauci, A. S., Lachmann, P. J., L'Age-Stehr, J., Ngu, J., Pinching, A. J., Rosen, F. S., Spira, T. J. and Wybran, J. (1984) AIDS – An immunologic revaluation. *N. Engl. J. Med.*, **311**, 1286–92.

Shearer, G. M., Payne, S. M., Joseph, L. J. and Biddison, W. E. (1984) Functional T lymphocyte immune deficiency in a population of homosexual men who do not exhibit symptoms of Acquired Immune Deficiency Syndrome. *J. Clin. Invest.*, **74**, 496–506.

Sheil, A. G. R., Flarel, S., Disney, A. P. S. and Mathew, T. H. (1985) Cancer in dialysis and transplant patients. *Transplantation Proceedings*, **17**, 195–8.

Simmons, R. L., van Hook, E. J., Yunis, E. J., Noreen, H., Kjellstrand, C. M., Condie, R. M., Mauer, S. M., Buselmeier, T. and Najarian, J. S. (1977) 100 sibling transplants followed 2 to 7 1/2 years. A multifactorial analysis. *Ann. Surg.*, **185**, 196–204.

Singal, D. P., Joseph, S. and Ludwin, D. (1985) Blood transfusions, suppressor cells and anti-idiotypic antibodies. *Transplantation Proceedings*, **17**, 1104–7.

Solheim, B. G., Flatmark, A., Halvorsen, S., Jervell, J., Pope, J. and Thorsby, E. (1980) The effect of blood transfusions on renal transplantation. Studies of 395 patients registered for transplantation with a first cadaveric kidney. *Tissue Antigens*, **16**, 377–86.

Stiller, C. R., Lockwood, B. L., Sinclair, N. R., Ulan, R. A., Sheppard, R. R., Sharpe, J. A. and Mayman, P. (1978) Beneficial effect of operation day blood transfusions on human renal allograft survival. *Lancet*, **i**, 169–70.

Suciu-Foca, N., Reed, E., Rohowsky, C., Kung, P.and King, D. W. (1983) Anti-idiotypic antibodies to anti-HLA receptors induced by pregnancy. *Proc. Natl Acad. Sci., USA*, 80, 830–4.

Suthanthiran, M., Catto, G. R. D., Kaldary, A., George, K., Garavoy, M. R., Strom, T.

B. and Carpenter, C. B. (1979) Differential antibody responses to AgB (A region) and Ia (B region) antigens during enhancement of rat renal allografts. *Transplantation*, **28**, 4–9.

Taylor, I. (1985) Relation between cancer of the colon and blood transfusion. *Brit. Med. J.*, **290**, 1516.

Taylor, C. and Faulk, W. P. (1981) Prevention of recurrent abortion with leukocyte infusions. *Lancet*, **ii**, 68–70.

Terasaki, P. I., Kreisler, M. and Mickey, R. M. (1971) Presensitisation and kidney transplant failure. *Postgrad. Med. J.*, **47**, 89–100.

Tung, K. S. K., Koster, F., Bernstein, D. C. Kriebel, P. W., Payne, S. M. and Shearer, G. M. (1985) Elevated allogeneic cytotoxic T lymphocyte activity in peripheral blood leukocytes of homosexual men. *J. Immunol.*, **135**, 3163–71.

Unander, A. M., Lindholm, A. and Olding, L. B. (1985) Blood transfusions generate/increase previously absent/weak blocking antibody in women with spontaneous abortion. *Fertility and Sterility*, **44**, 766–71.

Vilmer, E., Rouzioux, C., Vezinet-Brun, F., Fischer, A., Cherman, J. C., Barre-Sinoussi, F., Gazengal, C., Dauguet, C., Manigne, P., Griscelli, C. and Montagnier, L. (1984) Isolation of new lymphotopic retrovirus from two siblings with haemophilia B, one with AIDS. *Lancet*, **i**, 753–7.

Weiss, S. H., Mann, D. L., Murray, C. and Popovic, M. (1985) HLA DR antibodies and ELISA testing. *Lancet*, **ii**, 157.

Werner-Favre, C., Jeannet, M., Harder, F. and Montandon, A. (1979) Blood transfusions, cytotoxic antibodies and kidney graft survival. *Transplantation*, **28**, 343–6.

Williams, K. A., Ting, A., Cullen, P. R. and Morris, P. J. (1979) Transfusions: their influence on human renal graft survival. *Transplantation Proceedings*, **11**, 175–8.

Witkin, S. S. and Sonnabend, J. (1983) Immune responses to spermatozoa in homosexual men. *Fertility and Sterility*, **39**, 337–42.

Wolff, H. and Schill, W. B. (1985) Antisperm antibodies in infertile and homosexual men. Relationship to serologic and clinical findings. *Fertility and Sterility*, **44**, 673–77.

Yamauchi, J., Yamada, Y., Otsubo, O., Takahashi, I., Sugimoto, H., Kusaba, K., Sakai, A. and Inou, T. (1983) Prolongation of kidney transplant survival by donor specific blood transfusion. *Transplantation Proceedings*, **15**, 923–34.

7

Serological tests

— *Philip P. Mortimer* —

7.1 INTRODUCTION

It is now accepted that AIDS is one of many clinical and pathological manifestations of an increasingly widespread infection due to the retrovirus, Human Immunodeficiency Virus (HIV). To understand the impact of this new virus on blood transfusion and blood products it is essential to realize that infection with HIV is persistent both in the individual and the community, and that the virus has already, within 5 years, attained epidemic proportions in sections of Western society, as well as in whole populations in Central Africa. There is also evidence that the infection is spreading rapidly in parts of South America, and reports that it has established itself in Eastern Europe and in Asia. As a result, any rational approach to the problem of HIV infection in blood and blood products must be grounded on a sound, up-to-date knowledge both of the natural history of HIV infection in the individual and of its epidemiology in the community from which the blood has been derived. In view of the very diverse origins of plasma used in the commercial manufacture of blood products the nearly universal spread of the virus is a particularly significant development. As will be shown in this chapter, screening tests for antibody to HIV (anti-HIV) have reached a remarkable level of accuracy and these tests go some way in ensuring the safety of blood and blood products; but they remain an indirect and insecure means of screening for HIV infection. No laboratory test, however sensitive, will remove the basic obligation in blood procurement to select donors who are fit and, wherever possible, to treat the products of donated blood in such a way as to make them safe. At its best the use of blood is a potentially risky business. In the face of the AIDS epidemic unstinted efforts must be made to make blood safe by every possible means.

Those responsible for the therapeutic use of blood are therefore obliged to acquaint themselves with all aspects of the pathology and epidemiology of

HIV infection. HIV is by far the most important recognized infection transmitted by blood and, without its timely discovery as the cause of AIDS in 1983 and 1984, it would by now have totally disrupted blood transfusion and the provision of blood products. Moreover, HIV may yet cause havoc in blood transfusion unless careful measures are applied and continuous vigilance shown. In various ways the virus continues to threaten the composure and well-being not just of blood recipients and donors, but of the professionals whose job it is to procure, process and supply blood and its products. The problems HIV poses are soluble if extra resources and dedication are applied, but any attempt to cut corners technically, or to relax the stringent measures increasingly coming into force to select donors will prove very costly in the longer run. HIV is going to persist as a serious problem for the individual and community as a whole, and therefore for blood donors and recipients.

7.2 THE TECHNICAL CHALLENGE

Screening of blood donations for virus infection has until recently been dominated by the now familiar transfusion hazard of hepatitis B virus (HBV), and it is instructive to compare the problems of HBV and HIV diagnosis. Most infections with HBV are accompanied by the production in gross excess of the surface protein, HBsAg. HBsAg, unlike antibodies to it or to the other main antigenic proteins of HBV, is already present in blood at an early stage of infection, before clinical or liver function abnormalities appear and even if the infection proves to be totally subclinical. In almost all cases HBsAg continues to be detectable for as long as the individual remains infectious. Rarely is a blood donation that is HBsAg negative by the most sensitive tests found capable of transmitting HBV infection and, if this does happen, antibody to the core or the 'e' protein of HBV is detectable in the donation. In contrast, recognition of HIV infection in blood donations has not attained the accuracy of hepatitis B testing. The underlying reason for this is not any lack of technical sophistication, but the differences in the nature of the markers of infection generated by HIV.

A virus may leave its footprints in the cells it infects, be free in body fluids or release products which can be detected in those fluids. It can also elicit specific, measurable responses from the immune system in the form of antibodies. Though data is sketchy for HIV, it appears that only a few specialized cells are infected with HIV at any one time, that free virus is not abundant and that viral antigens are not easy to detect or persistent, probably because they are complexed with antibody. Of the possible viral markers only the anti-HIV response is readily detectable, and it is far and away the most useful sign of infection. However, its absence does not guarantee freedom from HIV infection, and no matter how good anti-HIV tests have and may become they will never alone be as effective in detecting HIV infectivity as are HBsAg tests in detecting HBV infectivity (CDC, 1986).

The point can be illustrated by considering the natural history of HIV. With the exception of recipients of clotting factor concentrates (whose antibody response to HIV infection is often delayed (Ludlam *et al.*, 1985), a composite view of the way that individuals respond to HIV infection has begun to emerge. A week or two after exposure a viraemia begins which is detectable by reverse transcriptase production when buffy coat cells are cultured *in vitro*. Viraemia is also implied by the presence of viral antigen (probably mostly core protein, p24) in blood collected soon after exposure (Goudsmit *et al.*, 1986). Four to six weeks after exposure anti-HIV typically becomes detectable. The precise specificities of the early immune response have not been well characterized. Using Western blot analysis some workers have detected antibody to the envelope proteins (p120, p160) first, but others antibody to core protein fragments, especially p24. The order in which these antibodies seem to appear may depend upon the sensitivity of the various tests used to detect them and their ability to discriminate between them; but discrepancy may also arise from the problem of transferring high molecular weight viral proteins to nitrocellulose strips for Western blotting. If these are not represented on the strips antibody to them cannot be detected. There may, too, be real differences between infected individuals. The specific reactions also have to be distinguished from other Western blot findings, usually single bands at the p24 position, that are non-specific (Biberfeld *et al.*, 1986). A month or two later in true infection a characteristic pattern of other antibodies appears, demonstrable by Western blot or radio-immunoprecipitation tests. At the same time the antibody response is increasing in titre so that the signal in all types of antibody test is becoming stronger. Thus for a period of at least six months the anti-HIV response increases, making the recognition of specific infection more definite and the diagnosis more secure.

In the course of most virus infections the molecular size of specific immunoglobulin molecules changes. IgM antibodies appear earliest, quickly attain maximum concentration in serum, and then disappear or persist only at low titres. IgM anti-HIV has begun to be investigated, particularly as it might be indicative of the early stage of HIV infection, and preliminary evidence suggests that its appearance precedes other anti-HIV immunoglobulins (Parry and Mortimer, 1986); but IgM is technically quite demanding to measure. Moreover, because exposure to, and primary disease associated with HIV is often hard to recognize with precision it is difficult to correlate IgM anti-HIV with the development of infection or even to establish the specificity of tests used to measure it. The importance of specific IgM is that it might allow infectious blood to be identified before it could be detected by tests for other HIV antibodies.

There is now incontrovertible evidence that the blood of HIV-infected individuals is persistently infectious. This is based on epidemiological observation and on continual isolation of virus from many subjects. It is also known that anti-HIV is continuously present, though neither in the case of virus nor antibody is there good data about changes in titre. Viral titres, in particular, may be fluctuant and it has been suggested recently that viral antigen and probably infectiousness may be more prominent early in infection and when AIDS has developed (Lange, *et al.*, 1986). If true, this implies that a strong and diverse antibody response may limit infectiousness. While this may have little effect on the transmissibility of HIV in large volumes of blood, it has some bearing on transmission by inoculation, by sexual exposure and through the administration of blood products in which any virus present will have been depleted by manufacturing processes. The presence of anti-HIV also hampers laboratory attempts to measure viral antigens.

In summary, then, the markers of HIV infection are the virus itself, its antigens, and antibodies to them of various classes and specificities. Of these the most readily measurable and persistent, albeit indirect markers, are antibodies. These are present in several body fluids but their titre is highest in serum and plasma which, to the blood transfuser at least, are readily accessible fluids to do diagnostic tests on. The challenge to him is to establish in his laboratory the best means of detecting these antibodies. For this reason, this chapter mostly deals with the detection of anti-HIV in serum and plasma: the methods, their accuracy, and the way that they should be applied. Where they are of actual or potential importance, however, diagnostic tests other than those for antibody will be touched upon.

7.3 TESTS FOR ANTI-HIV

7.3.1 Sources of antigen

Common to all antibody assays is the need for a reliable and plentiful source of antigen. In the case of HIV this was first provided by a continuous line of human T lymphocytes growing in suspension culture infected with an HIV strain by Popovic and colleagues. They refer to the line as H9/3 and to the HIV virus as Human T cell Lymphotropic Virus III (Popovic *et al.*, 1984). More recently lymphocyte lines such as CEM have been persistently infected with other strains of HIV, such as lymphadenopathy associated virus (Barré-Sinoussi *et al.*, 1983) and AIDS associated retrovirus (Levy *et al.*, 1986). 'In house' and commercial assays for anti-HIV have been based on antigens prepared from these infected cell lines. There is no evidence of significant strain variation that would make it difficult to detect an antibody to one HIV strain with an assay based on antigen prepared from a different strain (though refer to the section below on new types, HTLV-IV, LAV-II, etc). Moreover the antigenic yield from these infected cell lines is, generally speaking, good; but it is difficult to purify HIV antigens from cell lines and at the same time preserve the full range of viral proteins. Purification involves a range of high speed differential centrifugations and other protein separation procedures, and usually entails chemical inactivation. During these stages viral protein concentrations are diminished, and particular proteins may be lost. What is more, chemical treatment will modify antigenic structure and the end product will contain small amounts of cellular proteins that may act as antigens.

Another approach to this problem of antigenic purity is to use antibody to HIV, and especially monoclonal antibody, to select out the relevant antigens from crude preparations of virus grown in cell culture. Some of the solid phase assays described below adopt this approach, though the problems of antigenic purity and specificity are not wholly avoided thereby. In fact, they are merely transferred to the 'capture' anti-HIV, which must be purely or at least predominantly specific for HIV.

A third possible approach to antigen preparation is to use recombinant DNA techniques to clone parts of the HIV genome in prokaryotic or eukaryotic cells and get expression of proteins that will act as HIV antigens. Partly because the same avenue is being used to produce candidate vaccine proteins, cloned HIV protein antigens are beginning to be made. Once again, there must be reservations. These proteins are probably antigenically incomplete, narrower in spectrum than antigen derived from cell culture and, though free from tissue culture antigens, likely to be contaminated with vector proteins, e.g. antigens of *Escherichia coli*.

The differences in the performance of apparently similar commercial kits for anti-HIV are probably attributable in large part to differences in antigen production. Commercial production procedures are not freely discussed and this is one of the most difficult features of HIV testing to control. In addition, there are many sources of antigen: various producer cell lines infected with different isolates of HIV, cloned proteins, and new novel human retrovirus types including some associated with AIDS-like disease (Kanki *et al.*, 1986; Clavel *et al.*. 1986). These differences between antigens introduce many variables and, from the point of view of the blood transfuser, diversity that is confusing and unwelcome. The transfuser may well take the view that a single versatile antigen is needed to use in one comprehensive test. Unfortunately, however, the trend is at present away from this, and is likely to continue in this direction at least until the whole antigenic spectrum of AIDS viruses and the antibody responses to them have been teased apart. At that point it may be possible to reassemble the antigens of HIV and related retroviruses and make them available to the transfusion community in a single, simple, screening assay.

7.3.2 Anti-HIV test methodology

A broad understanding is easily acquired of the way that anti-HIV assays are built, the order in which the reagents are applied and the method by which the signal is read, and this will be invaluable to those who have to choose between commercial kits and resolve the conflicts that arise when discrepancies occur. Most commercial and non-commercial assays are based on reactions on a polystyrene or other surface ('solid phase' assays), and these assays can be allotted to four types according to their structure (Fig. 7.1).

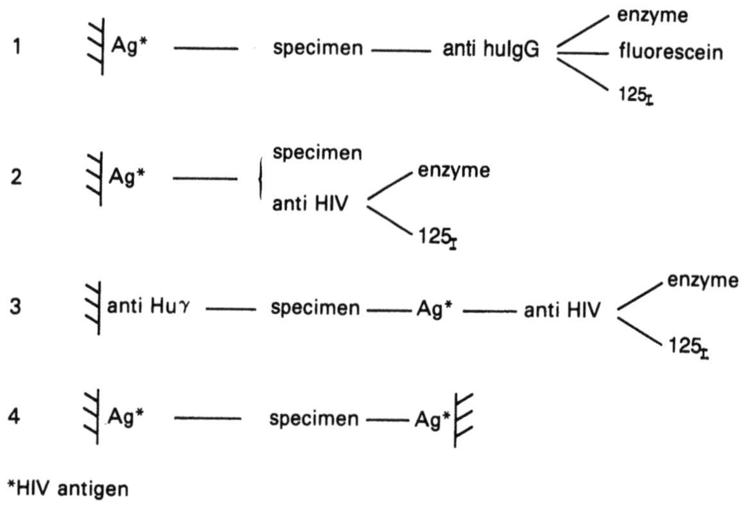

Figure 7.1 Four types of assay for anti-HIV.

7.3.3 Type I assays

In type I assays, virus antigen is immobilized on a solid phase, a serum specimen is applied and washed off, and then an antibody to human immunoglobulin G (anti huIgG) is added that has been tagged with fluorescein, an enzyme, or a radioactive isotope (Fig. 7.1). This gives a signal in ultra-violet light, in the presence of a chromogenic substrate, or by the measurement of bound radioactivity. In its simplest form the type I assay is a cytoplasmic immunoflourescence (IF) assay done on HIV infected cells dried and acetate-fixed onto glass slides. Another form of IF assay is done in live cells ('membrane' immunofluorescence) in which case antigenic sites on the cell surface are the target for anti-HIV in the specimen. A variation of fixed cell IF that has attracted some interest because the assay can be read by the naked eye, employs a peroxidase tagged anti huIgG reagent or a peridoxasetagged staphylococcal A protein to detect the binding of huIgG (Karpas *et al.*, 1985).

The advantages of IF, especially of fixed cell IF and its peroxidase based alternative, are speed, cheapness and convenience (Table 7.1). Though commercial IF kits have been devised, most diagnostic virus laboratories can prepare these slides from their own resources and use them to detect anti-HIV. However, there are drawbacks. Non-specific fluorescence is common, and though the pattern of fluorescence may be different it needs skilled eyes to recognize this. Non-infected cell controls can be used to avoid false positive findings, but some reactions are then indeterminable. The method is also less sensitive than those described below, and its reliance on subjective reading is a considerable drawback both because of potential inaccuracy and because of the need, in blood transfusion practice, to examine large numbers of specimens.

Table 7.1 Characteristics of HIV assays

	Cost	Sensitivity	Specificity	Ease of use	Objective/ subjective
EIA type I	moderate	very high	moderate	moderate	0
EIA type II	moderate	very high	high	high	0
EIA type III	moderate	high	high	moderate	0
Passive agglutination, type 4*	moderate	high	high	high	S
Immunofluorescence	low	moderate	moderate	high	S
Western blot	very high	high	moderate	low	S
Radioimmuno-precipitation	very high	high	?	low	S

*Preliminary observations only.

At present the mainstay of anti-HIV screening in almost all countries is the type I solid phase enzyme immunoassay (EIA). In contrast to IF, the virus antigens are purified, solubilised and coated onto polystyrene, which has an affinity for protein molecules. The polystyrene may be in the form of a bead, or be the internal surface of a well of a polystyrene multiwell plate. In the final stage of the assay anti huIg-enzyme bound to the specific reaction complex on the polystyrene is allowed to act on a colour generating substrate such as ortho-phenylene diamine (OPD). Optical densities can then be read in a spectrophotometer. The chief advantages of these EIAs are their high sensitivity and their objectivity (Table 7.1). Though the commercial market is now very competitive they are not cheap, and they are prone to extraneous effects that may lower their specificity. These include cross reaction with anti-HLA (Kuhnl, Seidl and Holzberger, 1985), storage of specimens in unsatisfactory conditions (Biggar *et al.*, 1985) and the heating of specimens, often done as a safety measure. Timing and the dilution of reagents may also be critical. These EIAs detect only IgG anti-HIV and not IgM, but they are the sheet-anchor of HIV screening, as or more sensitive than any alternative tests. They have evaluated and compared by several independent, non-commercial laboratories (Mortimer, Parry and Mortimer, 1986; Courouce, 1986; Reesnik *et al.*, 1986; Waldman and Calmann, 1986) and the continued close scrutiny of a multiplicity of users will probably ensure that their quality is maintained. In testing blood donors in a low incidence area they give an initial false positive rate of about 0.75% (Waldman and Oleszko, 1986). Except for the first few weeks after exposure, however, it seems that they are rarely falsely negative.

The third sort of type I test is Western (or immuno-) blot. Western blot differs from other type I assays in that the viral antigens are separated according to their molecular weight into bands on strips of nitrocellulose paper. Antibodies in the specimens are allowed to react with corresponding antigens on the strips, and once they have been 'developed' by applying anti huIgG-enzyme (or sometimes staphylococcal A tagged anti huIgG or a biotin/avidin based amplification of the anti huIgG step), the strips are read. The chief advantage of this method is the discriminating picture it gives of the antibody reponse. The patterns on the strips depend upon the stage of infection and are various; but very typical patterns are recognizable with experience. A chronically infected individual will have demonstrable antibodies to the main env (envelope) products, p120 and p41 and to the main gag (core) products, p55 and p24, together with other viral proteins, p18 and p65. However, Western blot is expensive, complex and slow. Partly for these reasons, it has been less rigorously evaluated than EIA, particularly on large numbers of specimens that may be presumed to be anti-HIV negative. Until effective machine reading of the strips can be developed, Western blot is also subjective and it is gradually being realized that the subjective reading and other features of the assay limit its specificity (Biberfeld *et al.*, 1986b; Courouce, Muller and Richard, 1986). For those who wish to screen out infected blood, as opposed to studying the development and the intricacies of the anti-HIV response, the Western blot has little value. The rapid transfer of this technology from the research laboratory to the routine of screening and diagnostic laboratories has, in the author's opinion, been ill-advised and largely unnecessary.

7.3.4 Type II assays

Diagnostic procedures are often transferable, and the methodologies for type II, as also for type III and type IV anti-HIV assays, have been borrowed from existing methods for hepatitis A and B virus antibodies. In competitive tests for anti hepatitis A and anti hepatitis B core the specimen and labelled specific antibody are allowed to react simultaneously with the solid phase. In the type II anti-HIV assays the same competitive principle is used. This was first described as a radioimmunoassay (Cheingsong-Popov *et al.*, 1984), the anti-HIV being labelled with ^{125}I, but has now been realized commercially as an EIA (*Wellcozyme*), the anti-HIV being conjugated with peroxidase. In a more recent development of the competitive principle, the antigen-coated solid phase has been modified. *Abbott Laboratories* have prepared solid phases bearing cloned envelope (p4l) and core (p24) protein so that anti env and anti gag may be determined separately. Tedder and colleagues have used monoclonal anti-HIV to bind antigen to the solid phase (Oldham *et al.*, in press). These two developments are likely to increase both the specificity (already high) and the sensitivity of type II assays.

The advantages of the type II assays are convenience, speed, high specificity, and a sensitivity which is probably as good as the type I assays. They mostly measure undifferentiated anti-HIV, however, and type II assays are not very sensitive in detecting IgM anti-HIV. Moreover, there is a some evidence, so far not confirmed, that they become positive a little after type I assays when an early infection is being investigated, and that they are insensitive to antibodies to HIV variants (HTLV-IV, LAV-II, see below). In the United Kingdom, unlike North America and the rest of Europe, the type II assay predominates as the screening test for blood donations. This choice was made by individual transfusion centre directors on the basis of the accuracy and convenience of the *Wellcozyme* assay. It requires and is receiving close surveillance to ensure that the type II assay is as effective as the type I in identifying HIV infected blood donations.

7.3.5 Other assay types

Other configurations for solid phase anti-HIV tests are much less widely used than the type I and II assays, but deserve to be mentioned. The method for the type III assay (Fig. 7.1) has also been derived from other viral diagnostic procedures. In it, antibody of particular Ig classes (IgM, IgG, IgA) is 'captured' from the specimen onto a solid phase coated with anti human μ, γ or α. The specificity of the captured immunoglobulin is determined by adding HIV antigen and then tagged anti-HIV. Although these procedures have not yet been developed commercially they do provide a means of detecting class specific HIV antibody. They are also independent of some of the non-specific effects that may dog type I assays, and provide a methodologically independent procedure for detecting anti-HIV that is more specific though not quite as sensitive as those assays. An interesting variant of the type III assay has been described by Schmitz and Grass (1986) which may share the same advantages of specificity and methodological independence that make these assays useful diagnostic and confirmatory procedures.

A further possible methodological variation is here referred to as the type IV assay (Fig. 7.1). This covers any assay in which anti-HIV in a specimen is detected by 'sandwiching' it between HIV antigens. The approach is the same as has been used in a sensitive radioimmunoassay for antibody to HBsAg (*Ausab, Abbott Laboratories*), and the availability of purified and/or cloned HIV antigens is likely to make similar assays for anti-HIV realizable. A passive agglutination assay for anti-HIV in which minute particles of gelatin coated with purified HIV are agglutinated by anti-HIV positive specimens (*Serodia, Fujirebio*) is spatially merely a variation of the type IV solid phase sandwich assay illustrated in Fig. 7.1. If passive agglutination proves accurate it may be a very useful additional assay for anti-HIV, simple to perform, and probably sensitive to IgM as well as IgG anti-HIV. Preliminary observations in the author's laboratory suggest that passive agglutination is both sensitive and specific, except when plasma (which may cause non-specific agglutination) is tested.

A further anti-HIV assay, which does not fit easily into the above classification, is radioimmuno-precipitation (RIP, Schneider *et al.*, 1984). For this assay, HIV infected cells are grown in the presence of radiolabelled amino acid which is thereby incorporated in the cells. A cell lysate is prepared in which labelled viral proteins are present. A serum specimen is added to this and immune complexes are formed which are then precipitated and separated in a polyacrylamide gel according to the molecular weight of the viral proteins. The pattern on the gel resembles that seen in Western blotting onto nitrocellulose strips, though the high molecular weight viral proteins are better represented. RIP is a comprehensive and apparently accurate method of demonstrating the presence of HIV antibodies; but even though less cumbersome, less complex RIP methods are now being applied (Lange *et al.*, 1986) it remains a specialist procedure. For this reason, its accuracy has not been investigated with the rigour that has been applied to most of the solid phase assays.

7.4 APPLICATIONS OF ANTI-HIV ASSAYS TO BLOOD DONATION SCREENING

The appropriate use of anti-HIV assays is often a matter of hot debate. A web of scientific and commercial interest envelopes the subject, though attempts are being made to achieve national and international consensus (Medical News, 1986). It has to be realized that the functions of research, diagnostic, and blood donor screening laboratories are separate and that their requirements of an anti-HIV assay differ. The research laboratory seeks maximum information about the quality of the anti-HIV response. The diagnostic laboratory needs an accurate test with an emphasis on specificity and access to follow up specimens. The transfusion laboratory requires a highly sensitive, rapid, objective and (because very many tests have to be done) a cheap assay. These last requirements are, in fact, the most exacting made by any kind of laboratory. There is as yet no simple anti-HIV assay that fulfils them all and consequently the blood donation screening procedure has to be broken down into an initial sensitive assay and detailed confirmatory testing of suspected donations. It hardly needs to be said that it is insufficient to test donors from time to time. Every donation must be separately screened.

Two patterns of operation have been developed to accomplish the procedures of screening and confirmation in the blood transfusion laboratory. In the first pattern a type I assay is used as the initial screening test. Up to 1% of tests may be positive and they are usually repeated twice because it has been shown that these reactions, if unrepeatable, are usually due to technical error. In most donor populations about 0.25% of donor specimens are *repeatedly* positive when type I assays are used. These specimens are then tested by Western blot and those that are positive regarded as confirmed. Those negative by Western blot may either have been reactive in the type I assay because of non-specific factors, or they may be only very weakly anti-HIV positive. The latter, less common situation is often identified when, on follow up, higher titres of anti-HIV are found. The main drawback of this confirmatory pathway is that Western blot testing is often outside the competence of the blood transfusion laboratory. Over time, this approach also leads to the accumulation of large numbers of EIA positive, Western blot negative blood donors whose anti-HIV status is indeterminate and whose donations cannot be used.

An alternative confirmatory pathway which does not depend so entirely on the complicated and subjective Western blot test and promises to be applicable within the blood transfusion laboratory is to make fuller use of the various types of EIA solid phase assay that are methodologically independent and give an objective signal. It is within the capability of these laboratories to use any of these assays. The constraint on them is their availability. It seems likely that many laboratories could, in the future, use type II and/or type III or IV assays to confirm type I screening assays, or type I, III or IV assays to confirm type II screening assays (Fig. 7.2). The former option, in particular, seems logical, depending as it does on the application first of a highly sensitive, then of more specific assays. The speed, cheapness and convenience of these procedures would make them attractive alternatives to the use of Western blot as a confirmatory test. In many parts of the world commercial sources of types I, II and IV assays are established. Transfusion laboratories should now avail themselves of them.

From the work of anti-HIV confirmatory centres in the United Kingdom it is evident that though most true anti-HIV positive results can be confirmed by

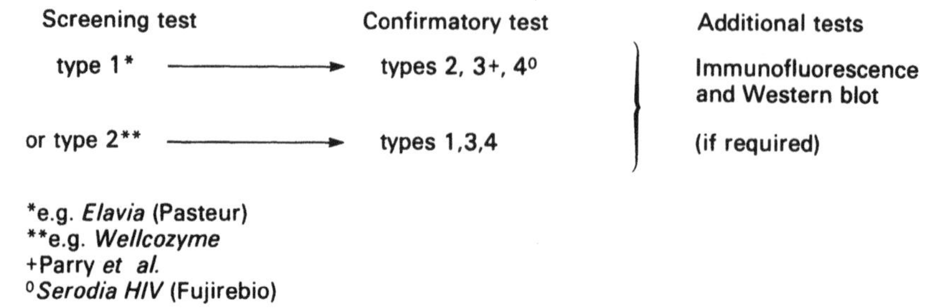

Figure 7.2 Confirmatory pathways in anti-HIV screening.

positive findings in all types of solid phase there will, as with Western blot confirmatory testing, be specimens that give discrepant results. Only experience will show which combinations of discrepant results are likely to be significant, which can be elucidated by follow up tests and which turn out to be non-specific effects. Specimens only reactive in a type I assay, which worldwide is the most used donor screening method, rarely emerge as true positives. However, it is essential to follow up these donors over a period of at least 3 months.

7.5 MISCELLANEOUS BUT IMPORTANT CONSIDERATIONS

Achieving the goal of effective blood donor screening does not just depend on the quality of the anti-HIV test: a number of other factors are important. The specimen itself must be suitable. Both serum and plasma can be used, but plasma may form unwanted clots and also cause non-specific effects, and serum is therefore preferable. Serum, if heated to reduce its infectivity, may yield weak false positive reactions (Mortimer, Parry and Mortimer, 1985). Pooled plasma products may give misleading results, both positive and negative. The rule in that case is that the individual constituent donations should be tested. Various chemical factors – even fumes around the laboratory bench from a jar of hypochlorite solution used as disinfectant – may interfere with enzyme reactions. Human error may occur at every stage, particularly in transferring specimens, adding reagents and transcribing results.

An invaluable aid to blood donor screening is a computerized read out of spectrophotometer results which flags specimens that fall outside the main distribution of negative results in the screening assay, whether or not these specimens are actually positive according to the manufacturer's criteria. The fact that large numbers of uninfected individuals are being tested in donor screening procedures provides an added and valuable control of the assay, and a relatively cheap microcomputer allows full benefit to be derived from this. Some manufacturers offer this facility with the spectrophotometer they supply, and most spectrophotometers are computer-compatible. If the laboratory has a microcomputer enthusiast on the staff he may arrange for spectrophotometer and computer to 'talk to' each other and generate a flagged print out, perhaps with a graphic representation of the distribution of results from uninfected donors (Fig. 7.3).

7.6 FUTURE DEVELOPMENTS IN HIV SCREENING

The near future holds both problems and potential benefits. To take the problems first: it is obvious that where HIV spreads outside particular risk groups or where, as in Central Africa, it has never been so confined, encouragement of donor self-selection to protect the blood supply is ineffective. In too many contexts (for instance plasma collection) it is scarcely being applied at all, and in others its efficiency has been compromised by the reluctance of many who are involved in blood transfusion to burden donors repeatedly with intimate and apparently impertinent questioning. As risk groups become everywhere less well-defined reliance on laboratory screening tests is bound to increase and they must therefore become even more accurate. Not only must the assay be capable of detecting all anti-HIV antibodies, no matter how weak in titre, but testing may become necessary for antigens or other viral products. The prospect of having to use more than one test to screen for the same infection is not attractive and ways of combining these tests in a single procedure will, if possible, have to be found. It seems unlikely that any test will replace current anti-HIV EIAs, and they themselves are probably not susceptible to very significant improvements in accuracy. Whether, however, an antigen or other direct test for virus is feasible, and whether it is needed as an adjunct that will detect infection in the first weeks after HIV exposure and in the apparently rare infected individual who never makes an antibody response, cannot yet be decided.

The future should also hold some prospect of cheaper, simpler assays to allow screening in the developing world, pre-eminently in Central Africa where prevalence of antibody in blood donor samples in several cities has been found to be as high as 18% (Melbye *et al.*, 1986). This is just one facet of the appalling predicament of some parts of Africa and it shows that entire blood transfusion services have been compromised. As well as Africans it threatens Westerners who, for business or professional reasons or as tourists, visit Central Africa. Indeed the 'pick-up' rate from donor screening in some Western countries is so small (about 25 per million donations are found anti-HIV positive in the United Kingdom, H. H. Gunson, personal communication) that at present a greater benefit might accrue to the West from it paying to screen African donors than from screening its own donors. It would protect Western nationals there, sustain diplomatic and business interests,

Controls
Strong positive/s at : F 1
Weak Positive/s at : C 1, D 1, E 1
Negatives at : A 1, B 1

	1	2	3	4	5	6	7	8	9	10	11	12
A:	949	158	823	828	869	815	846	774	863	778	834	841
B:	983	198	820	805	813	877	849	807	809	791	799	783
C:	526	92	888	637	858	806	746	788	851	807	891	782
D:	448	39	843	894	828	786	887	852	794	836	797	945
E:	449	34	800	747	837	733	785	773	807	793	833	757
F:	76	941	807	822	813	723	843	790	795	771	865	849
G:	1141	310	821	780	789	808	807	781	773	818	812	413
H:	280	39	848	850	790	774	829	907	761	854	828	967

A:	–	+	–	–	–	–	–	–	–	–	–	–
B:	–	+	–	–	–	÷	–	–	–	–	–	–
C:	?	+	–	–	–	–	–	–	–	–	–	–
D:	+	+	–	–	–	–	–	–	–	–	–	–
E:	+	+	–	–	–	–	–	–	–	–	–	–
F:	+	–	–	–	–	–	–	–	–	–	-	–
G:	–	+	–	–	–	–	–	–	–	–	–	+
H:	+	+	–	–	–	–	–	–	–	–	–	–

DISTRIBUTION GRAPH

PLATE NO. 15/01

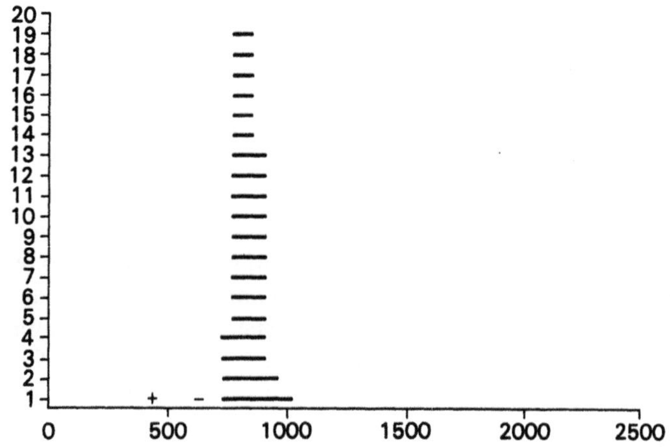

CUTOFF = 521

NEGATIVE RESULTS —
MEAN = 816.2025
RANGE from 637 to 967

STANDARD DEVIATION = 48.2 N = 79

Figure 7.3 This illustration shows the 12 × 8 microtitre plate format used for the Wellcozyme (type 2) anti-HIV assay. In the first two columns (1,2) the positive and negative control sera distributed as a panel to UK Blood Transfusion Service centres by the Public Health Laboratory Service have been tested. In the remaining columns and be a humane gesture at a time when African suspicion of Western political motives runs high. This contrast between Africa and the West also emphasizes the need to keep under review the cost/benefit position regarding the use of any HIV test in very low risk situations.

7.7 HTLV-IV, LAV-II AND TRANSFUSION

The more or less simultaneous but independent reports of HIV-like retroviruses in parts of West Africa by Kanki and colleagues and by Clavel and colleagues are still of unknown significance to blood transfusion. The virus described by the former group and referred to as HTLV-IV has only very recently been related to AIDS-like disease (Biberfeld *et al.*, 1986a), but the virus described by the latter group as LAV-II is definitely associated with AIDS and AIDS associated illness. It has not been proved that these two retroviruses form a single type but, on that assumption, they have collectively been referred to as HIV-II. In the view of Kanki *et al.* (1986) the virus is closely related to a previously described simian virus, STLV-III, and more distantly related to HTLV III (i.e. HIV).

Blood transfusers are now hoping for a synthesis of the rather disjointed evidence on this virus group and asking themselves what the significance of it is to them. Unfortunately, it is not easy to evaluate or simplify the data available, though some features of it are of obvious importance. It is of concern that increasing numbers of West Africans are being found infected with HIV-II, usually through their being tested for it in various centres in Europe where they live or are visiting. This underlines the need in the West to exclude from blood donation African donors and those who have recently travelled in Africa. It should be noted that HIV-II, like HIV, is likely to be spread by sexual contact and in blood, and that its association with immunodeficiency and wasting disease also recalls HIV and AIDS. Finally, it seems that no antibody test for HIV, least of all one based on the competitive principle (type II), will reliably detect anti-HIV-II.

At the time of writing (late 1986) there is insufficient evidence to justify routine screening of blood donations for anti-HIV-II. However, two things

---

blood donors' sera have been tested, including one weakly positive specimen (G12). This has been flagged (+) in the array of signs below the OD values and appears as a cross on the distribution graph. The graph also shows that there was one specimen (C4) lying ›3 standard deviations below the mean of the seronegative donors. This specimen was retested.

This analysis of spectrophotometer readings was done with computer software supplied by Sanguine Computing Ltd, Hillgrove, Burton on Trent, DE15 ORD, UK. I am grateful to Dr. H. H. Gunson, Director, N.W. Regional Blood Transfusion Centre, Manchester, for allowing me to show work done in his laboratory.

need to be done. Firstly, better collaboration between scientists in West Africa, Europe and North America has to be established so that the status of these viruses becomes better understood. Secondly, as many Westerners as possible who have recently been in West Africa, together with their sexual contacts, should be offered tests for anti-HIV-II. Blood donors who defer themselves because of African connections ought especially to be tested, even though their blood cannot be used for transfusion. In this way some assessment can be made of the likelihood of HIV-II spreading into indigenous Western populations and of the need to introduce HIV-II screening there. Those concerned with blood transfusion should take active steps to get a resolution of this question. They cannot expect to be given an answer and the means, if it proves necessary, to test for the new virus unless they co-operate actively in attempts to define and monitor the problem.

7.8 CONCLUSION

The HIV epidemic is constantly growing and its pattern changing rapidly. Those responsible for maintaining a safe blood supply must remain alert and flexible in their attitude to HIV as to other virological threats to the practice of blood transfusion and product manufacture. However cleverly HIV tests are modified and however minutely the anti-HIV response is dissected, what is being sought is still the easiest way to answer the question 'Will this donation transmit infection?' At present it seems unlikely that tests other than those for antibody have a role in answering this question. As to the anti-HIV assay chosen, it should be one whose antigens conform as closely as possible to the natural viral proteins, have the widest possible spectrum (including, if necessary, HIV-II) and are free from extraneous proteins. It remains to be seen whether these requirements will be met through refinement of existing screening technology or through innovation. Current EIAs for anti-HIV are some of the most accurate virological assays ever devised, and whether they will be displaced by a new generation of tests seems at present very much open to question.

REFERENCES

Barré-Sinoussi, F., Cherman, J. C., Rey, F., Nugeyre, M. T., Chamaret, S. C., Rozenbaum, W. and Montagnier, L. (1983) Isolation of a T-lymphotropic retrovirus from a patient at risk for acquired immunodeficiency syndrome (AIDS). *Science*, **22**, 868–71.

Biberfeld, G., Bottiger, B., Bredberg-Raden, U., *et al.* (1986a) Findings in four HTLV-IV seropositive women from West Africa. *Lancet*, ii, 1330.

Biberfeld, G., Bredberg-Raden, V., Bottiger, B., *et al.* (1986b) Blood Donor sera with false positive Western blot reactions to Human Immunodeficiency Virus. *Lancet*, ii, 289–90.

Biggar, R. J., Melbye, M., Sarin, P. S., *et al.* (1985) ELISA HTLV-retrovirus antibody reactivity associated with malaria and immune complexes in healthy Africans. *Lancet*, **ii**, 520–3.
CDC (1986) Transfusion-associated HTLV III/LAV-associated virus infection from a sero negative donor – Colorado. *Morb. Mort. Wkly Rpt*, **35**, 389–90.
Cheingsong-Popov, R., Weiss, R. A., Dalgleish, A., *et al.* (1984) Prevalence of antibody to human T-lymphotropic virus type III in AIDS and AIDS-risk patients in Britain. *Lancet*, **ii**, 477–80.
Clavel, F., Guetard, D., Brun-Vezinet, F. *et al.* (1986) Isolation of a new human retrovirus from West African patients with AIDS. *Science*, **233**, 243–346.
Courouce, A. M. (1986) Evaluation of eight ELISA kits for the detection of anti LAV/HTLV III antibodies. *Lancet*, **i**, 1152–3.
Courouce, A. M., Muller, J. Y., Richard, D. (1986) False positive Western Blot reactions to human immunodeficiency virus in blood donors. *Lancet*, **ii**, 921–2.
Goudsmit, J., de Wolf, F., Paul, D. A. *et al.* (1986) Expression of human immunodeficiency virus antigen (HIV-Ag) in serum and cerebrospinal fluid during acute and chronic infection. *Lancet*, **ii**, 177–80.
Kanki, P. J., Barin, F., Boup, S. *et al.* (1986) New human T-lymphotropic retrovirus related to simian T-lymphotropic virus type III (STLV-III). *Science*, **232**, 238.
Karpas, A., Gillson, W., Bevan, P. C., Oates, J. K. (1985) Lytic infection by British AIDS Virus and development of rapid cell test for antiviral antibodies. *Lancet*, **ii**, 695–7.
Kuhnl, P., Seidl, S., Holzberger, G. (1985) HLA DR4 antibodies cause positive HTLV III antibody ELISA results. *Lancet*, **i**, 1222.
Lange, J. M. A., Paul, D. A., Huisman, A., *et al.* (1986) Persistent HIV antigenaemia and decline of HIV core antibodies associated with transition to AIDS. *Brit. Med. J.*, **293**, 1459–62.
Levy, J. A., Hoffman, A. D., Kramer, S. M., Landis, J. A., Shimabukuro, J. M. (1986) Isolation or lymphocytopathic retroviruses from San Francisco patients with AIDS. *Science*, **225**, 840–2.
Ludlam, G. A., Tucker, J., Steel, C. M. *et al.* (1985) Human T lymphocytotropic virus type III (HTLV III) infection in sero negative haemophiliacs after transfusion of factor VIII. *Lancet*, **ii**, 233–6.
Medical News (1986) Consensus on AIDS Screening. *Brit. Med. J.*, **293**, 1509.
Melbye, M., Njelesani, E. K., Bayley, A. *et al.* (1986) Evidence for heterosexual transmission and clinical manifestations of human immunodeficiency virus infection and related conditions in Lusaka, Zambia. *Lancet*, **ii**, 113–15.
Mortimer, P., P., Parry, J. V., Mortimer, J. Y. (1985) Which anti HTLV III LAV assays for screening and confirmatory testing? *Lancet*, **ii**, 873–7.
Oldham, L. J., Moulsdale, H. J., Mortimer, P. P., Tedder, R. S., Morgan-Capner, P. (1987) How sensitive are the commercial assays for anti HTLV III/LAV? *J. Med. Virol.* **21**, 75–9.
Parry, J. V., Mortimer, P. P. (1986) The place of IgM antibody testing in HIV serology. *Lancet*, **ii**, 979–80.
Popovic, M., Sarngadharan, M., Read, E. *et al.* (1984) Detection, isolation, and continuous production of Cytopathic Retroviruses (HTLV-III) from patients with AIDS and pre-AIDS. *Science*, **224**, 497–500.
Reesnik, H. W., Lelie, P. N., Huisman, J. G. *et al.* (1986) Evaluation of six enzyme immunoassays for antibody against Human Immunodeficiency Virus. *Lancet*, **ii**, 483–6.
Schmitz, H., Grass, F. (1986) Specific enzyme immunoassay for the detection of

antibody to HTLV III using rheumatoid factor – coated plates. *J. Virol. Methods.*, 13, 115–20.

Schneider, J., Yamamoto, N., Hinuma, Y., Hunsmann, G. (1984) Sera from adult T cell leukaemia patients react with envelope and core polypeptides of adult T cell leukaemia virus. *Virology*, 132, 1–11.

Waldman, A. A. and Calmann, M. (1986) Serum screening for anti-HTLV-III antibodies. II: Screening tests. *Lab. Management*, 24 (8), 31–4.

Waldman, A. A., Oleszko, W. R. (1986) Serum Screening for Anti-HTLV-III Antibodies. III: Confirmatory Tests. *Lab. Management*, 24 (9), 45–51.

8

Donor screening for HIV in the United States

—— *Roger Y. Dodd* ——

8.1 INTRODUCTION

As the first country to recognize AIDS, the United States was inevitably the first to develop and implement measures to reduce the transmission of the disease by blood transfusion. In essence, the problem has been attacked at three levels; first by the selection of low risk donor populations; secondly by use of laboratory test procedures and finally, by inactivating viruses in products derived from pooled plasma. The sensitive social issues associated with AIDS, along with the uniform fatality of the disease, generated numerous ethical, social and medical problems which had to be resolved during the development of the screening programmes. At the same time, laboratory tests for the identification of potentially infectious donors were developed, commercialized and implemented in a remarkably short time span. In fact, within two years of the initial recognition of the AIDS virus, donor testing was uniformly in place. It is reasonable to claim that these activities have prevented a significant number of cases of transfusion associated AIDS cases, as testing alone has identified several thousand infected and potentially infectious donors during its first year. Major milestones in the management of transfusion AIDS in the United States are outlined in Table 8.1. Even so, it must be remembered that only 2% of AIDS cases in the United States are due to transfusion and the major problems of this epidemic are yet to be solved.

AIDS was first recognized in 1981 as an unusual epidemic of the rare tumor, Kaposi's sarcoma, and/or an outbreak of opportunistic infections, occurring among male homosexuals (CDC, 1981a,b). Subsequently, the disease was identified among intravenous drug abusers, recent entrants to the United States from Haiti and haemophilia patients treated with factor VIII

Table 8.1 United States: key events in the development of donor screening policies

Date		*Action*	*Reference*
June	1981	AIDS first reported	CDC (1981a,b)
July	1982	AIDS reported in 3 haemophiliacs	CDC (1982a)
Dec.	1982	First report of presumed transfusion-associated AIDS in an infant	CDC (1982b)
Jan.	1983	Joint statement by US Blood Collection Agencies recommending precautions to limit transfusion-associated AIDS	
March	1983	US Public Health Service interagency recommendations to reduce the spread of AIDS. Included recommendations on deferral of blood donors at risk	CDC (1983)
May	1983	LAV reported as an AIDS-associated virus	Barre-Sinoussi *et al.* (1983)
Jan.	1984	Publication of follow-up studies on transfusion AIDS	Curran *et al.* (1984)
		US Blood Collection Agencies joint statement recommends strengthened donor screening and donor designation of units as inappropriate for patient support	
May	1984	Recognition of HTLV III as potential AIDS agent	Gallo *et al.* (1984)
		Description of ELISA test. Transfer of technology to industry for test development	Sarngadharan *et al.* (1984)
Jan.	1985	US Public Health Service interagency recommendations for screening blood and plasma for antibodies to HTLV III	CDC (1985a)
March	1985	First commercial test kit licensed in USA	
July	1985	Testing uniform throughout USA	
Sept.	1985	Revised definition: any male who has had sex with another male since 1977 should refrain from donating blood	CDC (1985b)
June	1986	First report of transfusion association HIV infection after implementation of donor anti-HIV testing	CDC (1986a)

concentrates. The incidence of the disease increased rapidly and, by May 1987, some 36 000 cases had been diagnosed. AIDS appears to be uniformly fatal, with an extremely low survival rate two years after diagnosis. A number of lines of evidence suggested that AIDS was indeed a new disease, rather than a newly recognized, or more extreme form of an existing pathology. There was considerable speculation about the aetiology of AIDS, with two major hypotheses: a transmissible agent, or a dysfunction stemming from immunologic overload. The latter concept was not strongly favoured and became unacceptable once the aetiologic agent was identified.

The epidemiologic pattern of AIDS and, in particular, its restricted occurrence in distinctive risk groups, suggested that the aetiologic agent was a blood-borne infectious agent like heptatitis B virus. This model led to predictions that additional risk groups for AIDS would be identified – in particular, recipients of blood or components. In fact, it was not long before the first apparent case of transfusion-associated AIDS was observed in an infant which had received an exchange transfusion (Amman *et al.*, 1983). Subsequently, extensive investigation of persons with AIDS showed that a small proportion – of the order of 1% – had, as their only apparent risk factor, a history of blood transfusion in the 5 years preceding diagnosis of AIDS (Curran *et al.*, 1984; Peterman, Jaffe and Feorino, 1985). Careful follow up studies showed that in almost all cases, at least one of the donors to each patient had an AIDS risk factor, or showed abnormalities of T cell subset ratios characteristic of AIDS (Peterman, Jaffe and Feorino, 1985). These findings engendered considerable concern, not only that blood recipients were at risk of AIDS, but also that this population might be a conduit allowing the disease to affect the general population. As a result, a number of measures were introduced in order to reduce the risk of transmission of AIDS by blood transfusion, even before it was clearly demonstrated that the disease was caused by a virus.

8.2 DONOR SELECTION

In March, 1983, the United States Public Health Service issued the first set of guidelines to reduce the transmission of AIDS (CDC, 1983); in addition, the Food and Drug Administration provided more detailed recommendations pertaining to the safety of the blood supply. These recommendations were based upon the concept that AIDS was caused by a virus and that persons with risk factors for AIDS were likely to be infected with that virus. Specifically identified as being at increased risk of AIDS were persons with: 'symptoms and signs suggestive of AIDS; sexual partners of AIDS patients; sexually active homosexual or bisexual men with multiple partners; Haitian entrants to the United States; present or past abusers of IV drugs; patients with haemophilia; and sexual partners of individuals at increased risk of

AIDS' (CDC, 1983). Existing donor selection policies already excluded drug abusers, persons with residence in, or recent travel to Haiti (an area endemic for malaria) and those with a history of recent treatment with blood products. The recommendations suggested specific efforts to educate individuals and designated risk groups about AIDS and its potential for transmission by blood. Persons with risk factors were required to refrain from donation. Also, additional questions were incorporated into the donor medical history, in order to identify AIDS-related symptomatology, such as involuntary weight loss, night sweats, etc. Further, measures for preventing the transfusion of products from such donors were proposed. Finally, somewhat more stringent criteria were introduced for source plasma collection, including the maintenance of donor weight records.

These recommendations were accepted and implemented by blood collecting agencies. Educational activities were undertaken at both the community and individual levels. In particular, in many areas, considerable effort was made to identify and interact with the organized gay community. In addition, blood collection agencies in the United States provide prospective donors with a leaflet containing information about the donation process. This leaflet in fact represents a component of an informed consent procedure, which is completed when the donor signs the registration card and specifically acknowledges having read and understood the leaflet. The description of AIDS risk factors was therefore incorporated into this leaflet and blood collection personnel were trained to draw the donor's attention to the leaflet and its contents at all stages of the registration process. The recommended additional questions about AIDS symptoms and contact with AIDS patients were also incorporated into the medical history. However, there was no move to question the donor about his or her sexual orientation.

There was evidence that these measures did have some effect on the structure of the presenting donor population, at least in some localities. Pindyck and her associates in New York compared the structure of the donor population in comparable 9-week periods in 1982 and, after implementation of the measures described above, in 1983 (Pindyck *et al.*, 1985). Overall, there was a small, but statistically significant decrease in the proportion of male donors, from 62.6% to 61.5%. However, blood is collected over a variety of localities in the greater New York region and it is particularly important to note that there was a 6.1% decrease in the number of male donors including a 12% decline among males 21–35 years old in the area with highest risk for AIDS, New York City. The effects of the expanded medical history were also evaluated and reported in the same study (Pindyck *et al.*, 1985). On implementation of the additional health questions, deferrals for respiratory symptoms – namely persistent coughing, increased from 1.3% to 2.9%. Questions relating to AIDS-associated symptoms resulted in the rejection of an additional 0.4%. The lack of specificity of these measures is illustrated by the fact that 46.9% of the additional rejections were among women. Similar data have also been reported from Los Angeles (Kleinman, Thompson and Kaplan, 1984). There was also an intriguing report from Philadelphia, that the frequency of HBsAg positive donations decreased among repeat donors, and there may also have been a concomitant decrease in the incidence of postransfusion non-A, non-B hepatitis (Dahlke, 1984) on implementation of these donor screening measures.

The success of this approach to screening is dependent upon the ability of the donor to understand the educational materials, to recognize and acknowledge his or her own risk status and to avoid giving blood. Each of these steps may cause problems but the last of them caused the greatest initial concern. More specifically, the recruitment of donors in the United States depends to a great extent on peer and affinity groups, particularly in the workplace. Since almost 90% of AIDS patients have been identified as homosexuals or drug abusers, it is understandable that a potential donor might feel socially vulnerable if he or she were to decline to donate, particularly in this time of increased awareness about AIDS. In recognition of this potential, blood centres developed procedures to allow donors to reconsider the consequences of completing the donation process. Two methods are in use. The first is a simple call-back, in which the donor is provided with the blood centre telephone number and is encouraged to make a confidential phone call if, after donation, he or she feels that the blood may be unsuitable. In New York, a more stringent approach was taken, in which the donor is required to make a specific designation, on a confidential form. The donor must read about AIDS risk factors and must then specify whether the donation should be used for patient support, or for other purposes ('studies'). The form is coded only with the identification number of the collected blood unit. Designation of the unit for studies, or failure to designate at all, results in withdrawal of the unit. In New York, this procedure has resulted in about 1.4% of donations being specifically excluded and a further 1.6% being discarded on the basis of incompleted forms (Pindyck *et al.*, 1985). Although a significant proportion of the self-excluding donors do not appear to be at risk of AIDS, there is a clear increase in the prevalence of infection markers, including antibodies to the AIDS virus, among the excluded units. Although the process clearly has some effect, not all high risk donors exclude their units. There is also some controversy about self-exclusion, since it does provide a mixed message to the donor inasmuch as the initial approach places full responsibility on the donor to avoid donation at all, while the designation program implies that it is, nevertheless, acceptable to give.

Donor screening and self-exclusion measures were not fully effective, as evidenced by the continued occurrence of transfusion-associated AIDS, plus the detection of a number of cases in which patients developing AIDS acknowledged a history of donation, even after March 1983. In addition, approximately 90% of donors with confirmed positive results for anti-HIV acknowledge the presence of known risk factors for AIDS (Schorr *et al.*, 1985). As a result of these findings, donor exclusion criteria were made more stringent, with a specific prohibition of donation by males who had ever had sex with another male since 1977 (CDC, 1985b). Data suggest that the proportion of seropositive donors decreased markedly after this criterion was added to the donor selection process (Kalish, Cable and Roberts, 1986), although other factors may have contributed to this change.

Coercive or legislative approaches to the selection of safe donors have not been accepted in the United States. Legal or criminal sanctions against high risk individuals who knowingly give blood have been proposed in a number of States, but have never been ratified. The nature of the voluntary donor population, the implied and specific contract between the donor and the blood centre and respect for individual rights all contribute to this. The legal liability of blood collection and transfusion centres is also generally restricted to circumstances where negligence can be demonstrated. At the same time, there is increasing concern about the need for effective means to screen potential donors, specifically illustrated by the finding of seronegative, but infectious individuals (Mayer *et al.*, 1986) and the transmission of HIV from an apparently seronegative donor (CDC, 1986a). It seems likely that additional educational efforts will have to be undertaken and donors may be required to specify, by their signature, that they consider themselves free of AIDS risk factors. One area of developing concern, however, is the spread of the infection into populations with new, or ill-defined risk for AIDS, primarily by heterosexual routes.

8.3 LABORATORY TESTING

8.3.1 Surrogate tests

Because of continued concern about the safety of the blood supply, additional screening measures were sought. Surrogate testing – that is, the use of non-specific laboratory markers – gained some attention prior to the recognition of the causative agent of AIDS. Surrogate testing was based upon two distinct concepts. First, that persons in the early stages of AIDS might not have symptoms, but would be infectious and would have detectable laboratory abnormalities characteristic of the disease. On this basis, one university blood blank implemented a policy of measuring T lymphocyte subset ratios on all donors. There was also discussion, but no implementation, of tests for elevated levels of beta 2 microglobulin or thymosin alpha-1. The other, and more popular approach to surrogate testing was to use a marker which was frequent among populations with, or at risk for, AIDS. Anti-HBc, a marker of infection with the Hepatitis B virus, was considered most appropriate, and was widely adopted in the San Francisco Bay area. As with other non-specific tests, there were clear problems with specificity and sensitivity. For example, in retrospect, only about 40–50% of donors with anti-HTLV III also have anti-HBc.

8.3.2 Tests for antibodies to the AIDS virus

In 1983, Montagnier and colleagues reported on the isolation of the lymphadenopathy associated virus, LAV, from a patient at risk for AIDS (Barre-Sinoussi *et al.*, 1983). Subsequently, Gallo and colleagues reported on the isolation of a retrovirus, termed human T-lymphotropic retrovirus type III (HTLV III) from a number of patients with AIDS and ARC (Gallo *et al.*, 1984). He postulated that the virus was the causative agent of AIDS. At the same time his group also reported on the development of methods for the large-scale culture of the virus and the production and use of a procedure for detecting antibodies to the virus (Popovic *et al.*, 1984; Sarngadharan *et al.*, 1984). Although it was possible to isolate the virus from only a proportion of patients with AIDS or ARC, the antibody could be shown, by a combination of methods, to be present in essentially 100% of such patients (Sarngadharan *et al.*, 1984). Since the virus is a retrovirus, infection results in integration of a genome copy into the infected host cells and infection is persistent. Consequently, the presence of antibody not only defines prior infection, but also the potential for presence of the HTLV III and infectivity. As a result, it was suggested that an enzyme-linked immunoassay (ELISA) test for anti-HTLV III should be used to screen blood donors in order to detect those who might transmit the agent to recipients. One other set of isolates of the AIDS virus, termed AIDS-associated retrovirus (ARV) was reported by Levy and colleagues (Levy *et al.*, 1984). It is now clear that LAV, HTLV III and ARV are the same virus and it has been suggested that the virus be named Human Immunodeficiency Virus, HIV (Brown, 1986). This term will be used throughout, unless it is necessary to identify specific isolates.

All tests for antibodies to HIV which are currently available in the United States are based on the same mechanism. That is, whole virus is lysed and coated onto a solid phase, which is either a plastic bead or the inside of a well on a microtitre plate. The solid phase is exposed to a dilution of the sample to be tested. If antibody to the viral components is present in the sample, it adheres to the solid phase, where it is subsequently detected with an enzyme labelled antiglobulin probe. The presence of probe is detected by means of a chromogenic substrate. In the United States, blood collection and processing is regulated by the United States Food and Drug Administration. This agency also regulates the procedures which are used in the testing of collected blood. Consequently, anti-HIV tests have to achieve and maintain designated levels of performance before they are licensed as 'Biologics' and are made available for use. The procedures required for licensure include extensive clinical trials on patient and donor populations. The results of such trials define the product claims made by each manufacturer. In the case of tests for anti-HIV, the tests have been defined as qualitative screening tests and claims are made for sensitivity and specificity; where sensitivity was defined as the proportion of persons with diagnosed AIDS found positive in the test, and specificity was the proportion of normal donors found non-reactive in the test. While it would be anticipated that all AIDS patients should be positive, the definition of sensitivity is dependent upon the accuracy of diagnosis and may also be affected by the finding that anti-HIV may not be detectable late in the disease. Seven commercial tests are currently licensed by the FDA. All but one of these tests are based upon Gallo's HTLV III isolate, while the seventh is derived from the Montagnier isolate, LAV. Product claims for the tests reflect a range of sensitivity from 98.3 to 100% and specificity of 99.2–99.8%, as shown in Table 8.2. Published and unpublished information suggests that these tests all have a similar capability to detect true positives, and that the major differences lie in the specificity of the tests (Fang *et al.*, 1986; Kuritsky *et al.*, 1986).

There is an essentially common pattern of use of the tests, following guidelines and regulations established by the United States Public Health Service (CDC, 1985b). In general, a sample of each blood or plasma donation is tested. Any sample giving an absorbance value greater than that defined as the cut-off of the test is regarded as initially reactive. However, because the test format is susceptible to false reactive readings caused by minor procedural variations, each initially reactive sample is subjected to repeat testing. Usually, two additional tests are performed, one on the original sample and another on a sample drawn directly from the original blood collection bag. If either or both of these repeat tests generates a reactive value, then the blood unit is defined as repeatably reactive, or 'positive' in the ELISA test and

Table 8.2 Tests for anti-HIV licensed for use in the United States – manufacturers' product claims

Manufacturer	*Sensitivity*	*Specificity*
Abbott	98.3	99.8
DuPont	99.3	99.7
ENI	99.6	99.2
Genetic Systems	100.0	99.8
Litton*	98.9	99.6
Ortho	99.3	99.7
Travenol Genentech	100.0	99.2

*Now Organon Teknika.
Data derived from the manufacturers' labelling (product inserts) for each procedure.

cannot be used for transfusion. If both repeat tests are non-reactive, then the initial result is regarded as a laboratory error and the blood unit may be issued for transfusion. Extensive studies on samples that are reactive only on the initial test show that this policy is safe and reasonable (Ward *et al.*, 1986). The major reason for using two different samples for the repeat test is to detect any problems caused by misidentification of the test sample. This clearly implies that extensive efforts should be made to resolve any differences in the results of the two repeat tests.

The policy of discarding all blood units which are repeatably positive in the ELISA test is considered to provide the maximum available safety to the blood supply. The role of confirmatory procedures is to assure the donor that he or she will not be incorrectly notified of a positive test result. Therefore, at least in the blood bank, the purpose of a confirmatory test is to identify those ELISA positive results which are clearly due to the presence of antibodies directed against the gene products of the AIDS virus. There are a number of available methods to do this, although most of them are in the nature of research level procedures, rather than routine laboratory tests. Confirmatory tests should use a methodology independent of the primary test and must clearly have a higher inherent specificity.

The signal level of the ELISA test itself may be indicative of the true nature of the reactivity of the sample. In general, those samples which give a high absorbance reading in the direct test are more likely to be found specific for anti-HIV and conversely, the majority of samples with signal levels close to the cut-off are found to be non-specific. However, exceptions do occur, and this approach is not an acceptable basis for donor notification (Ward *et al.*, 1986). Similarly, at least one manufacturer has developed a test which identifies the presence of antibodies directed against antigens found in the cells used to grow the virus. Such an 'exclusionary' test provides guidance that at least some positive test results are a result of non-viral reactions, but the procedure is not considered rigorous enough for routine confirmation.

The Western blot procedure has been extensively used as a means of evaluating the specificity of ELISA positive samples. Unfortunately, it is expensive, complex, time-consuming and subjective. In brief, the procedure consists of disrupting the virus and separating the components electrophoretically on polyacrylamide gel. After separation, the characteristic pattern of viral polypeptides is electrophoretically transferred (blotted) to a nitrocellulose sheet. This sheet is cut into strips, which are exposed to the test sample. Antibodies in the test sample, if reactive with the viral components, adhere to the polypeptides trapped on the nitrocellulose. The presence of the viral antibodies is then detected by an anti-immunoglobulin preparation, labelled with an enzyme or with radioactive tracers. The reactions are then visualized by an appropriate procedure (Sarngadharan *et al.*, 1984). If the antibodies in the test sample are reactive to the viral components, then they will be found in characteristic positions on the blot. Currently, the presence of antibodies to the p24 polypetide component of the *gag* gene product, and/or to the gp41 glycopeptide of the *env* gene product are regarded as definitive evidence for anti-HIV reactivity. However, it is important to recognize that some patterns which are observed may be misleading, and considerable skill is required to interpret the blot patterns, particularly in the context of donor notification. Some authorities suggest that lines should not be interpreted as positive except in the presence of an overall pattern which is compatible with infection by HIV. The finding of a single reactivity in the p24 region is particularly troublesome, since it may indicate early infection with HIV, or may be a non-specific reaction, or an artifact, especially among donors. A recent recommendation suggests that p24 in the absence of gp41 should be ignored unless there is also reactivity against the p55 parent *gag* protein (Burke and Redfield, 1986). Currently, in the absence of diagnostic information, bands must be present at p24, p31 (a product of the *pol* gene) and gp41 or 160 in order to assign an unequivocal positive interpretation.

8.3.3 Results of donor testing in the United States

Approximately 12–13 million whole blood collections are completed annually in the United States and there are an additional 8 million plasmapheresis procedures. The anti-HIV test became available in March of 1985 and testing started immediately and was uniformly in place by the end of June that year. Consequently, a large amount of information is available on the results of testing among donors. Schorr *et al.* (1985), reporting on approximately 1 million tests, and representing about half of the whole blood collection capacity of the country, indicated that 1% of all tests were initially reactive, 0.17% were repeatably reactive in ELISA and that confirmation by Western blot indicated a true positivity rate of 0.038%. The population of Western blot positive donors was predominantly (92%) male and, in 41 cases where interviews had been completed, 36 of the Western blot positive donors were found to have risk factors for AIDS. It was of interest that regional variations in the prevalence rate of Western blot-confirmed anti-HIV correlated directly with variations in the incidence of AIDS. In contrast, there was little, if any, epidemiologic significance in the ELISA test results themselves, confirming the value of the Western blot as a measure of true positivity for anti-HIV. Other studies have generated similar data, using different test procedures (Kuritsky *et al.*, 1986). Current trends suggest a significant decrease in the frequency of Western blot positive test results, presumably as a result of elimination of positive donors from the population of repeat donors, and to strengthening of the donor selection procedures.

The implementation of testing in the United States has apparently been entirely successful inasmuch as there have been no cases of transfusion-associated AIDS attributable to transfusions conducted during the 18 months after the implementation of the test programme. However, it must be recognized that, at least among adults, the mean incubation period for transfusion AIDS may be as long as 4–5 years (Lui *et al.*, 1986) and that, although the incubation period for transfusion AIDS among paediatric patients is much shorter, there are relatively few such cases. Consequently, the absence of diagnosed AIDS among transfusion recipients may not be a very effective, or sensitive measure of the efficacy of current screening mechanisms. In fact, the first documented case of seroconversion in a recipient transfused after the implementation of testing has just been reported (CDC, 1986b); the infectious product was apparently collected just prior to the donor's seroconversion.

There is much additional evidence in support of the overall value of screening donors for anti-HIV. In every transfusion-associated AIDS case retrospectively evaluated by the CDC, at least one of the implicated donors was shown to have anti-HIV and each of the seropositive donors yielded virus when lymphocytes were subjected to appropriate culture procedures (Peterman, Jaffe and Feorino, 1985). Similarly, in studies on blood donors identified as a result of anti-HIV screening in Atlanta, virus could be isolated from about 63.9% of those donors positive by ELISA and confirmed by a Western blot procedure to identify antibodies to the p24 *gag* and or gp41 *env* components of the virus (Ward *et al.*, 1986). In contrast, no virus could be isolated from ELISA negative donors, although two ELISA positive, Western blot negative donors did have isolatable virus. Initial evidence suggests that recipients of seropositive blood or components are at extremely high risk of being infected by HIV (Alter *et al.*, 1985) and a seroprevalence study in a transfused paediatric population, performed prior to test implementation, showed that the infectivity rate was compatible with the subsequently measured seropositivity rate in the local donor population (Williams *et al.*, 1985). In other words, infectivity for HIV appears to be uniformly associated with the presence of anti-HIV, as detected by ELISA and confirmed by Western blot procedures. Mounting evidence suggests that ELISA positive tests which are not supported by the presence of characteristic patterns of reactivity in Western blot are false positives, due to a number of causes, including antibodies directed against host-derived components of the AIDS virus (Kuhnl, Seidl and Holzberger, 1985; Fang *et al.*, 1986; Sayers, Beatty and Hansen, 1986). The overall frequency of the confirmed presence of anti-HTLV III in the donor population was 0.038% in August of 1985 and has declined somewhat since (Schorr *et al.*, 1985). Thus, even in the first year of testing, several thousand potentially infectious donations have been identified and eliminated. However, none of these studies provided any information about the sensitivity of testing or the possibility of transmission from seronegative donors.

8.4 POLICY AND OPERATIONAL ISSUES

8.4.1 General

Implementation of screening for antibodies to HIV generated a number of complex, ethical, legal and operational issues which had to be resolved in the context of current bioethical principles. Recognition of the rights of the individual donor resulted in policies requiring that donors specifically consent to the test itself. Such considerations also prompted the decision to notify those individuals with a positive test and to make arrangements for their referral to competent sources of medical advice. Developing information indicates that the majority of donors with Western blot confirmed antibodies are actively infected and presumably infectious (Ward *et al.*, 1986), so this notification policy does have a public health dimension. Notification policy also generated the need to establish sites when persons could obtain a test result in confidence and without the need to donate a unit of blood.

Issues of confidentiality of test results and donor referral registries were paramount and policies had to be developed to deal with requests for third-party notification of test results. The mounting numbers of donors with false positive test results is a matter of considerable concern, as yet unresolved. Implementation of testing has resulted in the realization that earlier, untested donations from seropositive donors may have infected recipients, who must now be told. Finally, considerable effort has been required to maintain the confidence of the general public, blood recipients and even donors themselves.

8.4.2 Donor consent and notification

In the United States, it is widely recognized that significant medical information cannot be withheld, or concealed from a patient. This guiding principle was applied on implementation of the anti-HIV test and it was generally accepted that a donor would have to be notified of a positive test result. However, it was also recognized that this information was extremely serious in nature, potentially reflecting the early stages of a uniformly fatal disease. Therefore, it was unacceptable to perform the test in the absence of explicit permission from the donor. As a result, an explanation of the anti-HIV (and other) tests to be performed on the blood was incorporated into the donor information leaflet, along with the statement that the donor would be advised of a positive result. The donor's signature then became an explicit consent for the test, and was a requirement for continuation of the collection process.

During the first several months of implementation of HIV antibody testing in blood centres throughout the United States, all blood products from donors who had reproducibly reactive results were withheld from transfusion. This period of time was viewed as a 'phase-in' period and blood donors were not informed of the test results. Donor notification of positive test results began at many centres in July, 1985, and was based on the following criteria: the sample was repeatedly reactive by a commercial ELISA and also was reactive following testing with another technique, such as the Western blot (Schorr *et al.*, 1985; Holland *et al.*, 1985; Osterholm *et al.*, 1985). A study done at the American Red Cross showed that all of the licensed tests were able to detect the same three Western blot positive samples in a population of 900 donor sera but that non-specific positive results also occur and appear to be directed against the cell substrate used to grow the virus. For these reasons, combinations of ELISA tests derived from the same virus/ substrate combination should not be used to define true positives (Fang *et al.*, 1986).

Donor counselling is a difficult task because the implications of a positive test are presently unknown. Studies to define the outcome of HIV infections in donors are currently under way. However, since most seropositive donors are now found to have known risk factors for AIDS, it seems likely that their prognosis is similar to that determined in follow up studies on high risk groups. In other words, a significant percentage – perhaps even up to 35% – may ultimately develop AIDS.

The plasmapheresis industry has pursued a slightly different approach in donor notification, largely for logistics reasons. Since donors may give up to twice a week, and ELISA positive donations cannot be used, it is considered important to identify and remove ELISA-positive donors from the population. Western blot tests are not used. Before entering a plasmapharesis programme, the donor is examined by a physician and told about HIV testing and its interpretation. Any units that are repeatedly reactive are not used; the donor is also informed of the result without additional testing. At the same time, the donor is reminded of the initial conversation during which time the ELISA was emphasized as a screening test which was designed specifically to determine plasma product suitability; further evaluation of test results is necessary to determine the significance to the donor.

8.4.3 Confidentiality

The confidentiality of test results is critically important, as it is widely recognized that a positive test result could have major implications for an individual's employability or insurability. In addition, although clearly inappropriate, it is possible that a positive test result could be interpreted as an indicator of the donor's life style. At the same time, it is accepted that future donations from individuals found to have antibodies to HIV should not be used, so some form of deferral record must be maintained. The dilemma of making a usable record while maintaining confidentiality has been resolved by maintaining a single listing of all donors considered permanently unsuitable for any reason, without listing the cause. Existing registers of this type already reference large numbers of individuals deferred for positive HBsAg tests or a history of hepatitis. It is also important to note that deferral registers are not used during interactions with the donor, but rather, to alert staff to the fact that a collected blood unit has been identified as being from a donor previously defined as unsuitable.

An additional problem in dealing with donor deferrals is that of false positive results. The current regulatory climate in the United States requires that a donor be permanently disqualified on the basis of repeatably positive ELISA test results – that is, two or more reactive results during the initial and repeat tests. The majority of these test results are not confirmed by Western blot and many of them are not even positive when retested in ELISA. It has been considered inappropriate to inform such donors that they have 'false positive' test results, since this concept cannot readily be presented without creating alarm. Consequently, the donor's identity is placed on a local deferral list and future donations are discarded. In the absence of a change in the regulatory position, it appears that it will also be necessary to notify these donors of their status.

Blood collection agencies have had to develop policies to deal with notification of anti-HIV test results to third parties, such as employers, public health agencies and insurance companies. In general, the position has been that the donor has a confidential, medical relationship with the blood centre medical director and that any release of information without the donor's express consent is unacceptable. In addition, the donor should be aware that release of such information should be undertaken with full knowledge of the potential consequences. In some circumstances, there is a legal requirement to provide HIV test information to specific agencies. For example, the United States Defence Department requires that, when blood was collected by civilian agencies on military bases, the names of HIV positive military personnel would have to be reported to the military medical authorities. Similarly, reporting of positive test results is legally required by some State public health agencies. In such circumstances, the potential donor is specifically advised as part of the informed consent procedure that positive test results will be provided to the specified agencies. Given the extent of the AIDS epidemic, the possibilities for heterosexual transmission and the fact that behaviour modification is the only effective preventative measure, it may be appropriate for public health agencies to be aware of the identities of any infectious individual. Therefore, provided that appropriate consent procedures are followed, and that public health agencies perform their duties ethically and confidentially, notification of HIV test results may be proper. In addition, knowledge that this will occur may deter donation by individuals with AIDS risk factors. Nevertheless, there continues to be concern that some persons exposed to HIV infections will continue to donate, even if only to obtain a test result. Thus, there is a need to maintain stringent measures to permit individuals with AIDS risk factors to defer themselves, or their donations (CDC, 1983, 1985a; Pindyck *et al.*, 1985). In addition, this potential problem has mandated the establishment of alternate sites where a person may seek testing and counselling under anonymity, or in confidence (Mason, 1985); available evidence clearly suggests that such establishments fulfil their purpose (Forstein *et al.*, 1985). Another approach, adopted by some States, was to prohibit the provision of test results to any person. In general, regulations of this type are relaxed at some specified time after the availability of the alternate test sites.

In May, 1986, the Centers for Disease Control reported on the overall results of the first year of operation of alternate test sites (CDC, 1986b). More than 79 000 persons were tested in 874 sites and 17.3% were found to be repeatably reactive in ELISA tests for anti-HIV. Certainly, some, if not all of these persons might have donated blood in order to obtain a test result in the absence of the alternate site programme.

8.4.4 Directed donation

Directed donation is the term used when a patient selects the donors of blood to be used, generally in support of elective surgery. Blood collection agencies in the United States have issued statements against this practice. The rationale for discouraging directed donations includes: the absence of demonstrated safety of directed donations; concern that unsuitable donors may conceal their status; concern that potential donors may 'save' their blood for friends and relatives and not give for community needs, and, perhaps most important, that the process is unethical, as it generates two levels of service. The issue is complex, emotional and controversial and there are a number of blood centres which do engage in directed donation programmes. Directed donations may be acceptable on the basis of medical need, and in special circumstances such as risk of serious psychological harm to the patient who is pathologically concerned about the safety of the community blood supply, and when parents give to their own infant. However, a better solution for individuals facing elective surgery, is the use of autologous (predeposit) donations along with intraoperative salvage of blood.

8.4.5 Recipient notification

Finally, at the inception of testing, a number of frequent donors have been found to be positive for antibodies to HIV. Clearly, there is a degree of concern that at least some prior donations from such individuals will have been positive and presumptively infectious. Should recipients of these earlier donations be informed? Current policy is that it is appropriate to advise the physicians responsible for the care of such recipients when there is significant risk that the blood product was infectious. These 'look back' programmes were started in the middle of 1986 and it is anticipated that a proportion of recipients will indeed be found to have been infected.

8.5 CURRENT AND FUTURE IMPACT

The AIDS epidemic has generated a high level of awareness and concern. This has been clearly expressed in public attitudes to blood transfusion. Specifically, opinion polls have shown that most individuals are aware that the disease can be transmitted by transfusion. Somewhat more surprisingly, 43% of those surveyed believed, incorrectly, that AIDS can be acquired by the act of giving blood. Even so, it seems that concern about transfusion-associated AIDS has not impacted either blood usage or supply to a great extent. Certainly, awareness of the risks of transfusion has prompted a more conservative attitude to this procedure and there is increased focus on autologous and directed donation. Actual utilization of blood in the United States has, however, only declined by a few percentage points. It is not clear to what extent such declines may also reflect changes in health care financing in the United States. Similarly, during the AIDS crisis, there have been occasions on which individual blood centres have experienced shortages of donors and in some cases, such shortages have been linked, anecdotally, with fear of AIDS.

The AIDS epidemic has ceased to be confined to the United States and as additional countries register initial cases, donor screening is implemented. Because of the lengthy incubation period of AIDS, it will be some years before the efficacy of these actions can be demonstrated. However, laboratory studies clearly indicate that, since most seropositive individuals do harbour virus, significant numbers of potentially infectious blood units are being eliminated. It is thus reasonable to assume that most potential transfusion-association AIDS cases will indeed be prevented. Additional research may focus on direct tests for infectivity, or on tests of improved specificity. In the absence of immediate prospects for vaccination against, or treatment of AIDS the major future preventative actions will be at the public health level and will focus on the 98% of cases which are not related to transfusion of blood and blood products.

REFERENCES

Alter, H. J., Esteban, J. I., Shih, J. W-K, Kay, J. and Tai, C. C. (1985) A prospective study of the infectivity of anti-HTLV III positive blood donors (abstract). *Transfusion*, 25, 479.

Amman, A. J., Cowan, M. J., Wara, D. W. and Weintrub, P. (1983) Acquired immunodeficiency in an infant: Possible transmission by means of blood transfusion. *Lancet*, i, 956.

Barré-Sinoussi, F., Chermann, J. C., Rey, F., Nugeyre, M. T. *et al.* (1983) Isolation of a T-lymphotropic retrovirus from a patient at risk for acquired immune deficiency syndrome (AIDS). *Science*, **220**, 868.

Brown, F. (1986) Human immunodeficiency virus (Letter). *Science*, **232**, 1486.

Burke, D. S. and Redfield, R. R. (1986) False-positive Western blot tests for antibodies to HTLV III. *JAMA*, **256**, 347.

CDC (1981a) Pneumocystis pneumonia-Los Angeles. *MMWR*, **30**, 250.

CDC (1981b) Kaposi's sarcoma and Pneumocystis pneumonia among homosexual men – New York City and California. *MMWR*, **30**, 305.

CDC (1982a) Pneumocystis carinii pneumonia among persons with hemophilia A. *MMWR*, **31**, 365.

CDC (1982b) Possible transfusion-associated acquired immune deficiency syndrome (AIDS) – California. *MMWR*, **31**, 652–4.

CDC (1983) Prevention of acquired immune deficiency syndrome (AIDS): Report of interagency recommendations. *MMWR*, **32**, 101.

CDC (1985a) Provisional public health service inter-agency recommendations for screening donated blood and plasma for antibody to the virus causing acquired immunodeficiency syndrome. *MMWR*, **34**, 1.

CDC (1985b) Update: Revised Public Health Service definition of persons who should refrain from donating blood and plasma – United States. *MMWR*, **34**, 547.

CDC (1986a) Transfusion-associated human T-lymphotropic virus type III/Lymphadenopathy-associated virus infection from a seronegative donor – Colorado. *MMWR*, **35**, 389.

CDC (1986b) Human T-lymphotropic virus type III lymphadenopathy-associated virus antibody testing at alternate sites. *MMWR*, **35**, 284–7.

Curran, J. W., Lawrence, D. N., Jaffe, H., Kaplan, J. E. *et al.* (1984) Acquired immunodeficiency syndrome (AIDS) associated with transfusion. *N. Engl. J. Med.*, **310**, 69.

Dahlke, M. B. (1984) Designated blood donations. *N. Engl. J. Med.*, **310**, 1194.

Fang, C. T., Darr, F., Kleinman, S., Wehling, R. H. and Dodd, R. Y. (1986) Relative specificity of enzyme-linked immunosorbent assays for antibodies to human T-cell lymphotropic virus, type III, and their relationship to Western blotting. *Transfusion*, **26**, 208.

Forstein, M., Page, P., Coburn, R., Corwell, R. C. *et al.* (1985) Alternative sites for screening blood for antibodies to AIDS virus. *N. Engl. J. Med.*, **313**, 1158.

Gallo, R. C., Salahuddin, S. Z., Popovic, M., Shearer, G. M. *et al.* (1984) Frequent detection and isolation of cytopathic retroviruses (HTLV III) from patients with AIDS and at risk for AIDS. *Science*, **224**, 500.

Holland, P. V., Richards, C. A., Teghtmeyer, J. R., Douville, C. M., Carson, J. R., Hinrichs, S. H. and Pederson, N. C. (1985) Anti-HTLV III testing of blood donors: Reproducibility and confirmability of commercial test kits. *Transfusion*, **25**, 395–7.

Kalish, R. I., Cable, R. G. and Roberts, S. C. (1986) Voluntary deferral of blood donations and HTLV III antibody positives. *N. Engl. J. Med.*, **314**, 115.

Kleinman, S., Thompson, P. and Kaplan, H. (1984) Evaluation of donor screening procedures for AIDS prevention in a high risk area (abstract). *Transfusion*, **24**, 434.

Kuhnl, P. S., Seidl, S. and Holzberger, G. (1985) HLA-DR4 antibodies cause positive HTLV antibody ELISA results. *Lancet*, **i**, 222.

Kuritsky, J. N., Rastogi, S. C., Faich, G. A., Schorr, J. B. *et al.* (1986) Results of nationwide screening of blood and plasma for antibodies to human T-cell lymphotropic III virus, type III. *Transfusion*, **26**, 205.

Levy, J. A., Hoffman, A. D., Kramer, S. M., Landis, J. A. *et al.* (1984) Isolation of lymphocytopathic retrovirus from San Francisco patients with AIDS. *Science*, **225**, 840.

Lui, K.-J., Lawrence, D. N., Morgan, W. M., Peterman, T. A. *et al.* (1986) A model-based approach for estimating the mean incubation period of transfusion associated acquired immunodeficiency syndrome. *Proc. Natl Acad. Sci. USA*, **83**, 3051.

Mason, J. O. (1985) Alternative sites for screening blood for antibodies to AIDS virus. *N. Engl. J. Med.*, **313**, 1157–8.

Mayer, K. H., Stoddard, A. M., McCusker, J., Ayotte, D. *et al.* (1986) Human T-lymphotropic virus type III in high risk, antibody negative homosexual men. *Ann. Intern. Med.*, **104**, 194.

Osterholm, M. T., Bowman, R. J., Chopek, M. W., McCullough, J., Korlath, J. and Polesky, H. (1985) Screening donated blood and plasma for HTLV III antibody. *N. Engl. J. Med.*, **312**, 1185–9.

Peterman, T. A., Jaffe, H. W. and Feorino, P. M. (1985) Transfusion–associated acquired immunodeficiency syndrome in the United States. *JAMA*, **254**, 2913.

Pindyck, J., Waldmann, A., Zang, E., Oleszko, W. *et al.* (1985) Measures to decrease the risk of acquired immunodeficiency syndrome transmission by blood transfusion: Evidence of volunteer blood donor cooperation. *Transfusion*, **25**, 3.

Popovic, M., Sarngadharan, M. G., Read, E. and Gallo, R. C. (1984) Detection, isolation and continuous production of cytopathic retroviruses (HTLV III) from patients with AIDS and pre-AIDS. *Science*, **224**, 497.

Sarngadharan, M. G. Popovic, M., Bruch, L., Schupbach, J. and Gallo, R. C. (1984) Antibodies reactive with human T-lymphotropic retroviruses (HTLV III) in the serum of patients with AIDS. *Science*, **224**, 506.

Sayers, M. H., Beatty, P. G. and Hansen, J. A. (1986) HLA antibodies as a cause of false-positive reactions in screening enzyme immunoassays for antibodies to human T-lymphotropic virus type III. *Transfusion*, **26**, 113.

Schorr, J. B., Berkowitz, A., Cumming, P. D., Katz, A. J. and Sandler, S. G. (1985) Prevalance of HTLV III antibody in American blood donors. *N. Engl. J. Med.*, **313**, 384.

Ward, J. W., Grindon, A. J., Feorino, P. M., Schable, C., Parvin, M. and Allen, J. R. (1986) Laboratory and epidemiologic evaluation of an enzyme immunoassay for antibodies to HTLV III. *JAMA*, **256**, 357–61.

Williams, A. E., Luban, N. L. C., Fang, C. T. and Dodd, R. Y. (1985) Serial development of anti-HTLV III and AIDS-related complex in highly transfused children (Abstract). *Transfusion*, **25**, 479.

9

Blood donor screening for HIV infection: introduction in the United Kingdom and Europe and its impact on transfusion medicine

—— *D. B. L. McClelland* ——

9.1 INTRODUCTION

The preceding chapters have dealt with the nature of the immunological tests which are available to detect HIV infection, and describe the blood donor screening programmes operating in the United States. This chapter reflects the experience of the first year of routine HIV testing of blood donors in the United Kingdom and gives a view, necessarily very incomplete, of the situation in some other European countries.

Although many aspects of the epidemic of HIV infection probably differ relatively little between Europe and North America, it is clear that events in the United States are 2–3 years in advance of those in Europe, with substantially larger numbers of cases of AIDS and of other HIV-related clinical problems, and in some areas of the country, strong evidence that much larger numbers of so far asymptomatic individuals are infected with this virus. Public anxiety about the problem was already at a very high level by the end of 1983 and early 1984 when the crucial scientific advances were made which permitted the culture of the virus in sufficient quantities to make practicable an antibody screening test to detect infected individuals.

It was inevitable that there would be overwhelming pressure to introduce screening of blood donors 'to make the Nation's blood supply safe', not least because this was and remains today one of the few relatively straightforward and rapidly achievable ways of reducing transmission of HIV. Thus the medical and epidemiological requirement for blood donor screening was backed by an urgent sense of the political necessity to take some form of decisive, visibly effective action.

Against this backdrop, the development from a research laboratory immunoassay into a mass produced screening test, within a matter of a few months was a remarkable technical achievement. Equally the nationwide introduction of donor screening over a period of weeks was an administrative tour de force. Inevitably there has been a penalty in terms of certain aspects of the performance of the first generation of screening tests, notably the problem of a relative lack of specificity, leading to a substantial number of false positive results arising from the donor screening programme. Although in historical terms, this problem of the first year of testing will be of little importance, it has led to immense short-term difficulties for the blood collection agencies employing these procedures and some of these problems have at times tended to dominate discussion perhaps to the exclusion of other very important issues which may prove eventually more difficult to resolve than that of test specificity and confirmation.

In Europe, although the necessity of screening of donors was in general rapidly accepted, several countries felt able to proceed under slightly less pressure, moving a pace or two behind the United States and so were able to reap some advantages from early American experience and to benefit from the opportunity to evaluate a rapidly extending range of screening procedures. In the case of the United Kingdom at least, the selection of a different type of procedure for most donor screening (Mortimer, Parry and Mortimer, 1985) has markedly altered the impact which the introduction of the screening programme has had on the blood collection services.

As Table 9.1 shows, the visible part of the HIV infection problem – clinical AIDS, or the 'tip of the iceberg' – is still relatively small in Europe when compared with the very large numbers of cases in the United States and with the catastrophic spread of infection in Africa. The number of cases of transfusion-associated AIDS in Europe appears so far to be quite small and these figures, taken together with the timing of the introduction of donor screening (also shown in Table 9.1) may suggest that Europe has moved sufficiently quickly to forestall the problem of transfusion-associated AIDS. Unfortunately, as in the United States there is good evidence that in some European countries at least, there was a significant prevalence of clinically silent HIV infection for some years before clinical AIDS became apparent. Even a completely successful donor screening programme operating from 1985 onwards leaves us with the problem of those who have been infected through transfusion before the start of screening.

There are several main aspects of the impact of the HIV epidemic on

Table 9.1 AIDS in Europe and programmes for donation testing

Country	Cases	*AIDS* Rate per million	Transfusion associated	*Donation screening* Recommended	Compulsory	*Methods for confirmatory testing*
Austria	34	4.5		6.85	1.86	ELISA + IB
Belgium	160	16.2	5		8.85	ELISA + IB or IF
Czechoslovakia	4	0.3				
Denmark	80	15.7	1		9.85	IB + IF
Germany (FDR)	457	7.5	6		4.85	IB + IF + ELISA
Finland	11	2.2			8.85	ELISA + IB
France	707	12.9	19		8.85	ELISA + IB
Greece	14	1.4			8.85	ELISA + IB
Hungary	0	0			11.85	ELISA + IF
Iceland	2	10.0				
Ireland	9	2.5				
Italy	219	3.8	4	7.85		ELISA + IB
Luxembourg	3	7.5			8.85	ELISA + IB
Netherlands	120	8.3	3	6.85		WB
Norway	21	5.0			8.85	ELISA + IF
Poland	0	0				
Portugal	24	2.3			9.85	
Spain	145	3.8				
Sweden	50	6.0		6.85		ELISA + IB
Switzerland	113	17.4			11.85	IB + IF
United Kingdom	340	6.0	4		10.85	ELISA + IB
Yugoslavia	3	0.1				

IB = immunoblot; IF = immunofluorescence.
Data from *WHO Weekly Epidemiological Record*, **61**, 5 1986 (January).
AIDS Surveillance in Europe No. 9, March 31st 1986 (WHO Collaborating Centre on AIDS, Paris).

transfusion which may be interesting to discuss from a European standpoint, although it must be said that between Europe and the United States, the difference in the approach to coping with the problem are differences of emphasis rather than of direction. This must be starkly contrasted with the situation in many African countries where the scale of the epidemic now threatens to overwhelm completely the resources available to fight it and the whole approach may require to be radically different.

9.2 INTERFACE OF DONOR AND BLOOD COLLECTION SERVICE – DONOR EDUCATION, VOLUNTARY DEFERRAL, SELECTION PROCEDURES AND ROUTES FOR OPTING OUT OF DONATION

From 1983 onwards, transfusion services in most European countries have taken steps to encourage voluntary self-deferral of donors in groups thought to be at high risk of being infected. Some countries including the UK have introduced the requirement for a donor to sign that he or she has read and understood the relevant information explaining the groups at risk. Most countries have modified the standard donor health questionnaires in an attempt to elicit symptoms which could indicate symptomatic HIV infection. Policies with respect to physical examination vary but in the UK there has been no attempt to introduce a clinical examination for lymphadenopathy or other features. In some centres an option has been introduced to permit donors to designate their blood for non-transfusion purposes, with some evidence that this is being used as a confidential opting-out mechanism by individuals in high risk groups (e.g. Contreras *et al.*, 1985).

However European experience seems generally to reflect that of the United States – there is continuing evidence that individuals in high risk groups do attend donor sessions and that virtually all donors who have positive HIV antibody tests confirmed are found on careful questioning to have a history of some form of behaviour which puts them at risk of infection. A typical analysis is given by Courouc é *et al.* (1986) (Table 9.2).

In the South East of Scotland, where the prevalence of confirmed HIV antibody in donors is considerably higher than elsewhere in the UK, virtually all HIV positive donors have on questioning given a history of intravenous drug misuse, reflecting the high prevalence of infection among drug misusers in the local community (Peutherer *et al.*, 1985).

Individuals in risk groups may attend to give blood for various reasons; for example they may wish to have a free antibody test, they may simply be convinced that they personally could not be at risk, they may fail to understand the warning messages given by the Transfusion Service, or they may be unable to read. The experience of most European Transfusion Services appears to be that donation purely with the intent to obtain a test is

Table 9.2 Characteristics of blood donors in France found to have HIV antibody confirmed by immunoblot or radioimmunoprecipitation assay (RIPA) (Study Group of the French Society of Blood Transfusion. Couroucé *et al.*, 1986)

60% positive for anti HBc
85% male
90% under 30 years
70% of males are homosexual or bisexual
15% of males are injecting drug users
50% of females contacts of above groups
40% injecting drug users
10% polytransfused or no risk factor found

unusual and that the other reasons given above account for most attendances by high-risk individuals.

There is therefore a continuing and difficult challenge for the blood collection services; how do we improve our ability to communicate the self deferral message to relevant individuals? There is an urgent need for more studies to identify the communication problems and to assist in the design of a more effective information campaign to support self-deferral.

Equally a more intrusive and direct form of interview with the donor must probably become a standard part of the donor's attendance. My own centre has recently introduced a two-stage process of questioning with, at the second stage, the donor being requested to read the card reproduced in Fig. 9.1 at the time of donation. The donor is offered the opportunity to indicate in

AIDS

PLEASE REMEMBER

1. ANY MAN WHO HAS HAD SEX WITH ANOTHER MAN SINCE 1977
2. ANYONE WHO HAS EVER INJECTED THEMSELVES WITH DRUGS
3. ANYONE WHO HAS EVER HAD A SEXUAL RELATIONSHIP WITH ANYONE IN THE ABOVE GROUPS

MUST NOT GIVE BLOOD

Figure 9.1 Additional information given to blood donors at the time of donation, with opportunity for confidential telephone callback.

confidence at the time of donation or by a confidential telephone call-back contact if he or she wishes the donation to be used for non-transfusion purposes only.

9.3 ALTERNATIVE TESTING SITES

The concern that high risk individuals would donate blood to obtain a free antibody test prompted moves in the United States to provide, at least temporarily, ways in which HIV antibody tests could be obtained confidentially and free of charge outside the blood collection agencies (CDC, 1986a). At the time of this report, 79 000 persons had been tested at these sites with a prevalence of HIV antibody of 17% (repeatably positive ELISA test).

In the UK, it was proposed that testing should be made available via sexually transmitted disease clinics or through family doctors. There is no information about the extent to which these opportunities have been taken up or how they may have influenced attendances of high-risk persons at blood donation centres. In Edinburgh, a self-referral open access clinic was established in the infectious diseases hospital to provide full pre-test counselling, HIV testing and post-test support free of charge to any person requesting it. This was introduced at the same time as HIV antibody testing on blood donors. A preliminary report has been published (Brettle *et al.*, 1986) of which relevant features are given in Table 9.3.

These findings suggest that this facility has been effective in reducing the number of drug misusers attending donor sessions. More effective marketing of this service would be likely to increase its efficacy in this respect. It is this writer's view that any serious attempt to offer effective alternative-site testing must ensure that the service is offered in a way which is readily and freely

Table 9.3 Attendances of an open access, self-referral clinic for HIV antibody testing

Attendances 10/85 to 6/86		*400*
Analysis of first 100 subjects		*No. with HIV Antibody*
Drug misusers (DM)	46	30
Sexual contacts of DM	21	1
Homosexual/bisexual	13	1
Others (e.g. African contacts, transfused)	20	1
Those who stated an intention to donate blood to obtain test if clinic facility not available	14	3

available in a neutral and confidential environment which should not be associated with, for example, a clinic for sexually transmitted diseases since this may well deter many individuals from attending. Experience in New York appears to suggest that the failure to offer such facilities may in an area of high AIDS incidence put serious pressure on blood collection agencies (Caiazza, 1985).

9.4 SCREENING TESTS AND CONFIRMATORY TESTS FOR ANTIBODY TO HIV: VARIATIONS IN SPECIFICITY AND THEIR EFFECT ON THE MANAGEMENT OF BLOOD DONORS

By definition, donor screening tests must have the greatest possible sensitivity; this is dealt with in Section 9.5. However, blood donor management is profoundly influenced by the extent to which the screening test used is specific and by the rapid availability of a reliable confirmatory test procedure. Table 9.4 is intended to help illustrate this statement with data from existing donor testing programmes. Attention is drawn to the following features of the data.

1. In certain programmes (e.g. USA, Germany) more than 0.3% of donors (3 per 1000) have repeatedly reactive screening tests. Only 5–10% of these results can be confirmed by additional procedures such as immunofluorescence, immunoblotting or RIPA. Therefore substantial numbers of donors accumulate who have positive ELISA tests which cannot be confirmed. This raises serious problems. Can this donor be accepted in the future? Must the donor be told the results of the tests? If told, what advice should be given about the clinical significance to the individual of the test results?

   These problems have recently been a central theme of a Consensus Development Conference at the National Institutes of Health (NIH Consensus Development Conference, 1986). In its draft consensus statement, the panel concluded that in a situation where a donor's blood test is repeatedly positive on an ELISA assay, but the Western blot confirmatory test is negative, the donor should be informed of these results and counselled appropriately that although the blood will not be transfused, the tests almost certainly indicate that the donor is not infected with HIV.
2. The scale of this particular problem is much smaller in the UK donor testing programme because the testing systems used lead to a much smaller number of positive screening results which cannot be subsequently confirmed. To illustrate this more clearly, Table 9.5 compares data from the UK centres using a competitive immunoassay system with data from a German centre using an antiglobulin type assay. In both

Table 9.4 Some reported data on blood donor testing for HIV antibodies

Country	*USA*	*UK*	*France*	*Germany–FDR (Hessen)*	*Germany–FDR (Bavaria)*	*Italy (Turin)*	*Sweden (Stockholm)*
Reference	*1*	*2*	*3*	*4*	*5*	*6*	*7*
Period of testing	3/85–2/86	10/85–5/86	8/85–3/86	4/85–10/85	5/85–12/85	8/85–1/86	6/85–12/85
Donations tested	5 500 000	1 700 000	2 800 000	82 400	140 500	22 000	175 600
Initially reactive	65 000(1.19*)	6959(0.4)			1551(1.1)		
Repeatably reactive	18 000(0.33)	642(0.03)		164(0.2%)	541(0.39)		
Confirmed positive	1675(0.03)	37(0.002)	1661(0.06)	(0.018)	10(0.007%)	(0.09)	5(0.002)

*Figures in brackets are % of the total sample tested.

References	*Tests used: Screen*	*Tests used: Confirm*
1 Presented by Dr G. S. Sandler, NIH Consensus Development Conference, Washington, July 7–9, 1986	Abbott	WB
2 Data from UK BTS Reporting Centre, Manchester (Dr V. I. Rawlinson)	Organon Wellcome	ELISA, WB, IF
3 Couroucé, A. M. *et al.* (1986)	Not stated	
4 Kuhnl *et al.*(1986)	Abbott Organon	WB
5 Jochen, A. B. B. *et al.* (1986)	Abbott	
6 Giachino, O. *et al.* (1986)	Abbott Organon	WB
7 Böttiger, M. *et al.* (1986)	Not stated	

Table 9.5 Donor testing results in two areas of low prevalence of HIV antibody: data selected to show the extent to which different testing performances may impact on a donor programme

	United Kingdom (all centres using competitive EIA) [1]	*Germany (FDR) (Bavaria)* [2]
Test procedure	*Competitive EIA (Wellcome)*	*Antiglobulin (Abbott)*
Testing period	12/85–5/86	5/85–12/85
Total donations tested	1027268	140500
Initially reactive	1865 (0.18%)	1551 (1.1%)
Repeatably reactive	70 (0.007%)	541 (0.39%)
Confirmed positive	26 (0.002%)	10 (0.007%)
Confirmed as % of repeatably reactive	37%	1.8%

[1] Data from V. I. Rawlinson UK Transfusion Services Reporting Centre, Manchester, reflecting all UK centres using competitive EIA procedure: routine testing programme December 1985 to May 1986 inclusive.

[2] Jochen, A. B. B. *et al.* (1986) Presentation at International Conference on AIDS, Paris, June 1986, Poster No. 391.

populations, the percentage of confirmed antibody positive donations is extremely low (0.002% and 0.007% respectively). However, there is a very large difference in the proportion of repeatedly positive ELISA screening tests which are subsequently confirmed (37% in UK, 0.18% in Bavaria). These data are intentionally selected to show the extremes which may be found in different test programmes and to emphasize the scale of the problems which may arise if the test specificity is low.

From the above there is no doubt that a screening test which is highly specific offers very substantial advantages in the following respects.

1. Avoids the distress caused to the donor by being informed of a positive screening result (even if careful reassurance is given, the donor will still be told that his blood is not transfusable).
2. Avoids a large workload of donor counselling.
3. Reduces the numbers of complex and expensive confirmatory test procedures required.
4. Reduces the number of donations discarded due to positive screening test results.

However, these advantages are irrelevant unless it can be demonstrated convincingly that there is no loss of test sensitivity as a penalty of high specificity, since detection of *all* infective donations must remain the only goal of the screening programme.

9.5 SENSITIVITY OF SCREENING TESTS FOR THE DETECTION OF HIV ANTIBODIES

9.5.1 Evaluations of test sensitivity

It is much more difficult to reach a definitive conclusion about the sensitivity of a screening test for HIV antibody than about its specificity. Specificity can be assessed by testing large numbers of healthy donor samples which are easy to obtain. Sensitivity assessment requires extensive panels of samples containing HIV antibody and especially containing the types of antibody response likely to be particularly difficult to detect. Sensitivity testing thus should include at least the following features.

1. All panel samples fully characterized by sensitive qualitative assays (immunoblot, radioimmunoprecipitation – RIPA).
2. Large selection of panel samples containing antibodies of restricted specificity (e.g. anti-core protein only), low affinity and low titre.
3. Serial samples obtained from persons during the course of conversion from seronegative to seropositive.

The third item is particularly important in the context of blood donor testing especially in areas of high prevalence of HIV infection since donors may be infected unknowingly, e.g. by sexual contact and attend for donation during the period (which some have termed the 'seronegative window') between exposure and the development of a strong, easily detectable antibody response. Blood obtained at this early stage of infection may well be highly infectious as demonstrated by the recent report of transmission of HIV by a seronegative blood donation from a donor who became antibody positive by three months after the donation (CDC, 1986b).

There is not yet sufficient data to state confidently how long this 'window' period may be but there are data to suggest that in some cases it may be much longer than the periods of a few weeks within which seroconversion occurs following the massive exposure caused by the transfusion of an infected unit of blood (Ludlam *et al.*, 1985; Huisman *et al.*, 1986a,b).

Table 9.6 summarizes data from some published and unpublished studies which have assessed the sensitivity of HIV antibody screening tests. This indicates some continuing problems in test sensitivity especially with samples reacting mainly with core proteins. It is difficult to summarize all aspects of the claims of the many investigators and manufacturers in relation to sensitivity and it may be unhelpful to do so since the rate of improvement in test performance is likely to outstrip the publication of this book. However some general conclusions about the present situation are necessary.

1. Most evaluations do not show great differences in overall test sensitivity.

Table 9.6 A Synopsis of some studies showing occasional failure of screening tests to detect antibody to HIV in human serum

Reference	*Tests examined*	*Evidence of failure to detect anti-HIV*
1	ENI, Abbott	Both missed one sample with anti p24 and anti p41
2	ENI, Abbott	Both missed 3 p24 only samples: 1 donor, 1 AIDS pt, 1 high risk patient. Each missed 1 further p24 only sample
3	Abbott, ENI Dupont, Litton Genetic Systems	One donor sample (p24, gp41, p55 and gp120 pos) detected only by Dupont
4	Abbott, Dupont, ENI	2 samples p24 only Dupont detected 4/5 ENI detected 2/5 Abbott detected 0/5
5	Abbott	Failed to detect 1 sample p24 + p55 6 samples p 24 only (IFA pos)
6	Abbott, Organon, Litton, Behring, Wellcome, Pasteur, Dupont	On p24, and p24 + 41 samples Wellcome gave highest detection

References
1. Holland, P. V. *et al.* (1985).
2. Carlson, J. R. *et al.* (1985).
3. Tregallas, W. M. *et al.* (1986).
4. Rubin, C. P. *et al.* (1986).
5. O'Shaughnessy, M. V. *et al.* (1986).
6. Reesink, H. W. *et al.* (1986).

Where there is a sensitivity advantage, it appears to favour some of the more recently released antiglobulin assays and the competitive ELISA system.

2. Samples which react strongly in the ELISA assays are almost always easily confirmed by immunoblotting.
3. Each test will find a selection of ELISA positive immunoblot-negative samples. There is relatively little overlap between the samples in this category which are detected by a range of different ELISA screening tests.
4. Most studies show that for any ELISA screening test, there is a small number of samples which are definitely positive by immunoblot and which cannot be detected by the screening test. These problems seem to occur more frequently with serum containing antibodies only to core proteins.
5. Clinical and epidemiological studies strongly indicate that in the great majority of cases blood which is ELISA positive and immunoblot negative is not infective and that virus cannot be isolated from such donors (Esteban *et al.*, 1985).

9.5.2 Studies on patients during seroconversion – performance of screening, testing and confirmatory tests for HIV antibody

Serial sampling from subjects in prospective studies on high-risk groups provides samples covering the period of seroconversion. Several studies (e.g. Lange *et al.*, 1986; Simmonds, Peutherer and McClelland, 1986) show that a consistent feature is that antibody to p24 is present in the first antibody sample with or without antibody to other bands (Fig. 9.2).

This suggests that a test to detect early seroconversion should have high sensitivity for antibody to core proteins. Simmonds, Peutherer and McClelland (1986); Ulstrup *et al.* (1986) and several other studies in preparation demonstrate that there are clear differences in the ability of present screening tests to detect early seroconversion with important implications for donor screening programmes.

What is the 'gold standard' for antibody detection tests? This philosophical question has exercised those responsible for screening programmes and although there will be no fixed answer, it is important to recognize that given a test of greatly increased sensitivity, our view of the performance of existing procedures could be greatly changed. Huisman *et al.* (1986a,b) showed that a radioimmunoprecipitation assay (RIPA) using virus exogenously labelled with ^{125}I was capable of detecting an IgG antibody to core proteins months before either immunoblot or ELISA. The findings were summarized in Table 9.7.

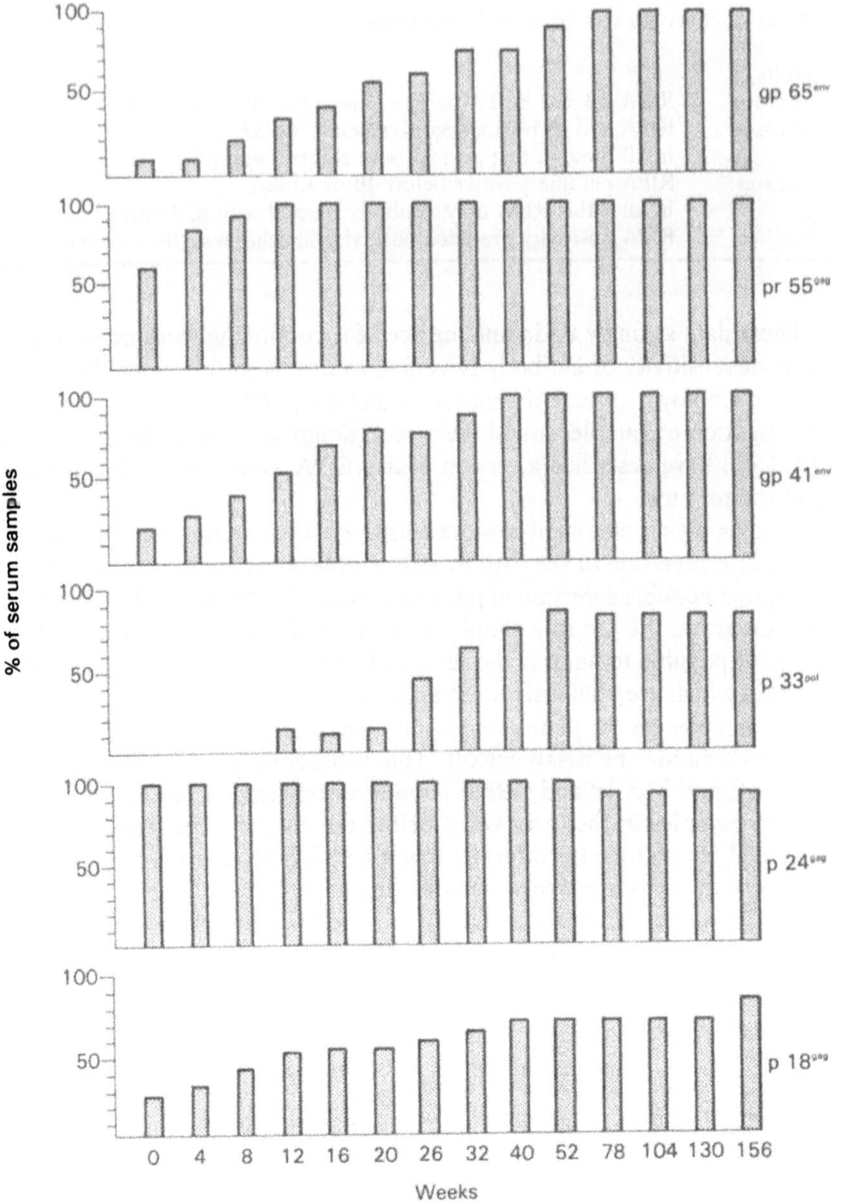

Figure 9.2 Percentage of serum samples reacting with different LAV/HTLV-III proteins by immunoblot analysis in relation to time. Although 15 subjects were studied not all were tested at each subsequent interval and not all were followed up for 156 weeks. At each interval shown, however, at least 6 subjects were tested (Lange *et al.*, 1986).

Table 9.7 Comparison of RIPA, Immunoblot (IB) and ELISA in the detection of onset of IgG antibody response, Huisman *et al.* (1986a,b)

Subjects: Sequential sera from 11 homosexual men	
Results	
4 cases:	RIPA, IB and ELISA became positive at the same time
2 cases:	RIPA and IB became positive before ELISA
	In all these 6, first positive sera reacted with p24
5 cases:	RIPA became positive before IB or ELISA
	In all 5 this RIPA-only antibody reacted with p24 only
	RIPA positivity preceded positivity in other tests by 3–5 months

These data strongly underline the need for continuing work on improvement of sensitivity of antibody screening assays. Also this work shows the need to employ a variety of procedures including RIPA in the confirmatory investigation of samples found reactive in donor screening. Huisman *et al.* (1986a,b) have described a version of this RIPA assay suitable for use as a confirmatory test.

Pending the development of more sensitive assays, attention must be given to the interpretation of the data from available screening tests to ensure the maximum possible detection of positive samples. In the case of the inhibition immunoassay, the use of a simple computerized data reduction procedure makes it possible to analyse the results of each plate to display clearly any samples which are obviously more reactive than the population of negative donor samples on the plate even though they may be less reactive than the samples defining the assay cut off. This procedure, described by Barclay, Hopcroft and McClelland (1986) permits an objective definition of a category of samples in the 'grey zone' below the cut-off value, which can be identified, quarantined and further investigated. It has already been demonstrated that weakly reactive samples including an early seroconversion specimen are rendered detectable by this modification of procedure (Simmonds, Peutherer and McClelland, 1986).

9.5.3 Does donor screening need assays which detect viral antigen or virally transformed cells in addition to antibody?

Preliminary studies using immunoassays to detect viral core protein show that in some patients these appear rarely in the course of infection, possibly in the absence of detectable antibody (Coutinho, 1986). It is too early to say whether assays of this type will offer advantages for routine donor screening. The use of a flow cytometry to detect peripheral blood cells expressing HIV coded antigens has been reported (Payne *et al.*, 1986). In 14 of 15 AIDS or PGL patients (all with HIV antibody) positive lymphocytes could be readily detected. It remains to be shown whether this method will be able to identify cells expressing viral antigens in patients who are antibody negative and also how these finding will relate to results of virus isolation attempts in these cases.

9.6 MANAGEMENT AND QUALITY ASSURANCE ASPECTS OF BLOOD DONOR SCREENING PROGRAMMES

9.6.1 The care of the blood donor

For the donor there are 4 possible outcomes of his voluntary informed participation in screening:

1. true negative result;
2. false negative result;
3. true positive result;
4. false positive result.

In the preceding sections the point has been made that attention to test performance can greatly reduce the problems for the donor and those responsible for the donor's welfare which can result from false positive results. In areas of low prevalence of HIV infection and given the good performance of existing screening tests, the number of false negative results will certainly be extremely small. The care and support of the donor who has to be informed of a true positive result is a major clinical responsibility and the correct discharge of this is a matter of great importance both to the individual donor and to the blood collection agency.

In the United Kingdom, in France and in several other European countries, the policy has been adopted that it is the responsibility of the blood collecting agency to inform the donor of a positive test result, to provide initial counselling and to ensure that appropriate long-term support and clinical care are provided. This has not been a general view in North America where both the commercial plasma collection industry and some parts of the non-profit blood collection system have felt that their responsibility should not extend beyond informing the donor of the test result. There is some evidence that this view may now be under reconsideration (NIH Consensus Development Conference, 1986).

In any case it is essential that the blood collecting organization has a clearly developed policy for the handling of positive screening test results to ensure that each incident is fully resolved to safeguard the interests of both donor and organization. An example of such a scheme, based on that used by the Scottish Blood Transfusion Service is shown in Fig. 9.3.

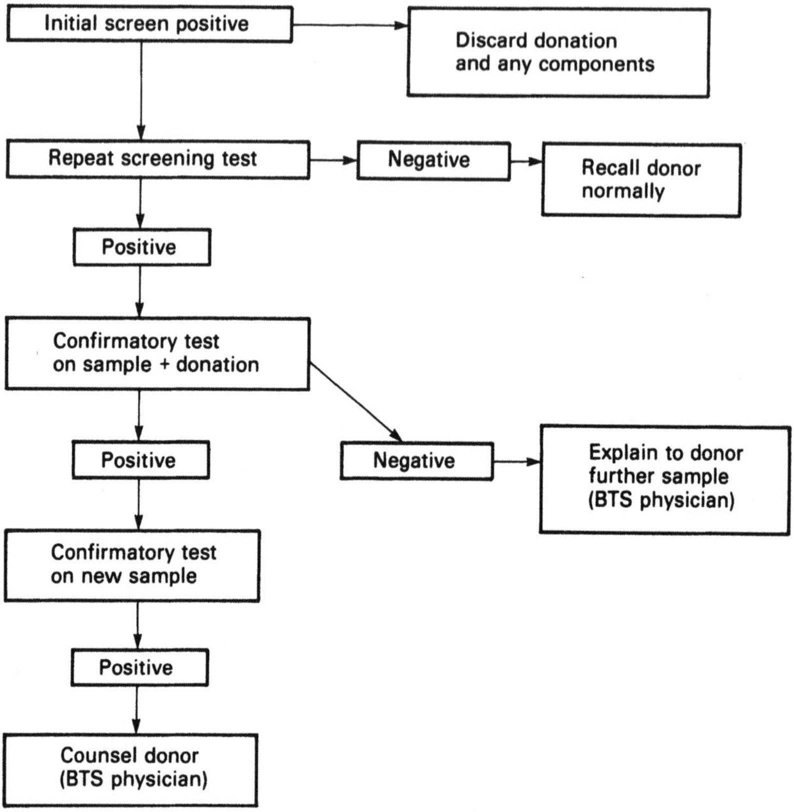

Figure 9.3 Flowchart for management of donor with initially positive HIV antibody screening test.

9.6.2 Quality control of the screening system

The experience of blood transfusion services over many years is that serious failures such as the transfusion of ABO incompatible blood, or the release of donations infected with Hepatitis B virus are more often the result of a human error than of an intrinsic inadequacy of laboratory procedures in use. There is no reason to suppose that this generalization would not apply to the screening programme for HIV antibody. Effort put into the correct performance of the available tests will contribute as much or more to patient safety as will the development of still more sensitive screening tests. Some of the features of an effective quality control structure are as follows:

1. nationally coordinated confirmatory procedures;
2. national external quality assurance schemes;
3. testing laboratories employ daily QA monitoring test performance of known samples;

4. testing laboratories run daily QA using coded unknown samples; correct results on these could be a release criteria for each batch of tests;
5. a management system which ensures that evidence of inadequate performances is immediately noted and leads to rapid corrective action.

In the writer's own laboratory, the use of daily 'blind' QA samples has been standard for some years in Hepatitis B testing as has the practice of retesting donor samples in a small pool (10 samples) to obtain the benefit of a duplicate test of slightly reduced sensitivity. Both these steps should be considered for a test of such importance as the HIV antibody screen.

9.7 RECIPIENT FOLLOW-UP

The decision has been taken in the UK and in several other European countries, as in the United States, that recipients of donations from HIV antibody positive donors should be traced and the responsible physicians informed so that necessary action can be taken in particular to help minimize the risk of further transmission of infection should the recipient prove to be infected. Several large studies in the United States have demonstrated that when donations known to be infected are given, a high proportion of recipients do develop HIV antibody; they may go on to develop AIDS although the number of post-transfusion AIDS cases is much smaller than might be predicted from the number of infected donations transfused before the introduction of testing (Alter, 1986).

Studies of unselected recipients of transfusions given prior to the introduction of testing can also indicate the magnitude of the risk of transmission of HIV by untested blood. An important study of this type in France has been reported by Mercadier *et al.* (1986). A group of 1000 highly transfused patients was identified who had received, before the start of testing, an average of 35 donations of cellular blood products. In this group the overall prevalence of HIV antibody was found to be above 3%. The seropositive recipients had no other risk factors but had received an average of 99 donations of cellular products each. In about one third of cases it had been possible to identify an infected donor.

9.8 CHANGES IN THE CLINICAL PRACTICE OF TRANSFUSION

9.8.1 Autologous transfusion and direct donations

Autologous transfusion, either of blood salvaged during operative procedures or of donations obtained and stored in advance of elective surgery clearly avoids the problem of HIV transmission. Although the scope for expansion of autologous programmes is limited because only a small proportion of patients is suitable, there has been a substantial increase in the United States. Kruskall (1986) reported that in one major hospital, 2% of all red cell transfusions and 7% of FFP transfusions were autologous even in 1983/84. This topic is under active consideration in the United Kingdom but as yet no overall transfusion service policy to develop autologous transfusion has resulted. The availability of improved red cell storage media, offering a 5 week shelf life under standard blood bank conditions should facilitate this development and further research in this area is definitely needed.

Directed donation, the practice of collecting blood from a donor designated by the patient or his relatives, appears to be rarely practised in Europe but has been the subject of fierce controversy in the United States. Several centres operate significant directed donation programmes in response to public pressure for this service which is perceived as offering safer blood. The arguments against this practice were reviewed by Kruskall (1986) and include the following:

1. These donors are not volunteers and may be subjected by relatives or friends to undue pressure to donate.
2. There is no evidence that such donors have a lower prevalence of Hepatitis B or HIV serological markers so there is no scientific basis for the practice.
3. Introduction of a directed donation programme can be interpreted as professional acceptance that blood obtained in this way is safer and therefore implies a lack of confidence in blood stocks obtained from conventional donor sources.
4. There are many serious practical problems in implementation.

9.8.2 Changes in the prescribing of blood and blood components

The most effective way of reducing HIV transmission by blood is to transfuse less blood and although there are exhortations about careful prescribing of blood in many official pronouncements, there is little evidence of systematic and effective efforts to exploit the clinical possibilities for minimizing patient exposure to donors. This must surely be the most important challenge to Transfusion Medicine and will involve the re-examination of many areas of clinical practice. Arguably the United Kingdom and other countries with a totally non-commercial blood supply system should play a leading role because the providers have no conflict between marketing requirements and the demands of safer clinical practice. The requirements for effective action include:

1. Prescribing clinicians must be offered accurate information about the risks of the products available and cumulative risks with numerous donor exposures in for example platelet therapy.

2. Clinical audit information on transfusion practice must be provided to ensure that prescribers are fully aware of their own practice in comparison with that of colleagues dealing with comparable clinical problems. Where substantial local or regional differences in blood usage are observed, these should be studied to determine their effects on patient outcomes.
3. Clinical criteria for transfusion decisions should be reviewed, e.g. what are appropriate haemoglobin levels to initiate transfusion in different clinical situations? Is there scope for wider use of intraoperative haemodilution procedures?
4. Prospective studies of transfusion recipients should be maintained to quantitate post transfusion infection problems.

9.9 CONCLUSIONS

The HIV epidemic will continue to have a profound influence on transfusion practice. HIV infection, once thought to be confined to 'high-risk groups' is becoming evident in a wider cross-section of the population. It is now reported that among US Military recruit applicants, the prevalence of HIV antibody is 1.5 per 1000 with a male to female ratio of 3:1 in contrast to the 13:1 ratio seen in all AIDS cases (CDC, 1986c). In a number of African countries, the prevalence of infection is already much higher than this and there are equal numbers of male and females infected. It will be increasingly difficult to rely heavily on the definition of high-risk groups and voluntary self-exclusion of these groups as donors so that dependence on a highly reliable donor testing programme will increase. If the prevalence of infection continues to rise in the community there may be increasing numbers of individuals in the early phases of infection where antibody is difficult to detect, so it will become increasingly important to have tests which reliably detect the earliest evidence of infection.

Continued awareness of these factors should exert strong pressure to review the indications for use of blood and blood components according to strict risk-benefit criteria.

Review completed June 1986.

REFERENCES

Alter, H. J. (1986) Transmission of LAV/HTLV-III by blood products, in *International Conference on AIDS*, Paris, June 1986 (Program and Abstracts), p. 6, Communication SP10.

Barclay, G. R., Hopcroft, W. and McClelland, D. B. L. (1986) What is an 'equivocal' negative HTLV-III antibody test in blood donors? *Lancet*, i, 912–13.

Böttiger, M. *et al.* (1986) Presentation at International Conference on AIDS, Paris, June 1986, Poster 662.

Brettle, R. P., Davidson, J., Davidson, S. J., Gray, J. M. N., Inglis, J. M., Conn, J. S., Bath, G. E., Gillon, J. and McClelland, D. B. L. (1986) HTLV-III antibodies in an Edinburgh clinic. *Lancet*, i, 1099.

Caiazza, S. S. (1985) Alternative test sites for screening blood for antibodies to AIDS virus. *N. Engl. J. Med.*, **313**, 1158.

Carlson, J. R. *et al.* (1985) *Lancet*, i, 1388.

CDC (1986a) Human T-lymphotropic virus type III/lymphadenopathy-associated virus antibody testing at alternate sites. *MMWR*, **35**, 284–7.

CDC (1986b) Transfusion associated human T-lymphotropic virus type III/lymphadenopathy-associated virus infection from a seronegative donor – Colorado. *MMWR*, **35**, 389–91.

CDC (1986c) Human T-lymphotropic virus type III/lymphadenopathy-associated virus antibody prevalence in U.S. Military recruit applicants. *MMWR*, **35**, 421–4.

Contreras, M., Hewitt, P. E., Barbara, J. A. and Mochnaty, P. Z. (1985) Blood donors at high risk of transmitting the acquired immune deficiency syndrome. *Brit. Med. J.*, **290**, 749–50.

Couroucé, A. M., Smilovici, W., North, M. L. and the Study Group of the French Society of Blood Transfusion (1986) Blood donors positive for anti-LAV antibodies in France: prevalence according to different criteria, in *International Conference on AIDS*, Paris, June 1986 (Program and Abstracts), p. 100, Communication 45.

Coutinho, R. A. (1986) The natural history of LAV/HTLV-III infection, in *International Conference on AIDS*, Paris, June 1986 (Program and Abstracts), p. 99, Communication 37.

Esteban, J. I., Wai-Kuo Shih, J., Tai, C. C., Bodner, A. J., Kay, J. W. D. and Alter, H. J. (1985) Importance of Western blot analysis in predicting infectivity of anti-HTLV-III/LAV positive blood. *Lancet*, ii, 1083–6.

Giachino, O. *et al.* (1986) Presentation at International Conference on AIDS, June 1986, Poster 389.

Holland, P. V. *et al.* (1985) *Transfusion*, **25**, 395–7

Huisman, H. G., Winkel, I., Lelie, N., Tersmette, M., Goudsmit, J. and De Lange, J. (1986a) Comparison of three different immunoassays in their ability to establish in human sera the onset of IgG antibody response to LAV/HTLV-III infection, in *International Conference on AIDS*, Paris, June 1986 (Program and Abstracts), p. 145, Poster 635.

Huisman, H. G., Winkel, I., Lelie, N., Tersmette, M., Goudsmit, J. and Miedema, F. (1986b) A LAV/HTLV-III radioimmuno-assay for confirmatory testing, in *International Conference on AIDS*, Paris, June 1986 (Program and Abstracts), p. 148, Poster 653.

Jochen, A. B. B. *et al.* (1986) Presentation on International Conference on AIDS, June 1986, Poster 391.

Kruskall, M. S. (1986) New trends in transfusion medicine: autologous transfusions and directed donations, in *NIH Consensus Development Conference. Impact of Routine HTLV-III Antibody Testing of Blood and Plasma Donors on Public Health*, Bethesda, July 1986 (Program and Abstracts), pp. 83–7.

Kuhnl *et al.* (1986), *Vox Sang*, **51** (Suppl. 1), 15–20.

Lange, J. M. A., Coutinho, R. A., Krone, W. J. A., Verdonck, L. F., Danner, S. A., Van der Noordaa, J. and Goudsmit, J. (1986) Distinct IgG recognition patterns during progression of subclinical and clinical infection with lymphadenopathy associated virus/human T lymphotropic virus. *Brit. Med. J.*, **292**, 228–30.

Ludlam, C. A., Steel, C. M., Cheinsong-Popov, R., McClelland, D. B. L., Tucker, J.,

Tedder, R. S., Weiss, R. A., Philp, I. and Prescott, R. J. (1985) Human T-lymphotropic virus type III (HTLV-III) infection in seronegative haemophiliacs after transfusion of factor VIII. *Lancet*, ii, 233–6.

Mercadier, A., Jullien, A. M., Guiard, J., Andreu, G., Noel, L., Courouсé, A. M. and the AIDS Study Group of the French National Blood Transfusion Society (1986) LAV/HTLV-III seropositivity among recipients of blood and blood components in Paris area, in *International Conference on AIDS*, Paris, June 1986 (Program and Abstracts), p. 102, Communication 58.

Mortimer, P. T., Parry, J. V., Mortimer, J. Y. (1986) Which anti HTLV-III/LAV assays for screening and confirmatory testing? *Lancet*, ii, 873–7.

NIH Consensus Development Conference (1986) Draft Consensus Statement: *Impact of Routine HTLV-III Antibody Testing of Blood and Plasma Donors on Public Health*, Bethesda, July 1986.

O'Shaughnessy, M. V. *et al.* (1986) International Conference on AIDS, Abstract 417.

Payne, B. C., Bishop, P., Rasheed, S., Gill, P., Levine, A. and Parker, J. W. (1986) The detection of HTLV-III/LAV associated surface antigens in human blood lymphocytes by flow cytometry, in *International Conference on AIDS*, Paris, June 1986 (Program and Abstracts) p. 144, Poster 633.

Peutherer, J. F., Edmond, E., Simmonds, P., Dickson, J. D. and Bath, G. E. (1985) HTLV-III antibody in Edinburgh drug addicts. *Lancet*, ii, 1129–30.

Reesink, H. W. *et al.* (1986) International Conference on AIDS, Abstract 426.

Rubin, C. P. *et al.* (1986) International Conference on AIDS, Abstract 420.

Simmonds, P., Peutherer, J. F. and McClelland, D. B. L. (1986) HTLV-III/LAV antibody testing: confirmation methodologies and future prospects, in *The Safety of Blood and Blood Products in Relation to AIDS. Proceedings of WHO Meeting*, Geneva (ed. J. Petricciani), April 1986, to be published 1986.

Ulstrup, J. C., Skaug, K., Figenschau, K. J., Ørstavik, I., Bruun, J. N. and Petersen, G. (1986) Sensitivity of Western blotting (compared with ELISA and immunofluorescence) during seroconversion after HTLV-III infection. *Lancet*, i, 1151–2.

10

Asymptomatic infection with human immunodeficiency virus

Gordon D. O. Lowe

10.1 INTRODUCTION

Asymptomatic infection by the human immunodeficiency virus (HIV) may be defined as follows:

Evidence of HIV infection

1. Presence of antibodies to HIV in serum (Melbye, 1986) or in other body fluids such as cerebrospinal fluid (CSF; Goudsmit *et al.*, 1986a); or
2. presence of HIV antigen in serum, or in other body fluids such as CSF (Goudsmit *et al.*, 1986b); or
3. isolation of HIV from stimulated peripheral blood mononuclear leucocytes, other tissues such as brain, or other body fluids (Barre-Sinoussi *et al.*, 1983; Gallo *et al.*, 1984; Vilmer *et al.*, 1984; Salahuddin *et al.*, 1985).

and current absence of symptoms attributable to HIV infection. HIV is lymphotropic and neurotropic: such symptoms include (Melbye, 1986; CDC, 1986a):

1. acute glandular fever-like illness;
2. acute encephalopathy, with or without lymphocytic meningitis;
3. persistent generalized lymphadenopathy (PGL) without other cause;
4. presenile dementia, myelopathy or peripheral neuropathy;
5. Acquired Immune Deficiency Syndrome (AIDS; CDC, 1985a), with secondary infections or cancers;
6. various persistent (over 3 months) clinical and laboratory features suggestive of immune disturbance, without other cause, which fall short of the

defined AIDS syndrome. Clinical features include fatigue, weight loss, fever, night sweats, diarrhoea, oral candidiasis (thrush), seborrhoeic dermatitis, folliculitis, herpes zoster, and hepatosplenomegaly. Laboratory features include anaemia, leucopenia, thrombocytopenia, lymphopenia, reduction in T-helper lymphocytes, decrease in ratio of T-helper to T-suppressor lymphocytes, hyperglobulinaemia, decreased lymphocyte responses to stimulation *in vitro*, and anergy to skin tests. Various combinations of these features have been defined as 'AIDS-related complex' (ARC) or 'lesser AIDS' (Goedert and Blatter, 1985).

In practice asymptomatic infection is usually detected by a positive HIV antibody test performed as a screening test on serum (Melbye, 1986; CDC, 1986a). Identification by antibody tests on CSF, by antigen tests on serum or CSF, or by viral isolation has only been achieved in a small number of asymptomatic persons in research studies. Screening of serum samples by blood transfusion centres, epidemiologists, and routine virology laboratories is usually performed by an enzyme-linked immunosorbent assay (ELISA): these colorimetric tests are simple, automated, rapid and cheap (Fischinger and Bolognesi, 1985; Melbye, 1986). They are sensitive and acceptably specific in Europe and the United States (Melbye, 1986), but are less reliable in renal dialysis patients (Peterman *et al.*, 1986; Neumayer, Wagner and Knesse, 1986) and in Africa (see below). False positive tests occur, due to non-specific reactivity, hence it is essential to perform a confirmatory test such as the more specific Western blot method (Fischinger and Bolognesi, 1985; Melbye, 1986). In this method, virus proteins are separated by electrophoresis blotted onto nitrocellulose papers; the test human serum is then applied. Positive sera form antigen–antibody complexes, which are identified by an enzyme labelled anti-human IgG with high binding affinity for such complexes. A profile of bands is therefore seen, representing all viral antigens, which is characteristic for HIV.

False negative tests also occur, i.e. negative serum HIV antibody tests in the presence of HIV infection, detected by positive viral antigen tests or viral isolation (Fischinger and Bolognesi, 1985; Melbye, 1986; Goudsmit *et al.*, 1986b). Some of these individuals are viraemic prior to seroconversion, which appears to take 4–16 weeks (Melbye, 1986; Goudsmit *et al.*, 1986b); some may never produce antibodies, as with hepatitis B (Melbye, 1986); and some may lose detectable antibodies, while remaining asymptomatic, before becoming symptomatic, or as clinical symptoms advance (Melbye, 1986).

The definition of 'asymptomatic' can be difficult. Studies of male homosexuals or multitransfused haemophiliacs with positive HIV antibody tests have shown that many do in fact have mild clinical abnormalities or abnormal laboratory tests. Some staging classifications of such paucisymptomatic patients have recently been proposed. The US Army (Walter Reed) Staging classification was adopted to provide uniformity for routine clinical evaluations (Redfield, Wright and Tramont, 1986). This classification is applicable only to adults, since young children have different functional T-lymphocyte indices. The stages are as follows:

- WRO — High risk contacts – recipients of blood products and sexual contacts of persons with documented HIV infection (antibody or virus isolation).
- WR1 — HIV infection (positive antibody by Western blot, or comparable antigen test or viral isolation). No lymphadenopathy, thrush or opportunistic infections; normal skin tests and T-helper lymphocyte count (over 0.4×10^9/litre).
- WR2 — Chronic lymphadenopathy, otherwise as WR1.
- WR3 — Reduced T-helper cells (under 0.4×10^9/litre), otherwise as WR1 or WR2.
- WR4 — Partial anergy to skin tests, otherwise as WR3.
- WR5 — Complete anergy to skin tests and/or oral thrush, otherwise as WR3.
- WR6 — Opportunistic infections.
- Suffix B — Fever, weight loss, night sweats or chronic diarrhoea.
- Suffix K — Kaposi's sarcoma.
- Suffix CNS — Neurological disease.
- Suffix N — Other neoplasm.

The Centers for Disease Control (1986a) have also recently produced a new classification for HIV infection, in which asymptomatic infection is Group II, PGL is Group III. Patients in these groups may be subclassified on the basis of laboratory evaluation. Such classifications may facilitate studies of the natural history of asymptomatic HIV infection.

10.2 IDENTIFICATION OF ASYMPTOMATIC INFECTED PERSONS

At present, persons with asymptomatic infection are usually identified by a positive HIV antibody screening test performed on their serum. This situation may arise in several ways.

10.2.1 Research studies

Epidemiological studies of high-risk groups for AIDS (male homosexuals with multiple partners, multitransfused haemophiliacs, intravenous drug abusers, sexual partners and babies of the above groups, and persons from sub-Saharan Africa) have shown high prevalences of serum HIV antibodies

(Melbye, 1986). Further epidemiological studies of serum HIV antigen are in progress (Goudsmit *et al.*, 1986b). Such epidemiological studies have been of great value in studying the natural history of HIV infection (Melbye, 1986). Similarly, epidemiological studies of health care workers or household members in regular contact with infected persons have provided valuable reassurance that viral transmission usually occurs only by congenital infection, sexual intercourse, parenteral inoculation with contaminated blood or blood products, or by receiving infected artificial insemination or transplanted organs.

Although valuable, these research studies raise the ethical question of what to do about positive test results. Results of tests in such studies apply to individuals: coding the sera avoids this reality and avoids facing the ethical issues (Welsby, 1986). It may be viewed as unethical to withhold the information of a positive test result from the individual and his doctors (Welsby, 1986). Considerable problems can result when an individual knows he has a positive result, including anxiety, depression, suicide, broken relationships, unemployment, and inability to receive life insurance, endowment mortgage policies, or optimal medical and dental care (Miller *et al.*, 1986a). Pre-counselling prior to test performance is therefore advocated increasingly (Miller *et al.*, 1986). If honest pre-counselling concerning the consequences of a positive test is given in research studies, it is likely that many of those approached will, understandably, refuse the test. If so, it is also likely that our information on the natural history and spread of HIV infection in populations will be less reliable.

10.2.2 Screening of donors

It is widely accepted that donors of blood, semen, and organs (e.g. kidneys, bone marrow, livers, hearts, lungs, corneas) be screened routinely for serum HIV antibodies, for the sake of the recipients and their contacts (Miller *et al.*, 1986). It would also be logical to screen donors of breast milk, since the virus has been isolated from the milk of three healthy carriers (Thiry *et al.*, 1985). Members of high-risk groups have been asked not to donate blood, semen or organs. However, as the prevalence of infection in the heterosexual, non-haemophiliac, non-drug-abusing population increases, so may the number of infected donors. Some blood transfusion services inform potential donors that HIV testing is performed routinely.

10.2.3 Screening of high-risk groups

The question of 'routine' screening of high-risk groups has recently been discussed by Miller *et al.* (1986) who generally oppose it, by Welsby (1986) who supports it, and by Acheson (1986).

(a) Planning of health care, and prevention of spread in the community

Welsby (1986) has argued for routine testing of intravenous drug abusers for HIV infection. Firstly, the information is required for planning of health care provision for this group (and other high-risk groups). Secondly, identifying and informing infected persons, contact tracing and screening, and counselling about the risks of transmission may reduce the spread of infection in the community. On the other hand, Miller *et al.* (1986) have argued that the advice is the same whatever the result of the test; and that since HIV infection appears to be for life, it may be unrealistic to suggest lifelong sexual abstinence. They also point out that sexual spread involves tacit compliance between two people, hence wider counselling of all at risk, rather than 'sources' of infection, may be more effective (Miller *et al.*, 1986). Whether knowledge of serological status alters behaviour is not yet known (Acheson, 1986).

(b) Protection of health care workers

Miller *et al.* (1986) have argued that the risk of infection of clinical and laboratory personnel is negligible, provided that basic standards appropriate for the care of all patients and samples are applied, i.e. avoidance of inoculation injury. They also point out that many infected patients will remain untested (especially if they fear suboptimal medical or dental care and therefore do not disclose membership of a high-risk group), and that false negative results occur. They suggest that patients in high-risk groups should be assumed to be seropositive and to use routine precautions (Miller *et al.*, 1986). Although testing of sera for HIV antibodies is not an infallible guide to infection, it now seems clear that a positive test is a strong pointer to infectivity, and that extra care is required for patients with positive tests when performing invasive procedures or handling blood. In haemophiliacs, for example, there is an increased risk of bleeding externally, and a regular need for venepunctures and laboratory tests, some of which require 'open' testing of blood or plasma. A stronger argument can therefore be made for 'routine' screening in this group, as has been accepted for some years for hepatitis B screening.

(c) Protection of the patient

Miller *et al.* (1986) have pointed out that there are strong arguments for screening for HIV antibody in two patient groups, for the patients' own sakes. In patients receiving haemodialysis, the use of therapeutic immunosuppressive drugs may lead to clinical deterioration: long-term haemodialysis or chronic ambulatory peritoneal dialysis may therefore be preferable to renal transplantation. In recent studies, Peterman *et al.* (1986) and Neumayer, Wagner and Knesse (1986) found that less than 1% of haemodialysis patients had positive HIV antibodies by Western blot. Women in high-risk groups who are contemplating pregnancy, or who are in early pregnancy, may benefit from screening, since pregnancy in seropositive women appears to accelerate maternal disease, as well as carrying a high risk of HIV infection and disease in their infants (Miller *et al.*, 1986).

10.2.4 Screening of exposed health care workers

Staff exposed to patients or specimens infected with HIV should be made aware that HIV antibody tests are now widely available. While staff can make personal arrangements for testing by their general practitioner or at a clinic, it is suggested that local occupational health services arrange to test, or to store for future testing on demand, serum of staff who request this in connection with their work. Staff who have an accident with the virus or contaminated material should promptly be offered the chance to have their serum tested, or stored for possible future testing. If they accept, an 'immediate' specimen is required, followed by further specimens at intervals thereafter. This should be an entirely voluntary procedure (Advisory Committee on Dangerous Pathogens, 1986).

10.2.5 Screening for legal purposes

There are prospects for compulsory screening for insurance, immigration or employment, which is currently being enacted in the United States and in Saudi Arabia (Miller *et al.*, 1986). It is likely that such screening will produce further cases of asymptomatic infection.

10.3 PREVALENCE AND OUTCOME

The Bureau of Hygeine and Tropical Diseases, London (Anon., 1986) reported that by April 1986, 22 780 cases of AIDS had been notified worldwide. It was estimated that for every case of AIDS there were about 100 more persons infected with HIV, i.e. 2.5–3 million persons worldwide. Of these, about 1.5 million were in the United States, and 0.5 million in Europe. The prevalence of both HIV seropositivity and of AIDS appears to be increasing exponentially worldwide.

Information on the outcome of asymptomatic HIV seropositivity is not easy to assess at present. The median latent period between estimated exposure or seroconversion and the development of AIDS in adults is about 30 months (Melbye, 1986), but this may reflect the timing of the introduction of the virus into the United States more than the biological process (Goedert *et al.*, 1986; Hunter and De Gruttola, 1986). Although it is likely that cofactors influence the progression of asymptomatic HIV infection to symptomatic disease, no clearcut cofactors have yet been established (Goedert *et al.*, 1986).

10.3.1 Haemophiliacs

Multitransfused haemophiliacs have the highest prevalence of asymptomatic HIV infection in developed countries. This reflects their frequent treatment with pooled donor plasma, either as cryoprecipitate (typically, one therapeutic infusion comes from about 20 donors) or as lyophilized clotting factor concentrates (typically, one therapeutic infusion comes from several thousand donors). Viral hepatitis is a constant finding after only one exposure to clotting factor concentrate (Editorial, 1986). Hence it is not surprising that haemophiliacs treated with factor concentrates between 1979 and 1984, during which time HIV infection started to spread in developed countries, frequently developed infection as measured by serum antibodies (Bloom, 1985). In surveys of European haemophiliacs, the prevalence of seropositivity was greater in users of commercial factor concentrates imported from the United States than in users of locally-produced volunteer donor concentrates, presumably due to the greater prevalence of infection in paid American donors (Melbye *et al.*, 1984a; AIDS Group of UK Haemophilia Centre Directors, 1986; Cheingsong-Popov *et al.*, 1986). It is hoped that future infection will be prevented by education and laboratory screening of blood donors; by heat treatment of factor concentrates; and by using low-risk treatments (cryoprecipitate, fresh frozen plasma, desmopressin, and eventually genetically-engineered factor VIII) where appropriate (*Lancet*, Editorial, 1986).

Because of their frequent bleeds and need for regular hospital attendance, severe haemophiliacs (factor VIII or IX level less than 2 IU/dl) are a well-defined population in developed countries. The similar number of moderately severe and mild haemophiliacs (respectively, 2–10 and 10–40 IU/dl) are also reasonably well defined. Haemophiliacs therefore probably constitute the best-defined database for study of the natural history of asymptomatic HIV infection. From approximately 4000 registered haemophiliacs in the United Kingdom, a survey in 1985 produced information on the most recent test for HIV antibody in 2609 (AIDS Group of UK Haemophilia Centre Directors, 1986). In factor VIII deficiency, the prevalence of seropositivity was 59% in severe cases, 23% in moderate, and 9% in mild cases. In factor IX deficiency, the corresponding figures were only 8%, 4% and 3%. The lower prevalence of seropositivity in factor IX deficiency may reflect the different preparation of the clotting factor concentrate (Bloom, 1985). In von Willebrand's disease, 5% were seropositive. In haemophiliacs as a whole, the prevalence of HIV antibodies was highest between the ages of 10 and 60 years (AIDS Group of UK Haemophilia Centre Directors, 1986).

The high prevalence of HIV infection in haemophiliacs may reflect not only the 'seed' (intravenous infusion of plasma fractions from many donors, and hence high risk of HIV contamination), but also the 'soil' (prior immunosuppression by regular infusion of non-HIV-infected plasma fractions). Many studies have reported immune disturbances in treated haemophiliacs, which do not always correlate with the presence of HIV antibody: these findings may reflect immune effects of plasma proteins, or possibly of other viruses (Bloom, 1985). Ludlam *et al.* (1985) reported that the probability of seroconversion in a group of haemophiliacs exposed to a batch of HIV-contaminated factor VIII concentrate was related to the severity of previous T-lymphocyte changes, and to the extent of total transfusion with factor VIII replacement therapy. It may be relevant that treated severe haemophiliacs had reduced skin test responses to a new antigen (DNCB), which was unrelated to their HIV antibody status, but which was correlated with the amount of factor VIII replacement therapy in recent years (Madhok *et al.*, 1986).

It has been suggested that positive HIV antibody tests in haemophiliacs may sometimes represent an antibody response to dead viral proteins in plasma factor concentrates (Bloom, 1985). However, progressive increase in antibody titre is invariably seen in serial studies of seropositive haemophiliacs (E. A. C. Follett, 1986, personal communication), suggesting active proliferation of the virus *in vivo*. While this has yet to be confirmed by isolation of the HIV virus from large numbers of haemophiliacs, there is no doubt that a percentage of haemophiliacs develop clinical evidence of HIV infection, and evidence of HIV infection is also seen in some of their sexual partners and children (see below). In the USA, Eyster *et al.* (1985) found lymphadenopathy in 70% of patients who had been seropositive for over 3 years, and in 10% of those who had been seropositive for less time. The 3-year incidence of AIDS in this cohort was 12.8% (Goedert *et al.*, 1986). In the UK 12.9% of 896 patients known to have positive antibodies in the August 1985 survey had been reported by June 1986 to have HIV-related illness. There were 23 cases of AIDS, of whom 13 had died. Three patients with ARC had also died, with a further death from haemorrhage after splenectomy for thrombocytopenia (J. Craske, 1986 communication to UK Haemophilia Centre Directors).

At present, therefore, the majority of haemophiliacs with positive HIV antibodies remain asymptomatic, despite evidence of infection for several years. However there is a long latency between infection and clinical AIDS (Goedert *et al.*, 1986), and the cumulative morbidity and mortality will only become apparent on long-term follow-up.

10.3.2 Homosexual and bisexual males

This group still accounts for the majority of AIDS cases in developed countries: risk factors for AIDS include sexual contact with men from high-risk areas, number of partners, and receptive anal intercourse (Melbye, 1986). Risk factors for HIV-seropositivity and for progression to PGL after seroconversion include episodes of other sexually-transmitted diseases (Weber *et al.*, 1986).

Initial studies of seropositive homosexual/bisexual men in New York City and in Denmark showed progression rates to AIDS of 6.9 per 100 patient-years and 7.7%/year respectively; however 49% of the New York patients had lymphadenopathy at entry to the study (Goedert *et al.*, 1984; Melbye *et al.*, 1984b). A more recent report of these cohorts, and of seropositive homosexual men in Washington, D. C., found that the 3-year incidence of AIDS, calculated by the Kaplan–Meier survival technique, was 34% in Manhattan, 8% in Denmark, and 17.2% in Washington (Goedert *et al.*, 1986). If the HIV virus entered the New York population before the other populations studied (as suggested by the high prevalence of lymphadenopathy at entry), then the long latency between infection and development of AIDS could account for the significantly higher AIDS incidence in the New York cohort (Goedert *et al.*, 1986). In another cohort of seropositive homosexual men in San Francisco, followed for 5 years, 6% developed AIDS, and another 26% developed other HIV-related disease (Jaffe *et al.*, 1985a). In a cohort of asymptomatic seropositive homosexual men in London, followed for 2 years, 12% progressed to AIDS, and another 48% progressed to PGL (Weber *et al.*, 1986). A cohort of high risk blood donors (mostly homosexual men) who had donated blood to patients with transfusion-related AIDS, showed similar progression rates to AIDS and PGL when evaluated 2 years after donation (Jaffe *et al.*, 1985b).

Current advice given to homosexual men as health education includes limiting the number of sexual partners (preferably to one) and discussing safer sex with them; avoiding anal and oral intercourse and other sexual practices which mix blood or body fluids; avoiding other sexually-transmitted diseases and drug abuse; and maintaining good mental and physical health.

10.3.3 Parenteral drug abusers

Clusters of intravenous drug abusers with high prevalences of HIV infection have been identified in the large cities of the USA and Europe. Transmission is probably largely by sharing of equipment (e.g. needles and syringes), but may also reflect sexual exposure: there is a strong link between drug abuse and prostitution (Melbye, 1986). The rate of progression to AIDS in seropositive parenteral drug abusers in New York City over a 3-year period was similar to that in homosexuals and haemophiliacs (Goedert *et al.*, 1986).

Advice given to parenteral drug abusers to reduce the risks of infection and progression to HIV-related disease may include stopping drug abuse; changing from parenteral to oral drugs; not sharing needles or syringes; and advice on sexual activity as above. Dispensing sterile needles and syringes free and on-demand to parenteral drug abusers has been advocated by some, but has been condemned by others since it may condone and increase parenteral drug abuse.

10.3.4 Sexual partners and babies of the above groups

Asymptomatic HIV-seropositivity and HIV-related disease have been reported in sexual partners and babies of members of the above high-risk groups. Several studies of the prevalence of HIV antibody in wives or sexual partners of seropositive haemophiliacs have been reported recently: in the largest study of 148 patients, 6.8% were seropositive (Allain, 1986). The clinical outcome in this group is not yet known. While this risk of heterosexual transmission from high-risk men to female partners is small, it seems reasonable to advise protection of vaginal intercourse with a condom, to avoid anal and oral intercourse (Melbye *et al.*, 1985); and to defer pregnancy at present. As previously discussed, females at high risk who are contemplating pregnancy or in early pregnancy should be offered screening for HIV infection, since pregnancy appears to accelerate maternal disease, as well as carrying a high rate of HIV-related disease in their babies. The incubation period for AIDS in babies with perinatal exposure is much shorter than in adults (Melbye, 1986).

10.3.5 Tropical Africa

HIV infection and AIDS are epidemic and spreading in tropical Africa: the topic has recently been reviewed by Biggar (1986) and by Pinching (1986). The clinical disease appears to be relatively new, with cases diagnosed retrospectively back to 1976. Some sera collected in the late 1960s in West Africa and Uganda were found to be reactive for HIV antibody by ELISA, and 5–20% of sera from recent healthy or hospital control groups in Tropical Africa are positive for HIV antibody by ELISA. However many positive ELISA tests are not confirmed by Western blotting: such false positive results may reflect effects of malaria and other parasitic diseases (Biggar, 1986; Greenberg *et al.*, 1986; Wendler *et al.*, 1986). This may not be due to serological cross-reactivity between antibodies to *Plasmodium* and antibodies to HIV (Greenberg *et al.*, 1986), and may reflect other antibodies or immune complexes (Biggar, 1986; Wendler *et al.*, 1986). Hence seroepidemiological estimates of the prevalence of HIV infection in Tropical Africa may be falsely high. A similar virus has been isolated from African green monkeys, hence the speculation has been made that the HIV virus may have originated in this species (Kanki, Alroy and Essex, 1985).

In contrast to the 19:1 male to female sex ratio in Europe and North America, the sex ratio of AIDS cases in Africa is equal. The age range is that of sexual activity, and AIDS is associated with sexual promiscuity. Hence heterosexual activity may be the commonest method of spread. This possibility is supported by recent evidence for male to female and female to male transmission in developed countries (Biggar, 1986; and see above). It is possible that 3–4% of current AIDS cases in developed countries have arisen from heterosexual spread (Pinching, 1986), hence sexually active heterosexuals should receive health education as well as homosexuals, to limit the spread amongst heterosexuals (Acheson, 1986; Pinching, 1986). Recent studies show a high prevalence of HIV antibodies in African prostitutes and their male clients (Van de Perre *et al.*, 1985). The high prevalence of venereal disease in tropical Africa may favour the spread of infection: there is little evidence that anal intercourse is a factor (Biggar, 1986; Pinching, 1986).

A prospective study of seropositive hospital employees in Zaire found a progression rate to AIDS of 1.3/100 patient years, and a progression rate to other HIV-related conditions of 10.4/100 patient years: these rates of progression appear similar to those reported in developed countries (Mann *et al.*, 1986). Further epidemiological studies are required to elucidate the natural history of asymptomatic HIV infection in Africa: however the governments in some countries may no longer allow these, for political and economic reasons.

10.3.6 Health care workers

Needlestick or scalpel injuries appear the most likely sources of occupational exposure to HIV in health care workers. The risk of seroconversion from an isolated parenteral occupational exposure to HIV-infected body fluids appears to be low – only three cases reported by early 1986 (Melbye, 1986). There is as yet no evidence that a health care worker has developed AIDS as a result of occupational exposure.

10.4 MANAGEMENT

The 'pros' and 'cons' of screening asymptomatic persons for evidence of HIV infection have already been mentioned. Given a positive result, how should the person then be managed?

10.4.1 Confirming the result

A positive serum HIV antibody test must be confirmed by a specific test such as Western blotting (Melbye, 1986). A second sample should be obtained and tested for confirmation before any result is given to the patient.

10.4.2 Informing and counselling the person or relatives

The present author believes that confirmed seropositive persons should usually be informed of their status, for the following reasons.

(a) They are sources of infection to others

It is their right to know this and to appreciate their responsibility, so that they can if they wish take appropriate precautions to reduce the risk of infecting their sexual partners, children, or persons who handle their blood and body fluids. In preventing the spread of HIV infection in the population, health education *for all* on sex, drug abuse and hygiene is crucial: however, informing and appropriate counselling of those found to be seropositive is also important. Such informing and counselling is already accepted practice for asymptomatic carriers of the similarly transmitted hepatitis B virus.

(b) HIV-seropositivity involves a definite future risk of HIV-related disease

Seropositive persons therefore have a right to know of this risk to their future health.

(c) It may be important that seropositive persons take actions which may reduce their risk of progression to disease

1. Avoidance of further HIV infection and of other sexually-transmitted disease, by reducing their number of sexual contacts and by using condoms. Episodes of other sexually-transmitted diseases were predictive of progression to PGL in one study (Weber *et al.*, 1986).
2. Avoidance of immune stimulation which might result in viral proliferation, e.g. vaccinations.
3. Seeking prompt medical advice in the event of deterioration in their health. This may result in earlier diagnosis and therefore in more successful treatment of opportunistic infections or tumours.

In the case of children, or adults who are incapable of understanding their status, it may be appropriate to inform and counsel the parent, guardian or next of kin, rather than the person themselves.

As previously mentioned, persons informed of their seropositivity may experience anxiety, depression, and broken relationships: several have committed suicide. Other sequelae have included unemployment, refusal of life insurance and endowment mortgage policies, and suboptimal medical and dental care (Miller *et al.*, 1986). Pre-counselling, prior to performing the test, is therefore advocated (Miller *et al.*, 1986). Informing seropositive patients of their result, and counselling them appropriately, is a challenging task which requires adequate privacy and time; empathy and consideration; and follow-up. Ideally one doctor and one trained counsellor or clinical psychologist should be involved. The approach may well differ for homosexuals, drug abusers, haemophiliacs, and heterosexuals without parenteral exposure. Counselling has been discussed in detail elsewhere (Miller, Green and McCreaner, 1986). In brief, the aims of counselling asymptomatic seropositive persons are as follows.

(a) To explain basic facts about the virus and the test result

- To explain that they have a positive antibody test, which means that they have been exposed to the HIV virus, which sometimes causes AIDS.
- To advise that they may decrease their chance of future ill-health by taking positive steps, e.g. good diet, avoiding other infections.
- To explain that although they will probably remain healthy, they can pass on the virus infection to others, who may then develop AIDS.

(b) To advise how to reduce the risk of infecting others

Sex

- Limit sexual partners, preferably to one. Discuss safe sex with them.
- Avoid anal and oral intercourse; protect intercourse with a condom; avoid other practices which mix blood or body fluids.

Blood

- Do not donate blood, organs (tear up donor transplant cards), sperm or breast milk.
- Their doctor, dentist and any other surgeons should be informed, in confidence (see below).
- Do not allow anyone who does not know that they are seropositive to take blood from them, or to perform other invasive procedures (avoid acupuncture and tatooing).
- Do not share razors, toothbrushes or other blood-contaminated instruments; do not have a shave by a barber.
- Do not share needles or syringes, if a drug abuser.
- Mop up blood spills with household bleach (one part to 10 parts water).

Reassurance

- Casual contact, handshaking, dry kissing, coughing and sneezing, and sharing eating utensils, towels and toilets have no risk of transmission.

(c) To discuss sexual and drug-abusing practices, and to ask for help with contacting and counselling sexual partners and needle-sharers

As previously discussed, this is especially important with female sexual partners or needle-sharers who are pregnant or contemplating pregnancy.

(d) To advise on their own health

- Avoid further HIV infection and other sexually-transmitted diseases by reducing numbers of sexual contacts and using condoms.
- Avoid vaccination without prior discussion with an expert.
- Seek prompt medical advice in the event of deterioration in health (e.g. persistent infections, skin spots, sore mouth, cough, diarrhoea).
- Explanation that symptoms of anxiety and depression are common initially, but improve with time and support.
- Arrangement of an early return appointment in the next few days, to go over the information, answer questions, and assess psychosocial reaction; arrangement of easy access by telephone or to clinic for questions to be answered.
- Advice for regular clinic follow-up (3 monthly), for health checks and further counselling and answering of questions.
- Advising that the person considers who of their family or friends they should confide in and receive support from; also consideration of National or community support groups, such as Haemophilia Society, Body Positive or other groups for homosexuals or bisexuals, or counselling groups for drug abusers.
- Advice that special care must be taken with blood tests, dentistry and other forms of surgery, but that necessary tests and treatment will be performed, and confidentiality respected.

10.4.3 Liaison with other health care workers

Advice to health care workers to prevent transmission of HIV infection during invasive procedures such as blood sampling, dentistry and surgery is now available (Advisory Committee on Dangerous Pathogens, 1986; CDC, 1985b, 1986b,c; Department of Health and Social Security, 1986; Dinsdale, 1985; Greenspan *et al.*, 1986). The most important principle is to handle blood, body fluids and mucous membranes from *all persons* with care, avoiding splashes on eyes, face or skin, and taking great care with needles, scalpels and other sharp instruments. However, particular care is appropriate for known HIV seropositive patients, who in general merit precautions as for carriers of hepatitis B virus.

It is important that all health care workers in close contact with patients, or their blood or other bodily material, are aware of the risk of infection, and take suitable precautions. However, information on HIV antibody positivity is confidential, and should not be disclosed for purposes other than health care. In hospital, patients need only be isolated in a single room if they are bleeding or likely to bleed externally, incontinent, have open or draining wounds, have disturbed consciousness, or have another infection requiring isolation.

10.4.4 Education and foster care of infected children

There is no evidence for transmission of HIV infection from infected children during casual contact in school, day-care or foster-care (CDC, 1985c; Department for Education and Science, 1986; Berthier *et al.*, 1986). It is recommended that school-age children should be allowed to have normal schooling, day-care and foster-care: a more restricted environment is advised for younger children, and for those who bite, lack control of body secretions, or have uncoverable, oozing lesions (CDC, 1985c). One domestic case of transmission to a sibling in the home may have resulted from biting (Wahn *et al.*, 1986). The number of persons informed of seropositivity should be restricted to the minimum required to assure proper care of the child and to detect increased potential for transmission (CDC, 1985c).

10.4.5 Follow-up

Regular follow-up (say, every 3 months) should be encouraged for several reasons: to support and advise the person; to detect HIV related disease early when treatment may be more effective; and to collect information on the natural history of the disease.

At each visit, counselling is continued concerning knowledge of HIV infection, precautions against transmission, psychosocial problems, and contacts. A full history and general examination is conducted, looking in particular for features of HIV-related disease. A proforma for serial recording of clinical features may be useful as a checklist and to show sequential changes clearly.

The patient's weight is recorded, and a throat swab taken to detect oral candidiasis. Blood is taken with appropriate precautions for blood count (in particular, haemoglobin, total and differential white cell count, and platelet count), to detect anaemia, neutropenia, lymphocytopenia, and thrombocytopenia. Other investigations are performed if clinically indicated. At baseline it may be useful to check hepatitis B antigen, to save a serum sample for comparison with later serology, and to perform a chest radiogram for subsequent comparison in the event of respiratory disease (e.g. *Pneumocystis carinii* pneumonia). Changes in numbers of T-helper lymphocytes are associated with changes in total lymphocyte count: hence in clinical practice it may not be necessary to add T-lymphocyte subset estimations to the total lymphocyte count (Weber *et al.*, 1986). While the lower limit of the reference range for the lymphocyte count is usually given as 1.5×10^9/litre, about 25% of healthy blood donors had levels below this in one study using an automated cell counter, and for such machines the lower limit is about 1.0×10^9/litre (Robbins, Henthorn and Brozovic, 1984).

Only by further, large, long-term follow-up studies will the natural history of asymptomatic HIV infection become apparent.

REFERENCES

Acheson, E. D. (1986) AIDS: a challenge for the public health. *Lancet*, i, 662–6.

Advisory Committee on Dangerous Pathogens (1986) *LAV/HTLV III – the causative agent of AIDS and related conditions – revised guidelines.*

AIDS Group of UK Haemophilia Centre Directors (1986) Prevalence of antibody to HTLV-III in haemophiliacs in the UK. *Brit. Med. J.*, 293, 175–6.

Allain, J. P., (1986) Prevalence of HTLV-III/LAV antibodies in patients with hemophilia and in their sexual partners in France. *N. Engl. J. Med.*, 315, 517–18.

Anon. (1986) The AIDS campaign. *Lancet*, ii, 353.

Barré-Sinoussi, F., Chermann, J. C., Rey, F. *et al.* (1983) Isolation of T-lymphotropic retrovirus from a patient at risk for AIDS. *Science*, 220, 868–71.

Berthier, A., Chamaret, S., Fauchet, R. *et al.* (1986) Transmissibility of HIV in haemophiliac and non-haemophiliac children living in a private school in France. *Lancet*, ii, 598–601.

Biggar, R. J. (1986) The AIDS problem in Africa. *Lancet*, i, 79–83.

Bloom, A. (1985) AIDS and haemophilia. *Biomed. Pharmacother.*, 39, 355–65.

CDC (1985a) Revision of the case definition of AIDS for national reporting – United States. *MMWR*, 34, 373–5.

CDC (1985b) Recommendations for preventing transmission of infection with HTLV-III/LAV in the workplace. *MMWR*, 34, 681–95.

CDC (1985c) Education and foster care of children infected with HTLV-III/LAV. *MMWR*, 34, 517–21.

CDC (1986a) Classification system for HTLV-III/LAV infections. *MMWR*, 35, 334–49.

CDC (1986b) Recommendations for preventing transmission of infection with HTLV-III/LAV during invasive procedures. *MMWR*, 35, 221–3.

CDC (1986c) Recommended infection-control procedures for dentistry. *MMWR*, 35, 237–42.

Cheingsong-Popov, R., Tedder, R. S., O'Connor, T., Clayden, S., Smith, A., Craske, J. and Weiss, R. (1986) Retrovirus infections among patients treated in Britain with various clotting factors. *Brit. Med. J.*, 293, 168–9.

Department for Education and Science (1986) Children at school and problems related to AIDS. Draft circulated to doctors in England with ref. CMO (86) 1.

Department of Health and Social Security (1986) AIDS: guidance for surgeons, anaesthetists, dentists and their teams in dealing with patients infected with HTLV-III. Letter circulated to doctors in UK, ref. CMO (86) 7.

Dinsdale, R. C. W. (1985) *Viral hepatitis, AIDS and dental treatment*. British Dental Journal, London.

Editorial (1986) Safer factor VIII and IX. *Lancet*, ii, 255–6.

Eyster, M. E., Goedert, J. J., Sarngadharan, M. G., Weiss, S. H., Gallo, R. C. and Blattner, W. A. (1985) Development and early natural history of HTLV-III antibodies in persons with hemophilia. *JAMA*, **253**, 2219–23.

Fischinger, P. J. and Bolognesi, D. P. (1985) Prospects for diagnostic tests, intervention and vaccine development in AIDS, in *AIDS – Etiology, Diagnosis, Treatment and Prevention* (ed. V. T. De Vita, Jr, S. Hellmann and S. A. Rosenberg), J. B. Lipincott Co., Philadelphia, pp. 55–88.

Gallo, R. C., Salahuddin, S. Z., Popovic, M. *et al.* (1984) Frequent detection of a human T-lymphotropic retrovirus, HTLV-III, from patients with AIDS and at risk for AIDS. *Science*, **224**, 500–3.

Goedert, J. J., Sarngadharan, M. G., Biggar, R. J. *et al.* (1984) Determinants of retrovirus (HTLV-III) antibody and immunodeficiency conditions in homosexual men. *Lancet*, ii, 711–16.

Goedert, J. J. and Blattner, W. A. (1985) The epidemiology of AIDS and related conditions, in *AIDS – Etiology, Diagnosis, Treatment and Prevention*, (ed. V. T. De Vita, Jr., S. Hellmann and S. A. Rosenberg), J. B. Lipincott Co., Philadelphia, pp. 1–30.

Goedert, J. J., Biggar, R. J., Weiss, S. H. *et al.* (1986) Three year incidence of AIDS in five cohorts of HTLV-III-infected risk group members. *Science*, **231**, 992–5.

Goudsmit, J., Wolters, E. C., Bakker, M. *et al.* (1986a) Intrathecal synthesis of antibodies to LAV/HTLV-III in individuals without AIDS or AIDS-related complex. *Brit. Med. J.*, **292**, 1231–4.

Goudsmit, J., De Wolf, F., Paul, D. A. *et al.* (1986b) Expression of HIV antigen in serum and CSF during acute and chronic infection. *Lancet*, ii, 177–80.

Greenberg, A. E., Schable, C. A., Sulzer, A. J., Collins, W. E. and Nguyen-Dinh, P. (1986) Evaluation of serological cross-reactivity between antibodies to *Plasmodium* and HTLV-III/LAV. *Lancet*, ii, 247–9.

Greenspan, D., Pindborg, J. J., Greenspan, J. S. and Schiødt, M. (1986) *AIDS and the Dental Team*, Munksgaard, Copenhagen.

Hunter, D. J. and De Gruttola, V. (1986) Estimation of risk of outcome of HTLV-III infection. *Lancet*, i, 677–8.

Jaffe, H. W., Darrow, W. W., Eckenberg, D. F. *et al.* (1985a) The acquired immunodeficiency syndrome in a cohort of homosexual men. *Ann. Intern. Med.*, **103**, 210–14.

Jaffe, H. W., Sarngadharan, M. G., De Vico, A. L. *et al.* (1985b) Infection with HTLV-III/LAV and transfusion-associated AIDS. Serologic evidence of an association. *JAMA*, **254**, 770–3.

Kanki, P. J., Alroy, J. and Essex, M. (1985) Isolation of a T-lymphotropic retrovirus related to HTLV-III from wild-caught African green monkeys. *Science*, **230**, 951–4.

Ludlam, C. A., Tucker, J., Steel, C. M. *et al.* (1985) Human T-lymphotropic virus type III (HTLV-III) infection in seronegative haemophiliacs after transfusion of factor VIII. *Lancet*, ii, 233–6.

Madhok, R., Gracie, A., Lowe, G. D. O. *et al.* (1986) Impaired cell mediated immunity in haemophilia in the absence of infection with human immunodeficiency virus. *Brit. Med. J.*, **293**, 978–81.

Mann, J. M., Bila, K., Colebunders, R. L. *et al.* (1986) Natural history of HIV infection in Zaire. *Lancet*, **ii**, 707–9.

Melbye, M. (1986) The natural history of human T-lymphotropic virus III infection: the cause of AIDS. *Brit. Med. J.*, **292**, 5–12.

Melbye, M., Froebel, K. S., Madhok, R. *et al.* (1984a) HTLV-III seropositivity in European haemophiliacs exposed to factor VIII concentrate imported from the USA. *Lancet*, **ii**, 1444–6.

Melbye, M., Biggar, R. J., Ebbesen, P. *et al.* (1984b) Seroepidemiology of HTLV-III antibody in Danish homosexual men: prevalence, transmission, and disease outcome. *Brit. Med. J.*, **289**, 573–5.

Melbye, M., Ingerslev, J., Biggar, R. J. *et al.* (1985) Anal intercourse as a possible factor in heterosexual transmission of HTLV-III to spouses of hemophiliacs. *N. Engl. J. Med.*, **312**, 857.

Miller, D., Jeffries, D. J., Green, J., Harris, J. R. W. and Pinching, A. J. (1986) HTLV-III: should testing ever be routine? *Brit. Med. J.*, **292**, 941–3.

Miller, D., Green, J. and McCreaner, A. (1986) Organising a counselling service for AIDS-related problems. *Genitourinary Med.*, **62**, 114–19.

Neumayer, H. H., Wagner, K. and Knesse, S. (1986) HTLV-III antibodies in patients with kidney transplants or on haemodialysis. *Lancet*, **i**, 497.

Peterman, T. A., Lang, G. R., Mikos, N. J. *et al.* (1986) HTLV-III/LAV infection in hemodialysis patients. *JAMA*, **255**, 2324–32.

Pinching, A. J. (1986) AIDS and Africa: lessons for us all. *J. Roy. Soc. Med.*, **79**, 501–3.

Redfield, R. R., Wright, D. C. and Tramont, E. (1986) The Walter Reed staging classification for HTLV-III/LAV infection. *N. Engl. J. Med.*, **314**, 131–2.

Robbins, G., Henthorn, J. and Brozovic, B. (1984) Reference range for lymphocyte counts in health. *Lancet*, **ii**, 1094.

Salahuddin, S. Z., Markham, P. D., Popovic, M. *et al.* (1985) Isolation of infectious human T-cell leukemic lymphotropic virus type III (HTLV-III) from patients with AIDS or AIDS-related complex and from healthy carriers: a study of risk groups and tissue sources. *Proc. Natl Acad. Sci. USA*, **82**, 5530–4.

Thiry, L., Sprecher-Goldberger, S., Jonckheer, T. *et al.* (1985) Isolation of AIDS virus from cell-free breast milk of 3 healthy virus carriers. *Lancet*, **ii**, 891–2.

Van de Perre, P. Clumeck, N., Carael, M. *et al.* (1985) Female prostitutes: a risk group for infection with HTLV-III. *Lancet*, **ii**, 524–6.

Vilmer, E., Barré-Sinoussi, F., Rouzioux, C. *et al.* (1984) Isolation of new lymphotropic retrovirus from two siblings with haemophilia B, one with AIDS. *Lancet*, **i**, 753–7.

Wahn, V., Kramer, H. H., Voit, T. *et al.* (1986) Horizontal transmission of HIV infection between two siblings. *Lancet*, **ii**, 694.

Weber, J. N., Wadsworth, J., Rogers, L. A. *et al.* (1986) Three year prospective study of HTLV-III/LAV infection in homosexual men. *Lancet*, **i**, 1179–82.

Welsby, P. (1986) Personal view. *Brit. Med. J.*, **292**, 954.

Wendler, I., Schneider, J., Gras, B., Fleming, A. F., Hunsman, G. and Schmitz, H. (1986) Seroepidemiology of HIV in Africa. *Brit. Med. J.*, **293**, 782–5.

11

Psychological and ethical implications of HIV screening

— Patricia Wilkie —

11.1 INTRODUCTION

Two groups of people may become identified as HIV sero-positive through testing in relation to blood or blood products. First there are those who come forward as blood donors and who are found to be sero-positive. Secondly there are those haemophiliacs who have been found to be sero-positive presumably after having received an infusion of infected blood products. These two groups have some similarities in that they are HIV sero-positive without necessarily showing symptoms of AIDS, but in other respects they are different. The source of the infection is different. The psychological and emotional responses may vary and therefore the type of long-term counselling and support they need may be different. While one must not underestimate the difficulties facing a non-haemophiliac sero-positive patient, the problems facing an HIV sero-positive haemophiliac are very great indeed because he also has haemophilia.

Section 11.2 discusses the first group in respect of their relationship with blood donations. Their subsequent counselling and treatment may be the same as that of any other non-haemophiliac found to be HIV sero-positive. Section 11.3 examines the problems of haemophiliacs.

There is a third group of people who may have become HIV sero-positive through contact with blood, namely those who have received transfusions of infected blood. As far as is known there are very few in this category and they cannot be readily identified. At a later date they may offer themselves as blood donors or be tested for HIV in other circumstances or they may develop symptoms of AIDS. In some cases the fact that the transfusion they received was contaminated may become known, and they may be traced. Again, their subsequent counselling and treatment is the same as that of any other person found to be HIV sero-positive. This small group is not discussed any further.

11.2 BLOOD DONORS

11.2.1 Screening

Screening for disease is familiar through the mass screening programmes for tuberculosis and more recently the programmes for breast and cervical cancer. The objective of such mass screening for disease is to discover those amongst the apparently well who are in fact suffering from an illness in order to treat them early and therefore more successfully. This procedure involves a departure from the usual doctor–patient consultative relationship in which the patient has a complaint and seeks an assessment of it from the doctor (Sackett and Holland, 1973). The criteria for introducing a screening programme have varied from study to study with the most frequently named criteria being:

1. the condition should be an important health problem;
2. there should be an accepted treatment for it;
3. the cost of finding each affected case should make sense in terms of medical expenditure.

Most authors have agreed that of all the criteria a screening test should fulfill, the ability to treat the condition adequately, when discovered, is the most important (Wilson and Junger, 1968).

A different set of criteria for screening applies when the disease is infectious and so presents a serious risk to society (McKeown, 1968). To protect society as a whole, the freedom of the individual may have to be restricted. Screening or follow up of suspected carriers and the notification of certain infectious diseases is required by law in various countries. Contact tracing of suspected carriers of sexually transmitted diseases operates from STD clinics. The main objective of notification of a disease is to enable rapid preventative action to be taken when appropriate, to bring the disease under control. In the United Kingdom the government has stopped short of making AIDS a notifiable disease since it considers that the condition is being effectively monitored (Daniels, 1985).

Screening of blood donors is again different in that the objective is to protect the supply of blood by ensuring that it is uncontaminated; this is effected by examining all blood donations for HIV antibody before they are used for transfusion or sent for fractionation and heat treatment. The main objective has not been to identify the HIV sero-positive person in the population. This identification has, however, occurred as a consequence of the testing. The dilemma for those in the blood transfusion service is that a person who has not sought investigation may be found to be positive, (Curran, 1985). Should he or she be informed of the diagnosis for a condition for which at the moment there is no cure? For an asymptomatic person it is the diagnosis not of a disease but of an asymptomatic state in which there is estimated to be a 1 in 20 chance of developing symptoms.

In recent years there has been heated debate amongst those working with genetically transmitted diseases as to whether or not the asymptomatic at risk person who has a high chance of developing a serious disorder for which there is no cure should be told of his or her risk (Sorenson, 1973; Twiss, 1974; Thomas, 1983). The most frequently cited reasons for not informing such individuals are that such knowledge may evoke anxiety, decrease job opportunities and diminish insurability (Suki, 1982). The same considerations apply to those who are found to be HIV sero-positive.

11.2.2 Blood donations in the UK

Screening in the UK of all blood donations by the Regional Transfusion Service began in October 1985. All blood donations are now routinely tested for HIV antibody. It is appropriate to inform all prospective donors of the reasons why this screening procedure is being carried out. At present all donors are asked not to donate blood if they belong to one of the known risk groups. Blood donations which are found to be HIV sero-positive are not used for transfusion and following the recommendations of the Chief Medical Officer of Health of the Scottish Home and Health Department all individuals who are found to have positive antibody tests receive counselling in order that they may understand the meaning of the results and the measure required to avoid transmitting the infection to others.

Since this programme started about 1 in 50 000 donations have been found to be HIV sero-positive. Blood transfusion services have not reported any reduction in prospective donors. This suggests that regular blood donors are not being put off by the possibility of HIV screening and this is not preventing them from donating blood.

11.2.3 Before donating blood

The blood transfusion service is in a unique position to inform a large section of the population about the transmission of the HIV virus and the methods of prevention. Ideally a member of staff should explain the reasons for screening and the implications of the results and should give the donor an opportunity to ask questions (Bove, 1985). The procedure for giving test results should be discussed at this point.

The present practice is to send no further communication to those who are found to be negative. This is presumably thought to be satisfactory and no expense is incurred. However, it can be argued that to notify that the test was negative would serve three functions: it would give a further opportunity for health education about the transmission of the virus; it would give immediate reassurance to those found to be negative; and it would encourage donors to return to give blood again. It would be necessary to make it clear that the person would not necessarily remain negative for life; the virus might be acquired at some later date.

11.2.4 After testing

All donors should know before donating blood whether they will be informed of a negative result or whether they will be contacted only when the result is positive, in which case no news should be interpreted as good news.

When a donors blood is found to be positive a second sample from the blood donated is tested for confirmation. If a donation is positive on retesting, and confirmed by Western blot analysis, a member of the medical staff contacts the donor so that he or she can be informed of the results and referred to an appropriate clinic. Donors who have one positive result and who are found to be negative on the retest are informed of this, but are nevertheless asked not to donate blood again.

11.2.5 Use of the Blood Transfusion Service for testing

The Blood Transfusion Service has been concerned that it may be used as a method of getting an HIV test and thereby attracting those who are high risk. It is hoped that by asking those at high risk not to donate blood and by the establishment of separate 'walk in' clinics where the public can be investigated and receive the appropriate counselling and advice, this problem will be overcome. An additional problem in those countries where blood donors are paid for their blood may be that certain categories of at-risk individuals – for example, drug abusers – may be attracted to transfusion centres for financial gain. Even greater care would need to be taken in the screening of blood in these circumstances.

11.3 HAEMOPHILIACS

11.3.1 HIV antibody testing and haemophilia

Haemophiliacs have now been identified as one of the major groups at risk of being infected by HIV, because they have received infected blood products. Their blood is in any case routinely tested and it has become routine to test for HIV antibody. The reason for testing haemophiliacs is not just for epidemiological and research reasons but because it is known that HIV sero-positive blood is infectious and is a potential danger to those who handle it, and also the patient may pass on the virus through sexual or blood contact.

Staff carrying out invasive procedures on those found to be sero-positive need to be alerted and to adhere to the same guidelines as for the control of hepatitis B infection. Gloves, masks and other additional protective clothing needs to be worn. Patients will be isolated for the carrying out of certain procedures. It is, therefore, not possible generally to conceal from the patient that specific precautions are being taken for him but not for the patient beside him; it is also not desirable to withhold this information because of the way in which the virus is spread in the community; and in any case there are strong arguments in favour of being honest with the patient.

The problem then becomes one of what to tell, how to tell it, and perhaps even who should tell. There are clearly conflicting aims: there is a desire to protect others and therefore to influence the patient's behaviour; but this has consequences for the patient which many, including the patient, may think are not to the patient's advantage.

11.3.2 Reaction to an HIV sero-positive diagnosis

There has been unprecedented media coverage about AIDS. The major at risk groups have been identified. Haemophiliacs are apprehensive about AIDS. It is our experience that the majority of patients want to know what their HIV status is, whether it is negative or positive. Such comments as 'it's my information', 'I need to know to stop it going any further' are not uncommon. Some patients state that they would not like to know if they were positive, but it is clear from their discussion that they 'know' what the result is; they have been informed by implication if not explicitly. Similar situations have been found in studies of cancer patients (Wakefield, 1970; McIntosh, 1974). The only solution is to treat all those who do not wish to know a positive result as if they were positive.

Confirmation of a positive HIV result produces quite explicit responses from the staff. From that point onwards blood samples and other body fluids will be treated as high risk and marked with biohazard signs. Staff carrying out certain invasive techniques, for example venepuncture, dental investigations and surgical procedure, will take specific protective precautions. For staff carrying out the procedures or handling samples, there is no doubt about diagnosis.

For the asymptomatic patient on the other hand, a positive HIV result brings very considerable doubt and uncertainty: 'What is the prognosis for the future?' 'Am I really infectious?' 'Will I always remain infectious?' 'Am I going to develop symptoms?' 'Will I ever develop symptoms?' 'Am I going to die of AIDS?' At the moment none of these questions can be answered with any certainty. As scientific and medical knowledge about AIDS is full of uncertainty, answers to patients' questions are invariably couched in the language of probability, from which is difficult for the patient to take constructive meaning even when the probabilities are well known. In the case of AIDS there is as yet insufficient evidence for anyone to make reliable estimates of the long-term probabilities of sero-positive persons developing the disease. Katz (1984) observes that 'medical and scientific uncertainty is seldom acknowledged when talking to patients'. The considerable uncertainty about AIDS makes it difficult to know what to say to patients and perhaps necessitates a different approach.

11.3.3 Control of infection

There are two major routes of transmission of HIV: blood and seminal fluids. It is not easy for the patient to conceal his infective status from others if he wishes to prevent the spread of infection. The HIV sero-positive haemophiliac has been asked to follow specific instructions when dealing with blood products (Jones, 1985; *Aids Center News*, 1986). Many haemophiliacs are already familiar with these precautions because of the risk of hepatitis so the instructions for the disposal of sharps and for dealing with blood and blood spillage seem to present little or no problem. Problems may arise if the patient moves away from home to shared accommodation, for example to university halls of residence. In these circumstances patients have expressed concern lest others interfere with their used sharps. The same patients find it difficult to know who to tell about their haemophilia. It has been observed that patients who carry their materials for home treatment on public transport now very carefully conceal any evidence of blood products and 'sharps' containers in double or treble bags.

Patients who have gone to hotels have expressed anxiety in case evidence of their haemophilia is discovered. Doors are locked when treating themselves and treatment is also locked away. In these circumstances and also when patients have travelled abroad, the used 'sharps' boxes may be brought back home in the hand baggage. This was done on one patient's own initiative; he thought 'it was the easiest solution'.

The state of being infectious can also be a state of isolation. For certain procedures requiring in-patient care patients will be nursed in single wards. As the situation of HIV sero-positivity is new, nursing staff may still be unfamiliar with the correct procedures. Sadly it may be easier to leave the patient on his own. In a general ward haemophiliacs wonder whether other patients notice that gloves are only worn when working with their blood.

The emotions associated with harbouring a contagious agent can cause the patient and his family to feel like an outcast, stigmatized and dirty. This has caused some patients to cut themselves off from friends and acquaintances because they are unsure of how to deal with the situation and how others will react to them.

In Western societies most infectious diseases are now treatable. It is unusual to have a state of infectiousness which as far as is known will last for the duration of the patient's life and where the patient may remain asymptomatic. The longer the patient remains free from symptoms the more difficult it may become for the patient to continue to believe that he is infectious and to continue to take precautions.

11.3.4 Sexual behaviour and relationships

Information about appropriate sexual practice is distributed to all haemophiliacs in the United Kingdom through the Haemophilia Society's Bulletin, and is available in other publications (Jones, 1985). The recommendations regarding sexual behaviour for HIV sero-positive haemophiliacs are straightforward – the use of the sheath on every occasion that the person has intercourse and an awareness of the dangers of oral and anal sex. In principle the use of a sheath is simple, but in practice there may be difficulties which will depend on such factors as stability of the relationship and whether other contraceptive measures have been used. It may be easier for a haemophiliac to discuss the implications of a positive diagnosis with a stable partner. It is more difficult for him to hide distress from someone who knows him well and there is less fear of his losing his partner.

This situation must be handled by a counsellor with tact and skill. Factual information about the methods of transmission can be given again as well as data about the incidence of HIV sero-positivity in sexual and household contacts. Testing of sexual partners can be offered, accompanied by an explanation of what the test involves and means. The couple should be given an opportunity to discuss whether the partner wishes to be tested. It is our experience that the majority of wives and stable partners of haemophiliacs wish to be tested. There are very few so far who have declined. It may be that it is sufficient to cope with the news that the patient is sero-positive. It may also be that those who have declined to be tested are the least sexually active couples because of the husband's haemophilia. The views of individual couples should be respected and they should know that the subject can be discussed again at any time.

11.3.5 Haemophiliacs who have no stable relationship

Haemophiliacs who have been sexually active but who do not have a partner at the time of the sero-positive diagnosis find it difficult to make a new relationship. They are aware of the risk of sexual transmission and of the need to use a sheath. Many young women use oral contraception and the young haemophiliac may fear that if the use of a sheath has not been discussed beforehand he may be ridiculed. On the other hand he may fear that if he tells a new partner too early in the relationship that he has haemophilia and that he is sero-positive the woman may decline to go any further. This fear has led some patients into transient relationships and 'one night stands'. They fear rejection, but they would like to be able to proceed on the basis of mutual confidence, and to make a steady relationship.

HIV sero-positivity has exacerbated the difficulties facing young haemophiliacs who have to come to terms not only with the normal emotions of adolescence but also with haemophilia and the chronic disability this entails. HIV sero-positivity brings yet more responsibility and restrictions on these patients at a time when they may not find it easy to deal with them. It has been reported that 'even once the information has been given some haemophiliacs are unwilling or unable to follow the health measures suggested – the use of a condom, limiting the number of sexual partners and modification of sexual practice' (Haemophilia and AIDS, 1985).

Our personal experience at Glasgow Royal Infirmary of counselling 16- to 20-year olds who have never had a sexual partner is that they are well aware of what precautions should be taken, and that they are very concerned that they should not be responsible for spreading infection. The easiest solution in the first place for all of them was to do nothing; 'I just stay at home and watch television – except programmes on AIDS' said one young man. The danger of this inaction on a permanent basis is that it may increase their isolation and encourage dependence on their family at a time when their peers are becoming more independent. To prevent the spread of infection sexually necessitates the use of a sheath. A very angry young patient declared that 'all the birds he knew were on the pill' and that he would feel 'a real Charlie' if he produced a sheath. A more experienced patient, finding himself in a similar situation, had said to his partner that 'he was into rubber; it turned him on'.

11.3.6 Reaction of the family

Haemophilia is a genetically inherited condition and the existence of a family member with haemophilia has an effect on all other members of the family. Indeed more than one son in a family may be affected. It is likely that a positive HIV diagnosis will also have a profound effect on the family. Two thirds of the haemophiliac patients treated at Glasgow Royal Infirmary are still resident at home, and several have haemophiliac brothers. The parents of adolescent patients have expressed great concern about HIV and consequently regular evening meetings for such parents have been arranged. Many interesting issues have been raised at these meetings. All parents have had experience of having a very difficult young man to deal with at the time of the diagnosis. This was manifested in various ways. Anger, bad temper and rudeness were common. The anger was directed at the government and at the homosexual population. In turn the parents felt annoyed with the medical profession particularly where they had younger haemophiliac sons. If a younger son was negative there was great concern lest he too became sero-converted. In one respect the reaction of the parents mirrored that of their sons who initially curtailed the use of their treatment in response to learning that they were sero-positive. Most parents have told their sons to cut back on the use of their treatment, and in some case this has been resented because of the implied interference with their son's life.

Parents are concerned too about the transmission of infection. They see sexual transmission as the greatest problem. Those whose sons have girlfriends have said to their sons that they hope he has told his girlfriend and that he is taking precautions. Parents grieve for their sons and for their girlfriends. All parents hope that their sons will not have children and they appreciate how hard this may be for their sons. They also express concern for the girlfriend, about how she copes with the situation, and about whether her family have been told.

Many parents have experienced guilt about having had a haemophiliac son, and some mothers may feel particularly guilty because she has 'caused' the disability, through being a carrier of the relevant gene (Hunt, 1976). It is likely that the parents of sero-positive sons may feel even more guilty. Some have shown this by their concern to have their daughters tested for carrier status. It is desirable for a counsellor to spend sufficient time with the parents before testing is carried out, so that they are better able to cope with a positive carrier status result.

Most parents want to protect their sons, but they are aware of the problem of over-protectiveness and its inhibiting effects on normal development. They want to help, but at the same time they want their sons to be independent. One mother said that she only felt happy when her son was at home. Concern for their affected son, fear of the future and of what may happen, concern for other children, and dislike of the publicity that AIDS has brought to haemophiliacs and to their families, all contribute to a very stressful situation. Some families have been unable to cope with it, and cases of marital breakdown attributed to problems associated with AIDS have been reported.

Other family members may be affected by a sero-positive diagnosis. They too are likely to be concerned, and the responsibility of discretion is considerable. Friends may comment. Indeed some younger sibs have said that they do not want to take their friends home any more, because their older brother is infected.

11.3.7 Pregnancy

It has been recommended to HIV sero-positive haemophiliacs that they delay starting a family because of the dangers of transmitting the infection to the fetus. This will be very dispiriting information for sero-positive haemophiliacs who have not yet had a family or for those who have not yet completed their family. It is not yet known whether this is a lifelong recommendation. Counselling, therefore, is to help the patient cope with this information. This is more easily achieved if the situation is discussed on a monthly basis or reduced to a manageable time limit. Many patients will not yet have been considering starting a family. These patients should know that if they were considering starting a family they can bring their partner to the clinic to discuss the situation in the light of the relevant information at that time.

The patient who says that he would like to start a family should be encouraged to bring his partner in for counselling. It is advisable in these circumstances that information is given when both partners are present. The principle is then to find out what both partners know and want. It may be that once the female has realized what the situation is she may not be prepared to take the risks of a pregnancy. The couple should be helped to examine the disadvantages of going ahead with a pregnancy when the husband is HIV sero-positive as well as the advantages. They will need information about the numerical risk to the fetus of becoming HIV sero-positive when a parent is positive. Will the couple be able to cope with the anxiety that this will raise? Also a daughter will necessarily be a carrier of haemophilia who in turn may be faced with difficult reproductive decisions in the future. On the other hand the fetus may not be infected and and the couple may have the pleasure of having a healthy child. Finally the choice of which risks to take has to be theirs.

11.3.8 Employment

Previous surveys of haemophilia (Markova, Lockyer and Forbes, 1977) indicated that difficulties in finding suitable employment remained one of the most serious problems for the haemophiliac. The difficulties in finding work can have psychological consequences resulting in a reduction in the person's self-esteem thus making it more difficult to seek employment (Markova *et al.*, 1980). With the advent of home therapy employment prospects for the haemophiliac should improve (Stuart *et al.*, 1980; Lineberger, 1981). Prior to home therapy recurrent bleeding resulted in significant loss of schooling and hence academic underachievement and also loss of time at work. Employment prospects also vary from region to region and reflect the current economic climate from time to time. In times of high unemployment there is a tendency for the chronic sick to lose their jobs early.

The long history of high unemployment for haemophiliac patients has resulted in a natural tendency to conceal their disability. In one survey one quarter of the patients had not told their employer that they had haemophilia

(Stuart *et al.*, 1980). However, in contrast, 78% of those who had taken their employer into their confidence considered that their employer was either very reasonable or helpful. In Glasgow Royal Infirmary, one quarter of sero-positive haemophiliac patients are unemployed and have been unemployed for at least two years. While knowledge of their sero-positivity is unlikely to help their employment situation, in their case it has not been the major cause or reason for their unemployment.

One third of our sero-positive patients are either full time students or recent school leavers in Youth Training schemes. Theoretically there is no reason why they should not continue into employment, assuming the availability of suitable work. However, if a future employer were to discover that an applicant for a job suffered from haemophilia, current prejudice about AIDS may cost the applicant the job. It is therefore, not surprising to hear haemophiliacs say 'I am not going to tell the firm about haemophilia. Least said soonest mended. It is none of their business'.

The sero-positive haemophiliac employee may feel that he is on the horns of a dilemma. On the one hand a sympathetic employer could assist in allocating suitable work and in making things more convenient for the employee in other ways. If his employer and work colleagues know that he has haemophilia, he is more likely to receive appropriate treatment in the event of an accident. Openness about his condition makes it easier for him to explain to his workmates the proper care to be taken in the event of blood spillage. On the other hand, he may find that an unsympathetic employer takes an opportunity to dismiss him, or that unsympathetic workmates shun him or revile him. If he conceals his infectiousness from his employer and workmates he may be concerned lest there should be an accident in which there would be a chance, albeit remote, of his infection of others through blood spillage. At the moment sero-positive haemophiliacs seem to prefer to live with the secrecy and the anxiety created by the latter choice.

11.3.9 Life insurance

Over the years haemophiliacs have encountered difficulties in acquiring life insurance. Better treatment and improved mortality and morbidity have made it easier for haemophiliacs to acquire life insurance and for increasing numbers of them to get a policy without an increased premium. However the insurance industry is by nature cautious and some companies may still refuse an applicant who states that he has haemophilia. Inability to obtain life insurance may also restrict one's ability to acquire a mortgage and therefore a home of one's own. It is clear that to be HIV sero-positive presents a serious problem for the individual who wishes to purchase life insurance. If such an individual discloses that he is sero-positive, his application will at present not be accepted. Life insurance companies are unable to underwrite risk where they have no way of assessing the numerical probability of a claim, which is the case with sero-positivity at present. It is understandable that there is a temptation for asymptomatic sero-positive individuals to withhold this information from their application. One of the principles on which insurance is based '*uberrima fides*' or 'utmost good faith' requires that no relevant information be withheld by either side.

An applicant who withholds the information that they are sero-positive, knowing that this information would alter the terms of the contract may find or (his executors) may find the policy is repudiated by the life office.

The life insurance industry in the United States has been affected by a number of very large claims from AIDS victims (*The Financial Times*, 7th May, 1986). The inference is that individuals at risk of contracting AIDS have been 'rushing to insure their lives for very high sums'. Life companies in the United Kingdom, anxious not to have a repeat of this situation, have been examining ways of identifying those who are likely to be at risk of contracting AIDS. The Life Insurance Company of the Association of British Insurers has recommended that an additional question such as: 'Have you received medical advice, treatment or a blood test in connection with AIDS or any AIDS related condition? If so, give details', be included in proposal forms of life insurance policies, and many companies have moved in this direction. This move by the life insurance companies has aroused considerable opposition from the Terrence Higgins Trust and the Campaign for Homosexual Equality. At the moment haemophiliacs are identifiable by several of the questions already asked in proposal forms for life policies, e.g. 'Are you at present suffering from any illness or physical defect or are you taking advice or treatment?' or 'Have you been ill or consulted a doctor within the past 5 years (ignoring minor ailments)?' Until all companies introduce specific questions about AIDS, haemophiliacs will remain the one at risk group who will invariably pay the price of their risk status.

A possible remedy for sero-positive haemophiliacs would be assistance from the blood transfusion service or effectively the government to enable them to obtain life insurance on reasonable terms. This would require cooperation between the life offices and the government with the government acting as guarantor or reassurer, so that life offices could offer sero-positive haemophiliacs insurance on the same terms as sero-negatives.

11.3.10 Confidentiality

Many articles and policy documents about AIDS stress the importance of maintaining the confidentiality of the patient. Whatever may be the case for those who have been infected through sexual contact, the same considerations do not seem to apply to haemophiliacs. Medical confidentiality is based on the ethical codes. The Hippocratic Oath states that '. . . whatever . . . I see or hear . . . which ought not to be spoken of abroad, I will not divulge.' This implies that there may be some information which it would be proper to divulge. The Declaration of Geneva alters this to: 'I will respect the secrets which are confided in me.' The word 'respect' does not necessarily imply an absolute prohibition.

The British Medical Association Handbook of Medical Ethics (1980) states that a doctor must preserve secrecy on all he knows, but it includes five exceptions to this principle:

1. The patient gives consent.
2. When it is undesirable on medical grounds to seek a patient's consent.
3. The doctor's overriding duty to society.
4. For the purposes of medical research . . .
5. The information is required by due legal process.

Of these five exceptions 'the doctor's overriding duty to society' is the least clear-cut, as it requires the doctor to take into account a balance between different priorities. As far as is known at present the danger to work colleagues or to the general public of an HIV sero-positive patient is small, so there is little reason for medical staff to inform an employer of the sero-positive status of their patient. On the other hand there is good reason to believe that other medical and hospital staff who may be carrying out invasive procedures or dealing with contaminated waste may be at risk, and so should be informed of sero-positivity.

Whether the wife or partner of a sero-positive patient should be informed of his sero-positive status without the patient's consent is a matter of dispute. One doctor has said that he would not tell the wife even if he knew she was considering pregnancy, since to do so would break the trust of his patient, a trust that he felt was essential if other at risk patients were to come to his clinic.

This issue is not peculiar to AIDS; it arises with other sexually transmitted diseases, and a similar problem arises with genetically inherited diseases, for example when one member of a family is found to be carrying an abnormal gene but is reluctant to allow this knowledge to be disseminated to other family members. The BMA suggest that 'consideration must be given to informing the spouse, or potential spouse of a carrier, because he may bear some responsibility for passing such genes on to future generations' because 'the importance of such information probably outweighs the importance of complete individual medical confidentiality, providing that the information is kept to the medical profession and to those entitled to it because of their potential carrier state' (BMA, 1980, p. 30). On the same grounds it can be argued that the partner or potential partner of an HIV sero-positive person who may be considering having children should be informed of the risk to herself and to the potential child.

A haemophiliac can scarcely conceal his haemophilia from his family, whether parents or spouse. There is little advantage to him in concealing a sero-positive status from them. Whereas in the case of sexually transmitted disease the source of the infection may cause at least embarrassment and at worst complete marital breakdown, a sero-positive haemophiliac need have no such fears. He may, however, find that his partner wishes to reduce her sexual contact with him. But since there is a real risk of infection to her unless proper precautions are taken, it may be considered only fair that she should be informed. It is hoped that any problems in this respect may be avoided by skilled and supportive counselling in the first place.

11.3.11 Counselling

Counselling and discussion about AIDS related issues for haemophiliacs may take place during a clinic visit or when the patient is attending the unit for other reasons. However it is important that a specific time is set aside for counselling for each haemophiliac. This should be on a separate occasion from clinical investigations and examinations and should take place in a quiet room where the counsellor is left undisturbed.

There are some general guidelines in counselling which are helpful:

- Discover what the patient knows about HIV and AIDS, by listening to what he says.
- Feed back factual information to fill in gaps in knowledge.
- Ask the patient if there are any aspects of his life that have been made difficult by HIV sero-positivity.
- Discuss one issue at a time giving the patient an opportunity to speak.
- Do not be afraid of silence; that can be beneficial.
- Get the patient to think what the important issues are: it might be helpful to write down the pros and cons of, e.g. taking a particular action; it may then become clear what is the best course of action for that patient.
- Find something positive about the patient's life and remind him of that; it may be something quite simple, e.g. that his garden is growing well or that that he is looking forward to a football match or that his team is winning.
- Keep the session to a clearly defined time; if it goes on too long everyone becomes tired.
- Make it clear that another appointment is available.
- Ask the patient if there is any information that he would like to have.
- If possible offer appointments out of normal working hours, when appropriate.

When counselling HIV sero-positive haemophiliacs, it is necessary to consider including the topics that have been discussed above:

- Control of infection from blood and the problems that that may bring.
- Control of infection transmitted sexually and the difficulties that that may bring.
- Problems regarding pregnancy if that is relevant.
- Relationships with the immediate family.
- Problems regarding employment and relationships in the work place.
- What to do about life insurance.
- Confidentiality – whether certain others need to be told of HIV status.

There is as yet no cure for AIDS, and as has already been discussed earlier in the chapter there is considerable uncertainty about if and when an asymptomatic sero-positive patient will develop symptoms and for how long he is likely to remain infectious. The information that is given about the prevention of the transmission of AIDS emphasizes the practice or behaviour that is not recommended. This may be overwhelming for the patient. Thus a main goal of counselling sero-positive haemophiliacs must be to help patients to deal with stress and to give them a sense of control over their lives. One way of doing this is to teach patients to be flexible and to redefine those goals that can be enjoyed and mastered with pride, thus increasing the patient's self-esteem (Wexler, 1979). It is necessary to find 'something positive'. For example while a pregnancy would not be recommended at the moment, it is possible to say to the patient that he can have an enjoyable and safe sex life.

Haemophiliacs continue to be dependent on blood products for their survival. There is evidence that some patients have cut back on treatment presumably for fear of future infection (Madhok *et al.*, 1986). They can be helped to keep a control over their lives by discussing their concern and working out an appropriate treatment programme with medical staff.

11.3.12 Conclusion

The problems faced by sero-positive haemophiliacs are compounded by their haemophilia. In this respect they differ from other groups in which sero-positivity is frequent, who nevertheless may have their own particular problems. It is important that these differences be more widely recognized and acknowledged by the medical profession, the press, and the public.

REFERENCES

Acquired Immune Deficiency Syndrome. AIDS Booklet 2. (1985) *Information for doctors concerning the introduction of the HTLV-III antibody test.* Scottish Home and Health Department.

AIDS Center News. April 1986 Vol 3 No 1. World Haemophilia Centre, Los Angeles.

Bove, J. R. (1985) How should we handle the ethical questions regarding information to donors etc. *Vox Sang.* **49**, 234–35.

British Medical Association (1980) *Handbook of Medical Ethics*. British Medical Association, London.
Curran, W. J. (1985) AIDS research and the 'window of opportunity'. *N. Engl. J. Med.*, **312**, No. 14, 903–04.
Daniels, V. G. (1985) *AIDS and the Acquired Immune Deficiency Syndrome*, STP Press, Lancaster. England.
The Financial Times. 7 May 1986.
Haemophilia Social Workers Special Interest Group (1985) Discussion paper: *Haemophilia and AIDS*.
Hunt, C. H. (1976) Psychological and social aspects. In *Comprehensive Management of Haemophilia* (ed. D. C. Boone) F. A. Davis Company, Philadelphia.
Jones, P. (1985) *AIDS and the Blood*. Haemophilia Society, London.
Katz, J. (1984) *The Silent World of Doctor and Patient*, Free Press, New York.
Lineberger, H. P. (1981) Social Characteristics of a Haemophilia Clinic Population. *General Hospital Psychiatry*, **3**, 157–63.
McIntosh, J. (1974) Processes of Communication, Information Seeking and Control Associated with Cancer. *Social Science and Medicine*, **8**, 167–87.
McKeown, T. (1968) *Validation of Screening Procedures Screening in Medical Care*, OUP, London.
Madhok, R., Campbell, D. and Gracie, A. *et al.* (1986)Changes in factor concentrate use subsequent to the publicity of AIDS in haemophiliacs. International Conference on AIDS, Paris 173.
Markova, I., Lockyer, R. and Forbes, C. D. (1977) Haemophilia: Survey on Social Issues. *Health Bulletin*, **35**, 177–82.
Markova, I., Lockyer, R. and Forbes, C. (1980) Self Perception of Employed and Unemployed Haemophiliacs. *Psychological Medicine*, **10**, 559–65.
Sackett, D. L. and Holland, W. W. (1973) Controversy in the Detection of Disease. *Lancet*, ii, 356–9.
Sorenson, J. R. (1973) Sociological and Psychological Factors in Applied Human Genetics. In *Ethical Issues in Human Genetics* (eds B. Hilton, D. Callahan, M. Harris, P. Condliffe and B. Berkley) Plenum Press, New York.
Stuart, J., Forbes, C., Jones, P., Lane, G., Ritza, C. and Wilkes, S. (1980) Improving Prospects for Employment of Haemophiliacs. *Bri. Med. J.*, **280**, 1169–72.
Suki, W. N. (1982) Polycystic Kidney Disease. *Kidney International*, **22**, 571–80.
Thomas, S. (1983) Ethics of a Predictive Test For Huntington's Chorea. *Bri. Med. J.*, **284**, 1383–4.
Twiss, S. B. (1974) Ethical Issues in Genetic Screening. In *Ethical, Social and Legal Dimensions of Screening for Human Genetic Disease* (ed. D. Bergsma) National Foundation March of Dimes. Vol. X. No. 6.
Wakefield, J. (1970) The Social Context of Cancer. In *What we Know About Cancer* (ed. R. C. J. Harris) Allen and Unwin, London.
Wexler, N. S. (1979) Genetic 'Russian Roulette'. The Experience of Being at Risk for Hungtington's Chorea. In *Genetic Counselling Psychological Dimensions* (ed. S. Kessler) Academic Press, New York.
Wilson, J. M. G. and Junger, G. (1968) *Principles and Practice of Screening for Disease*, World Health Organisation, Geneva.

12

The Future

—— *Louis M. Aledort* ——

12.1 THE PAST

If we were to look through a crystal ball and project what might happen in the future, we have to first look to see from where we came. Comprehensive care had become a key health care programme for haemophiliacs in many parts of the world. Home care, or self-infusion had become the ultimate goal of our patients, so they could be emancipated from emergency rooms and hospitals. By the 1970s, research and technology had transformed a generation of plasma dependent patients, to those capable of infusing cryoprecipitate or concentrated materials. The plasma industry grew enormously and could supply the world's needs by 1975. Plasmapheresis had become an established method of donor procurement and thousands of donors could be recruited for factor materials, such that by the 1980s, the average number of donors was 5000 for a single lot of material which reached approximately 100 recipients. In 1975, post-transfusion complications for chronically transfused haemophiliacs included hepatitis and liver disease, immune haemolysis, and inhibitors (Fratantoni and Aronson, 1976). Shortly thereafter, hepatitis B virus was identified and in rapid fashion, donor screening was initiated. Unfortunately, despite the great sensitivity and specificity of the test, hepatitis B continued to be transmitted by the factors. Not until a vaccine was available was there hope of total eradication of transfusion-induced hepatitis B.

Once over that hurdle, hepatitis virus non-A non-B reared its head as another threat to haemophiliacs. Quickly, we recognized its pathogenicity, its frequent clinical silence, and its common long-term sequelae. We now recognize that this virus may be even more important as a pathogen in producing liver pathology. The incidence of almost 25% of patients having either chronic active hepatitis or cirrhosis (Aledort *et al.*, 1985) had confirmed our fears that transfusion-induced disease was now a significant trade-off to the advances in therapy. We also have noted the high incidence of cytomegalovirus (CMV) and Epstein–Barr virus (EBV) infection in these chronically transfused recipients.

12.2 THE PRESENT

In 1982, a disease described as an aquired immune deficiency syndrome (AIDS), seen in homosexuals and drug addicts, was being recognized as a significant clinical problem. In that year, a haemophiliac was first diagnosed with such an immune deficiency syndrome. In June of 1982, the United States' HHS Department called a meeting to discuss this disease. It became clear that a common set of conditions existed in these three groups. They all had (1) a high incidence of abnormal liver function tests, (2) 90% markers for hepatitis B (5–7% were antigen positive and 85% were antibody positive), (3) high exposure to CMV and EBV, (4) elevated immunoglobulins, and (5) exposure to the body fluids of a large number of human beings. The homosexuals with large numbers of sexual partners, the IV drug abusers share needles, and persons with haemophilia are exposed to thousands of donors per year.

It took some time before the hypothesized viral transmission of this new disease was accepted by the scientific and medical community. It took careful and painstaking epidemiologic work by the Centers for Disease Control (CDC), reviewing transfusion-related AIDS, before this concept would gain acceptance. Finally, the identification of the causative agent was carried out and confirmed in rapid fashion. Its eradication or prevention, however, is far from being resolved.

Today haemophilia treaters can no longer feel the total sense of satisfaction that they felt before AIDS and non-A and non-B hepatitis was described. The very therapy that dramatically has made major changes in the health care delivery system, and emancipated the patient, has become an instrument for illness, and now AIDS being a uniformly lethal disease. We are currently dealing with an anxious, frightened patient population, and a group of guilt ridden treaters. In addition, mass hysteria over the general blood supply has led donors to believe AIDS can be contracted by giving blood. It is frequently believed by many that the mere presence of an AIDS or ARC patient in the room will lead to contamination.

The crystal ball has much inside. It needs to be turned in many directions in order to fully understand what the future must bring to relieve the lot of AIDS and potential AIDS patients.

Initially, I believe that nations will better understand the health care impact of AIDS. Already financial experts are estimating the cost of care. Institutions are recognizing and providing the appropriate services to deal with the medical and psychosocial aspects of this disease for the patient and his family. Cities with a high incidence of AIDS are starting to alter reimbursement mechanisms to help hospitals cope with the extraordinary costs of this disease. Communities are now demanding the availability of outpatient and appropriate long-term care facilities. Legal societies are being initiated to insure patients' rights, as well as sorting out the complex issues arising at employment sites. In the future there will be enough data on these issues so that countries will be able to provide a rational, affordable health care package for these individuals. Clinical experimentation and experience will also make it possible for us to deal with the serious psychosocial impact of this menacing disease. New techniques for stress management and coping mechanisms will be developed and refined to provide adequate counselling. Community, patient and health care team education will also reach a high enough level of sophistication, so that media hype will decompress, and the stigma and unwarranted fears will be dispelled.

The availability of HIV testing of donors of blood and plasma has been a major stride in the reduction of transmission of the retrovirus. How much greater an increment this will mean to eliminating HIV carriers, over the self-withdrawal of high-risk donors needs further study. Some HIV positive donors continue to donate despite their belonging to excluded high-risk groups because they do not perceive themselves in these categories.

Although the specificity and sensitivity of this test is extraordinarily high, there can be no doubt that some virus positive, negative tested bloods will be processed. The ability of such donors to transmit virus, resulting in either a recipient becoming antibody positive, developing clinical symptoms and/or disease, is now being studied. The NIH, NHLBI Transfusion Safety Study is currently studying, in a prospective fashion, recipients of HIV positive and negative blood units. Future research efforts will be able to identify the probable variants of HIV. The ability to identify the presence of antigen, as in hepatitis B, as a method of detecting active viral infection and/or infectivity of units will only be resolved by future research. Unfortunately, the inability to grow virus or identify it in either plasma or blood has substantially hindered this work.

12.3 THE FUTURE

In 1980 Factor VIII was purified, when several milligrams of it were extracted from 25 000 litres of cow blood. Dr Tuddenham and colleagues obtained purified human VIII, and Genetech and Genetics Institute sequenced a portion of this protein. Using this as a probe, a cultured cell line could be used. Factor VIII mRNA was found in the liver, kidney, spleen and lymph, with the liver being the most abundant source. Recombinant bacteria have been used to bioengineer small molecules. However, the complexity and size of factor VIII necessitated the insertion of the cloned gene into hamster cells. There were concerns that the bioengineered material would not be the full missing haemophilia piece, or would be an impurity or would not clot haemophiliac blood. Fortunately, none of these concerns were justified. The material clots human haemophilia blood and is equivalent to the protein now fractionated. The most significant impact of this bioengineered material is its application as replacement therapy for factor VIII deficient haemophiliacs. At this very moment plans are being made for clinical trials of this material. Hopefully, these will take place within the ensuing 2 years. When available, a truly safe, virus-free material will be on the market. Its supply and price are issues talked about but too premature for answers. Liver disease and AIDS might well be a concern of the past for haemophiliacs born in the next decade (Lawn and Vehar, 1986).

Factor IX by contrast is a smaller molecule whose sequence has been known for several years. Haemophilia B, factor IX deficiency is substantially less common than haemophilia A, factor VIII deficiency. There are a large number of genetic defects that occur in Haemophilia B in different families. A recent review of the structure, function and molecular defects of factor IX outlines the current state of the art related to this protein. Bioengineering of this material will be feasible and eventually marketed. It will be critical to have this material available in some proximity to factor VIII as the market for factor VIII is far greater than that for IX, and there will be little, if any, impetus to fractionate IX, if all the world supply of VIII is eventually bioengineered (Thompson, 1986).

The current supply and pricing of these factors has always been interdependent on the requirements for albumin. The market for albumin in general, has pushed the system in terms of plasma procurement and fractionation. Factors VIII and IX, except for a short period of time, represent by-products of fractionation for albumin. Currently, the way albumin is fractionated and treated prior to marketing has made it a safe product, not transmitting infectious disease, unless the approved process has been altered. Albumin has been shown to be able to be bioengineered. However, it has not been able to be made in large-scale production and appears currently not to be a viable product.

Fluorocarbons promised the possibility of treating bleeding or anaemic patients with synthetic, oxygen-carrying capacity without the hazards of transfusion induced disease. Recent clinical trials did not satisfy the FDA that these substances could truly serve as blood substitutes. Currently, investigations during surgical procedures may well show that transient use of fluorocarbons may be effective. A large amount of blood is used in the surgical setting and if approved for this indication one will be able to substantially reduce the high rate of transfusion-induced disease in this group. Many transfusion-associated AIDS cases were recipients of blood for surgery.

Mild and moderate haemophiliacs, and many von Willebrand patients are now treated exclusively with 1-desamino-D-arginine vasopressin (DDAVP), a synthetic analogue of vasopressin. It is currently given intravenously and can be given subcutaneously. In Sweden, the Ferring Company has now produced a premeasured nasal spray that delivers adequate amounts of DDAVP quickly and simply. The elevation of factors are similar to those achieved with intravenous administration. This will make control of menstrual bleeding in von Willebrand patients simple and a superb alternative to transfusion, D and C's and frequent requirements for iron replacement therapy. This new form of administration has made its use in plasma donors in Sweden easily acceptable and is now routine. The method has allowed fewer donors to be required for the production of fractionated products. Its wider application throughout the world might well make available small donor pool lots of plasma or cryoprecipitate for those patients who require little replacement therapy but cannot be treated successfully with DDAVP. Such an approach would substantially reduce the likelihood of transmitting hepatitis and HIV infection.

The marked success of vaccination with hepatitis B gives us all encouragement that such an approach will be viable for HIV. Current data however, suggest that because of frequent changing of the determinants on the envelope of the retrovirus, a quick solution to this problem seems unlikely. However, we can gain hope from history. When hepatitis B antibody was detected, we waited until we could identify the B antigen and test for a reduction in the transmission of this virus. Antigen testing has substantially reduced if not almost eliminated B virus transmission in single donor products. It took, however, almost 10 years before a vaccine was made, tested and proven to be effective in eliminating B transmission. HIV is a newly recognized virus. The presence of antibody is not protective most of the time. I feel that in the future, an effective vaccine will be available. However, it might well be another 3–5 years until high risk groups and their sexual partners would be able to be the first to receive this material.

Several years ago, the fractionation industry, heeding the concerns of haemophilia treaters, began to carry out research to determine ways to eliminate hepatitis B and non-A non-B from their large donor pool material. They extrapolated from the data that albumin, which is heated, does not transmit viral disease, and looked to heat treatment as a method of treating Factor VIII. Factor IX had already been successfully treated in Germany with UV light and ß-propiolactone to remove hepatitis B, but was not able to be used for Factor VIII. Factor VIII is a heat labile protein, and protecting the molecule by various methods were tried to keep Factor VIII yields at a financially viable level. Using the chimpanzee model, it appeared initially that hepatitis B and non-A and non-B could be either eliminated or attenuated. Heating in the dry or wet phase has been employed, as well as a sterilization process. When first tested in patients not previously exposed to replacement therapy, however, non-A non-B viruses were still viable and could transmit hepatitis (as measured by elevation of serum transaminases). Howe\ must be kept in mind that large donor pool material without treatmen transmits non-A non-B 100% of the time. Clinical trials are now underw determine if non-A non-B can be eliminated.

Encouraging reports in small studies make us feel sure that newer niques – heat, steam, and solvent detergent – may well eradicate this virus. Fortuitously, and at the same time it was recognized that the retrovirus HIV was a very heat labile substance. As with non-A non-B hepatitis virus, we had no markers for the measurement of virus in plasma. Therefore, one could only carry out experiments to define what would happen to added virus. It was rapidly discovered that the process of lyophilization could kill 1–2 logs of virus and heat 2–3 logs. It has been assumed that at worst guess, there would not be more than 5 logs of viruses in any given lot of factor material. Thus all would be killed by either heating, steam or solvent detergent. The estimation of maximum virus in the blood is, however, theoretical and at present cannot be tested. The sensitivity of testing for virus leaves approximately 1–1.5 logs of virus unaccounted for. This small amount, however, may be able to infect a recipient, particularly with repeated doses. Studies, however, of treated materials appear to have not transmitted HIV, except in several cases. Whether this was passive immunization or true infection is not known. The current studies involve few patients and repeated exposures are small and the follow-up time is short. The impetus for the research laboratories as well as the fractionation industry to devise means of eradicating HIV is great. I feel assured that this will happen soon.

Not all von Willebrand's and mild or moderate haemophiliacs respond to DDAVP. This leaves a substantial number of patients in the world who require transfusion infrequently. Treaters and patients alike are left with a great dilemma regarding the optimal and currently controversial approach to therapy. Concentrated factor materials rarely contain the appropriate amount of von Willebrand's factor to correct the deficiency in DDAVP unresponsive von Willebrand patients. These are treated with cryoprecipitate or plasma. These products are substantially less likely to transmit non-A non-B hepatitis. However, they cannot be assuredly depleted of HIV as compared to treated fractions. Mild and moderate factor IX and DDAVP non-responsive factor VIII also require replacement material, usually infrequently and in small amounts. Occasionally, following trauma or with surgical intervention, large amounts are required. The serious question facing the clinician is whether to use plasma or cryoprecipitate or concentrates. There are no current methods to successfully kill HIV in plasma and maintain factor activity. Thus we are left with the choice of either plasma and/or cryoprecipitate containing non-A non-B at lower frequency than concentrates, or concentrates with more non-A non-B but treated to minimize or eliminate HIV. It is as yet an unresolved dilemma because we cannot be sure whether AIDS or the sequelae of non-A non-B will produce the greatest morbidity and mortality to our congenital coagulation-deficient patients. Research is actively going on to find methods of eliminating HIV from plasma, and this will ease our decision making process.

AIDS reared its head as a transfusion related disease in 1982. The number of persons infected, clinically ill and dead are already more than we want to deal with. However, major advances are seen in the crystal ball. The epidemiologic studies quickly gave us much data. The research technology made recognition of the agent in record time.

The blood and blood-product supply is safer than ever, and the unanswered questions continue to decrease. Drugs for therapy, vaccines for prevention, financial underwriting of care are not too far off. Although AIDS may be here for many years to come, its incidence from blood transfusion will substantially decrease. Until we have all bioengineered products for haemophiliacs, our clinical challenge will be the reduction of viral transmission from blood products. Blood banking technology has mastered many challenges before and will undoubtedly make the blood supply safe.

REFERENCES

Aledort, L. M., Levine, P. H., Hilgartner, M., Blatt, P., Spero, J. A., Goldberg, D., Bianchi, L., Desmet, V., Scheuer, P., Popper, H. and Berk, P. D. (1985) *Blood*, **66**, 367–72.

Fratantoni, J. and Aronson, D. (eds) (1976) Unsolved therapeutic problems in hemophilia. Proceedings of a Conference Sponsored by Bureau of Biologics, FDA, NHLBI, National Hemophilia Foundation, held in Bethesda Maryland March 1–2, 1976, pp. 1–132.

Lawn, R. M. and Vehar, G. A. (1986) *Scientific American*, March, 48–54.

Thompson, A. R. (1986) *Blood*, **67**, 565–72.

Index